Beyond Fish Oil

Omega-3 and the Lipid Balance of the Body

First Edition: March 2026
ISBN: 978-1-966035-07-7
Published by Elite Nutrition Research
EliteNutritionResearch.com

ELITE

NUTRITION RESEARCH

Elite Nutrition Research is a science-driven health and education company dedicated to understanding and optimizing human physiology at its most fundamental level. Our work is built on an architecture-first approach—examining how nutrients interact with cellular systems, membranes, energy production, and signaling pathways to shape overall health and performance. Rather than following trends, we focus on first principles, combining biochemical insight, formulation precision, and practical application to create both advanced nutritional products and in-depth educational systems.

Through our books, courses, and formulations, Elite Nutrition Research aims to give individuals direct access to the mechanisms that govern their biology empowering them to think clearly, act intentionally, and build lasting health from the inside out.

To explore our full system of products, courses, and research, visit:
www.elitenutritionresearch.com

Table of Contents

Introduction 7

PART I - THE BODY AS A LIPID SYSTEM 11

Chapter 1 - The Lipid Architecture of the Human Body 13

Chapter 2 - Membranes as Decision-Making Surfaces 31

Chapter 3 - The Three Roles of Lipids 49

PART II - THE OMEGA SYSTEM 67

Chapter 4 - What Omega-3 and Omega-6 Really Are 69

Chapter 5 - Arachidonic Acid and the Initiation of Inflammation 85

Chapter 6 - Omega-3 as Resolution Substrate 101

PART III - SPMs: THE BIOLOGY OF RESOLUTION 117

Chapter 7 - What Are Specialized Pro-Resolving Mediators (SPMs)? 119

Chapter 8 - The Resolution Phase of Inflammation 135

Chapter 9 - Mechanisms of SPM Action 147

Chapter 10 - When Resolution Fails 161

PART IV - MEMBRANE COMPOSITION AND IMBALANCE 173

Chapter 11 - How Modern Diet Disrupts SPM Production 175

Chapter 12 - Membrane Composition Determines Resolution Potential 189

Chapter 13 - The Threshold Problem Revisited 203

PART V - EPA AND DHA THROUGH THE SPM LENS 215

Chapter 14 - EPA-Derived Resolvins (E-Series) 217

Chapter 15 - DHA-Derived Mediators (D-Series, Protectins, Maresins) 227

Chapter 16 - Functional Divergence: EPA vs DHA via SPM Output 239

PART VI - DISEASE AS FAILED RESOLUTION 251

Chapter 17 - Chronic Inflammation as Resolution Failure 253

Chapter 18 - Lipid Imbalance and Disease Patterns 263

PART VII - OMEGA-3 AND SPM-FOCUSED INTERVENTION 277

Chapter 19 - Why Most Omega-3 Supplementation Fails 279

Chapter 20 - Driving SPM Production Effectively 289

Chapter 21 - Direct SPM Supplementation vs Precursor Strategy 301

PART VIII - LIPID BALANCE AND SYSTEM RESTORATION 313
Chapter 22 - Resolution as the Foundation of Stability 315
Chapter 23 - Why Omega-3 Alone Is Not Enough 325
Chapter 24 - Restoring the Lipid-Controlled Body 337

Introduction

Omega-3 has been flattened into one of the most incomplete ideas in modern nutrition. It is usually presented as a simple health additive, a softgel associated with the heart, the brain, inflammation, and a vague category called wellness. That framing is too small for the biology involved. Omega-3 does not matter because it is a trendy nutrient class or because it can slightly improve a lab marker. It matters because it enters the deepest structural layers of the body. It becomes part of membranes. It changes what cells are physically made of, how receptors move, how signals are interpreted, how inflammation begins, and whether inflammation can end cleanly once it has served its purpose. This book is built on the position that omega-3 cannot be understood in isolation, because no lipid in the body operates in isolation. The body is a lipid-organized system, and once that is seen clearly, fish oil stops looking like a supplement category and starts looking like one small entry point into a much larger architecture. That architecture is the subject of this book. Its outline already centers that frame by moving from the body as a lipid system, into membrane decision-making, into omega-3 and omega-6 pathways, and then into the biology of resolution rather than simple suppression.

Most people have been taught to think about inflammation in only one direction. Something irritates the body, inflammatory pathways turn on, symptoms appear, and the goal becomes reducing those symptoms as quickly as possible. That model is incomplete because it treats inflammation as if it were only an activation problem. In reality, inflammation is a timed biological sequence. It starts, amplifies, performs work, and then must actively resolve. If that final phase fails, the system does not return to baseline. It stays partially activated, partially damaged, and metabolically expensive. This is where omega-3 biology becomes more important and more specific than the common conversation allows. EPA and DHA are not merely anti-inflammatory in the blunt sense of lowering output. They are upstream structural inputs for downstream resolution chemistry. They help create the conditions under which the body can stop recruiting unnecessary immune activity, clear debris, repair tissue, restore barriers, and exit inflammatory states without simply silencing the immune system. That is why this book goes beyond fish oil itself and into specialized pro-resolving mediators, failed resolution, membrane composition, and the threshold conditions required for the body to finish what it starts.

This shift in perspective changes more than the way omega-3 is described. It changes the way chronic disease is understood. When membranes are built from unstable inputs, when omega-6 initiation pressure remains high, when oxidative stress damages polyunsaturated fats before they can be used properly, and when the body lacks the structural reservoir needed to generate resolution signals at the right time, symptoms that look separate begin to reveal a common substrate. Cardiovascular dysfunction, metabolic syndrome, neuroinflammation, persistent pain, immune irritability, and slow tissue recovery stop looking like unrelated failures. They begin to look like the predictable behavior of a system that can still initiate defense but has lost closure. The problem is no longer that the body does too much inflammation. The problem is that it does not complete inflammation well. It cannot exit efficiently because the structural conditions required for exit are missing.

That is also why most omega-3 supplementation produces partial results. A person takes fish oil, notices modest improvement, and then plateaus. Another person feels nothing. Another feels worse and assumes omega-3 is overhyped or incompatible with their system. In many cases, the issue is not the concept of omega-3 itself. The issue is context. Omega-3 is being asked to enter membranes that remain damaged, energetically under-supported, and crowded by competing lipid signals. It is being expected to behave like a pharmacologic override when in reality it behaves more like a structural instruction set. Structural inputs require time, proportionality, and a compatible environment. They do not produce their highest effects when dropped into chaos and expected to fix it alone. That is why this book does not treat omega-3 as a magic bullet. It places omega-3 inside the wider lipid balance of the body, where saturated fats, phospholipids, membrane stability, oxidative protection, substrate competition, and resolution capacity all determine whether the signal carried by omega-3 can actually be received and used.

The title Beyond Fish Oil is therefore literal. This is not a consumer guide to capsules, brands, or simplistic dosage advice. It is an attempt to restore the real scale of the topic. Fish oil is only the commercial surface of a deeper biological reality. Underneath it is a lipid-based control system that governs membrane behavior, immune timing, receptor function, barrier integrity, neural stability, and long-horizon recovery. To understand omega-3 correctly, you have to understand the terrain it enters. You have to understand how modern diets distort membrane composition, why the omega-6 to omega-3 conversation became both oversimplified and distorted, how SPM biology fills in the missing half of inflammation science, and why resolution is not passive. It is built. It depends on stored material, enzymatic access, membrane placement, and enough physiological stability for the body to permit completion.

This book is written for the reader who is no longer satisfied with slogans. It is for the person who has heard that omega-3 is good for them but has never been given a serious explanation of what that actually means. It is for the clinician, coach, researcher, or patient who has watched inflammation remain chronically active despite years of symptom management. It is for anyone willing to replace the supplement model with the structural model. Once you do that, many of the contradictions disappear. Omega-3 stops being mysterious. The inconsistency of results becomes understandable. The apparent randomness of chronic inflammatory disease starts to look patterned. And the next step becomes clearer: stop asking what fish oil does in the abstract, and start asking what kind of body can actually use omega-3 to restore order.

PART I

THE BODY AS A LIPID SYSTEM

Chapter 1

The Lipid Architecture of the Human Body

The human body is usually explained from the outside inward. Bones create the frame, muscles generate movement, organs carry out specialized tasks, and food supplies the energy required to keep everything running. That sequence is familiar, but it hides the level where most biological behavior is actually decided. Life does not begin at the scale of the visible body. It begins at the scale of boundaries. Every cell survives by building a physical edge between what belongs inside and what remains outside. That edge is not a passive wrapper. It is an active material system made largely from lipids, organized into membranes with specific thickness, fluidity, curvature, charge behavior, and receptor placement. Before the body can think, contract, digest, detoxify, repair, or defend itself, it must first construct stable surfaces that can hold gradients, embed proteins, receive signals, and control exchange. The body is built from lipids in a much more literal sense than most nutrition language allows. Not because fat is merely stored in tissue or burned for fuel, but because lipid structure forms the basic material platform on which cellular function sits.

This changes the way anatomy should be understood. A cell is not simply a bag of fluid containing useful parts. It is a compartment made possible by membrane architecture. The mitochondrion does not generate energy in empty space. It depends on highly specialized membranes whose geometry and lipid composition allow electron transport proteins to sit in the correct position, pass electrons in sequence, and pump protons across a controlled barrier. The nucleus does not protect DNA through abstraction. It uses a membrane envelope with selective pores, anchored structural proteins, and tightly managed transport. Synapses, immune cells, endocrine glands, intestinal barriers, hepatocytes, and muscle fibers all depend on lipid-organized boundaries to decide what enters, what leaves, what binds, what activates, and how quickly the system responds once activation begins. The visible body is therefore the large-scale expression of countless microscopic interfaces. If those interfaces are stable, signaling becomes more precise. If they become distorted, oxidized, overly fluid, overly rigid, or compositionally disordered, function becomes noisy before disease becomes obvious.

Lipids are uniquely suited to this role because they solve a physical problem that proteins and carbohydrates cannot solve alone. They self-organize into bilayers because one end interacts with water and the other resists it. That amphipathic design creates separation without requiring external scaffolding. From that simple physical property, biological order becomes possible. A membrane can hold an electrochemical gradient because the lipid barrier slows uncontrolled ion movement. A receptor can detect an outside signal and convert it into an intracellular response because the membrane provides both anchoring and local organization. An enzyme can work efficiently because the surrounding lipid environment alters its orientation, mobility, and access to substrates. This is why the chemistry of lipids cannot be reduced to calorie value. A fat molecule is not important only because it can be oxidized for ATP. Its importance begins earlier, at the level of arrangement. Which fatty acids are present, where they are placed within phospholipids, how tightly they pack, how vulnerable they are to oxidation, and which neighboring molecules sit beside them all influence the behavior of the membrane that cell must live through.

Once this is understood, the old division between structure and signaling starts to collapse. In biology, structure is signaling. The membrane is not just the surface on which signaling occurs. It shapes which signals can occur, how strongly they propagate, how long receptors remain clustered, how channels open, how transporters cycle, and how inflammatory enzymes access their substrates. A receptor embedded in a stable, properly organized membrane does not behave the same way as that same receptor embedded in a disordered membrane loaded with damaged lipids or distorted by chronic metabolic stress. The protein may be identical, yet its performance changes because the physical environment around it has changed. The cell does not experience molecules as isolated concepts. It experiences them as material conditions. Thickness, viscosity, lateral mobility, oxidative load, lipid raft integrity, cholesterol distribution, and phospholipid saturation all alter what the cell can do in real time. This makes membrane composition one of the most overlooked determinants of system behavior across the entire body.

The term membrane often sounds flat and simplistic, as if it describes a thin film with a uniform job. Real membranes are more complex than that. They are dynamic assemblies containing phospholipids, cholesterol, sphingolipids, glycolipids, embedded proteins, peripheral signaling complexes, and localized microdomains that behave differently from the regions around them. Some parts of the membrane are more ordered and tightly packed. Some are more fluid. Some regions favor receptor clustering. Some favor vesicle formation, endocytosis, exocytosis, or immune synapse formation. The membrane is closer to a living surface than a generic envelope. It sorts activity spatially. It creates zones of probability. It determines whether molecules collide, whether enzymes find their targets, whether signaling stays local or spreads, and whether mechanical stress can be absorbed without tearing the underlying logic of the cell apart. When membrane composition drifts, the body does not merely become deficient in some abstract way. It begins making decisions through altered surfaces.

This is especially important in tissues that must signal rapidly or maintain strict discrimination. The nervous system depends on membranes that can support fast electrical behavior, synaptic vesicle cycling, receptor sensitivity, and long-range structural maintenance. The immune system depends on membranes that can detect threat, form immunological synapses, reorganize receptors during activation, and later generate the lipid mediators that help terminate inflammatory activity. The intestinal lining depends on epithelial membranes and junctional structures that preserve barrier function while still permitting selective absorption. The liver depends on membrane-intensive trafficking, packaging, detoxification, and bile production. Endocrine tissue depends on membrane receptor fidelity and transport precision. In each case, function emerges from architecture. Cells are not just using lipids in the background. They are behaving through them.

The body's internal communication network is therefore inseparable from lipid geography. Hormones can circulate through blood, neurotransmitters can cross synapses, cytokines can move through tissue, but the final effect of every one of those signals still depends on whether the target membrane can receive and translate the message correctly. Signal reception is not simply about ligand availability. It is about receptor conformation, receptor density, receptor mobility, membrane charge landscape, local cholesterol content, and the presence of neighboring lipids that either stabilize or distort the signaling platform. When people talk about receptor resistance, inflammatory sensitivity, or impaired cellular response, they often jump immediately to hormones, genes, or deficiencies. Those matter, but the membrane is where the instruction is either executed cleanly or degraded into noise. A cell can only respond with the precision that its structure allows.

Energy production follows the same rule. Mitochondria are often discussed as if they were little power plants floating inside the cell, generating ATP as long as nutrients arrive. That picture is incomplete because mitochondrial output depends on membrane architecture at every stage. The inner mitochondrial membrane holds the electron transport chain, maintains the proton gradient, and organizes the geometry required for oxidative phosphorylation. Cardiolipin and related membrane components help stabilize respiratory complexes and preserve cristae structure. If that membrane becomes compositionally damaged, oxidatively injured, or physically unstable, electron flow becomes less efficient, proton leakage rises, reactive oxygen species can increase, and ATP generation becomes more costly. The problem does not begin only at the level of fuel delivery. It begins at the level of whether the machinery has a coherent surface on which to operate. Biological energy is not produced by nutrients alone. It is produced by nutrients entering well-built structures.

Inflammation also has a structural dimension that is often ignored. Immune activation is not simply a matter of white blood cells releasing inflammatory molecules. It is built from membrane events, receptor assembly, arachidonic acid release, eicosanoid synthesis, vesicle trafficking, redox signaling, and later the generation of specialized pro-resolving mediators from omega-3 substrates. That means the inflammatory response inherits the strengths and weaknesses of the membrane systems that support it. A body with damaged lipid architecture may still initiate inflammation aggressively because initiation pathways are easy to trigger, but it may struggle to organize resolution once the acute threat has passed. The result is not just excess inflammation in the abstract. It is incomplete inflammatory sequencing. The system enters defense mode, spends resources, damages tissue, and then fails to exit cleanly because the underlying lipid environment does not support proper closure. The architecture of the membrane shapes the timeline of immunity.

This is one reason the phrase fat is fuel is too narrow to explain human biology. Fat can absolutely be used as fuel, and in many tissues it is an efficient and stable energy source. But if fat is discussed only in metabolic terms, the deeper logic is lost. Lipids are also insulation, signal precursors, barrier material, transport components, organelle-defining structures, and determinants of protein behavior. They influence mechanical resilience, oxidative vulnerability, membrane permeability, and the timing of inflammatory transitions. They participate in bile formation, myelin integrity, steroid hormone synthesis, and intracellular trafficking. When the nutritional conversation reduces fat to a question of caloric density, it strips away the reason lipid quality matters. Calories describe combustion potential. They do not describe membrane suitability. Two diets can deliver similar calories while building very different tissue behavior over time because the body is not made from calories. It is made from matter that must be arranged correctly.

The concept of lipid architecture also clarifies why chronic dysfunction often develops gradually and diffusely rather than through one clean failure point. A membrane can become slightly more oxidized, slightly more disordered, slightly less responsive, and slightly less capable of supporting receptor fidelity without producing an immediate dramatic symptom. Early changes appear as noise: slower recovery, less stable energy, mild inflammation, greater reactivity, poorer stress tolerance, altered mood, weaker barrier integrity, or reduced metabolic flexibility. Over time those small distortions compound across tissues. The nervous system becomes less stable. The immune system becomes less discriminating. The gut becomes more permeable. Mitochondria become less efficient. Endocrine responses become less predictable. None of these failures are fully separate because they are all being expressed through the same class of material surfaces. The body begins to behave like a system whose interfaces have degraded.

This chapter sets the foundation for everything that follows because omega-3 only makes sense within this structural frame. If the reader approaches omega-3 as a supplement that does things, the discussion stays shallow and eventually becomes contradictory. If the reader understands that omega-3 enters phospholipids, alters membrane behavior, changes substrate availability for inflammatory and pro-resolving mediators, and gradually modifies how cells organize signaling, then the subject becomes coherent. Omega-3 is not important because it produces a quick benefit. It is important because it changes the material conditions through which benefits become possible. That is a slower idea, but it is the more biologically honest one.

The human body is therefore not best understood as a calorie-processing machine with occasional structural needs. It is a structure-dependent system that uses energy to maintain organized matter. First the boundary has to hold. Then gradients can exist. Then proteins can work in place. Then signaling can become specific. Then tissues can coordinate. Then the organism can behave coherently across time. Lipids sit near the beginning of that chain. They are part of what makes a cell a cell, an organelle an organelle, and a tissue capable of organized function rather than biochemical drift. Once that is seen clearly, every later question about inflammation, metabolism, brain health, cardiovascular disease, immune regulation, and omega-3 biology can be asked at the right level.

The Body Is Built from Lipids

The body is commonly described as if its most important materials are obvious to the eye. Bone is treated as the frame, muscle as the engine, organs as the machinery, and food as the fuel supply that keeps the machinery running. That picture is not wrong, but it begins too late in the hierarchy. Before any organ can perform a task, before any tissue can specialize, and before any cell can maintain identity, the body has to solve a more primitive problem. It has to create boundaries that are stable enough to hold chemistry in one place, selective enough to control exchange, and flexible enough to change behavior without losing integrity. Those boundaries are built largely from lipids. Every cell depends on a membrane. Every organelle depends on a membrane. The body is not simply surrounded by fat, nor does it merely store fat for later use. It is assembled through lipid-based surfaces that determine where one biological space ends and another begins. Without those surfaces, there is no controlled metabolism, no electrical gradient, no receptor signaling, no mitochondrial output, no digestion, no immune discrimination, and no nervous system. There is only chemical mixing.

Lipids matter because they create organized separation in an aqueous environment. Water dominates the chemistry of the body, and that fact makes membrane formation necessary. A living system cannot function if all molecules move freely without compartmental control. The cell needs an inside that is chemically different from the outside. The mitochondrion needs an inner membrane that can hold a proton gradient. The nucleus needs an envelope that protects genetic material while still allowing controlled communication. Vesicles need lipid surfaces so cargo can be moved without being dumped into the wrong compartment. The intestine needs epithelial membranes that can absorb selected materials while refusing others. The nervous system needs myelin-rich lipid insulation and membrane surfaces capable of rapid electrical change. In each case, lipids are not background filler. They are the material solution that allows biological order to exist at all. The body does not first become alive and then add lipids as supporting accessories. It becomes organized because lipids make organized biological space physically possible.

This is why the usual nutritional framing of fat is too small. Fat is often reduced to energy density, body composition, appetite, or storage. Those categories are real, but they do not reach the deepest function of lipids in human physiology. A lipid is not important only because it can be oxidized. It is important because it can become part of a membrane, alter the packing of neighboring molecules, change permeability, modify receptor mobility, influence enzyme access, and serve as the stored substrate for later signaling molecules. A body built from unstable or poorly balanced lipids does not merely carry a bad nutrient profile on paper. It behaves differently. Receptors cluster differently. Inflammatory triggers spread differently. Immune cells activate and resolve differently. Mitochondria hold gradients with different efficiency. Barriers leak more easily or become harder and less adaptive. The quality of the material changes the behavior of the structure, and the behavior of the structure changes the behavior of the organism.

At the cellular level, this means function always sits on top of composition. Two cells can contain the same genes, the same proteins, and the same broad purpose, yet behave differently because their membranes are built differently. The physical environment surrounding membrane proteins changes how those proteins move, how they interact, and how reliably they transmit information. A receptor is not floating in abstraction. It is embedded in lipid matter. Its activity is shaped by membrane thickness, fluidity, saturation, cholesterol distribution, local curvature, and oxidative stability. Ion channels, transporters, docking machinery, inflammatory enzymes, and signal complexes all inherit the conditions of the membrane that holds them. When people think about health in terms of hormones, neurotransmitters, or immune messengers alone, they often miss the layer where those messages are actually interpreted. The cell reads the world through material surfaces. Change the surface, and you change the reading.

This structure-first perspective also explains why lipid biology reaches into every major system at once. The brain is enriched with specialized lipids because rapid signaling, synaptic plasticity, membrane excitability, and long-lived neural stability all require carefully built surfaces. The immune system depends on membrane reorganization to detect threat, build inflammatory synapses, release signaling molecules, and later transition toward resolution. The cardiovascular system depends on endothelial membrane behavior, lipoprotein transport, and vascular signaling that all emerge from lipid-organized interfaces. The liver packages lipids, modifies them, exports them, and uses membrane-intensive trafficking systems to manage the body's chemical load. The gut maintains a boundary with the external world through an epithelial surface whose composition influences permeability, immune tone, and nutrient handling. These are not separate stories. They are variations of the same underlying rule. Life is managed through boundaries, and biological boundaries are lipid structures under constant metabolic maintenance.

Once that is understood, the phrase the body is built from lipids becomes literal rather than metaphorical. It does not mean the body is made only of fat, and it does not mean every health problem reduces to one nutrient class. It means that lipids occupy a foundational position in biological organization because they help determine the architecture through which everything else operates. Proteins do work, but much of that work depends on being placed into the right membrane context. Genes encode instructions, but those instructions still have to be executed inside compartments defined by lipid surfaces. Energy can be generated from many substrates, but efficient energy production still depends on membranes that can hold gradients and organize electron flow. Even inflammation, which is often described as a purely signaling phenomenon, depends on lipid-derived mediator pathways and membrane events that decide how strongly a response begins and whether it can end cleanly.

This is the level at which omega-3 and the broader lipid conversation have to be approached. The question is not simply whether a given fat has benefits. The deeper question is what kind of structure that fat helps build over time. Does it strengthen membrane performance or weaken it. Does it improve signaling fidelity or increase instability. Does it support resolution chemistry or only add more susceptibility to damage if the surrounding environment cannot protect it. Does it enter a body already saturated with competing inflammatory substrates and oxidative stress, or does it become part of a coordinated reconstruction of membrane architecture. Those are structural questions, and they matter because the body expresses its health through the materials from which it is built. Long before symptoms become visible, the architecture has already been changing.

Membranes as the Foundation of Biology

Biology begins when matter is separated into controlled spaces. That separation is not philosophical and it is not optional. Without it, there is no cell, no organelle, no metabolism, no signaling sequence, and no stable life process that can persist long enough to become tissue, organ, or organism. The membrane is the structure that makes this possible. It creates an inside and an outside, but more importantly, it allows those two spaces to remain chemically different while still permitting selective exchange between them. That is the first real act of biological organization. A membrane holds gradients, localizes reactions, embeds proteins, and gives the cell a stable surface through which information can be received and acted on. Once that surface exists, the rest of biology can begin layering itself on top of it. Without the membrane, there is no meaningful distinction between environment and organism. There is only chemistry dispersing into chemistry.

This is why membranes should not be treated as passive wrappers or thin packaging around more important internal machinery. The membrane is part of the machinery. In many cases it is the condition that allows machinery to function at all. Ion channels require a membrane so ions can move across a meaningful barrier rather than through open fluid. Receptors require a membrane so outside information can be converted into intracellular action. Transporters require a membrane so nutrients, waste, and signaling molecules can be selectively moved rather than randomly diffused. Enzymes associated with the membrane often behave differently depending on the exact lipid environment surrounding them. A protein does not simply sit in a membrane like a bolt fixed into plastic. It exists in a material field that changes its position, motion, conformation, binding behavior, and access to substrates. The membrane is therefore not just where proteins are located. It is part of what determines what those proteins can actually do.

At the scale of the whole cell, membrane structure defines identity. A cell does not remain alive because it contains useful molecules. It remains alive because those molecules are organized within a bounded system that can maintain concentration differences, electrical gradients, pH differences, osmotic balance, and controlled traffic. The cell membrane prevents collapse into equilibrium. That matters because equilibrium in a living system is often death. Life requires maintained asymmetry. Sodium has to be kept in one distribution, potassium in another, calcium must remain tightly controlled, and metabolites must be directed rather than allowed to drift. The membrane is what gives the cell leverage over its own chemistry. It allows the cell to resist the passive tendencies of the surrounding environment and hold a state that is energetically costly but biologically useful. In that sense, the membrane is not merely a boundary. It is a tool for preserving non-randomness.

The same principle repeats inside the cell. The mitochondrion is not just a structure floating in cytoplasm. It is a membrane-built energy system whose inner membrane holds the electron transport chain and creates the proton gradient required for ATP production. The nucleus uses a membrane envelope to protect genetic material and control traffic between the genome and the rest of the cell. Lysosomes, peroxisomes, endosomes, secretory vesicles, and the endoplasmic reticulum all depend on membranes because each one performs chemistry that must be spatially separated from other chemistry. Once this is seen clearly, it becomes obvious that membranes are not a feature of biology. They are one of its core organizing laws. Life works by building compartments, and compartments only function when membranes are stable enough to preserve distinction while dynamic enough to support exchange and adaptation.

This turns membrane composition into a major determinant of physiology rather than a minor biochemical detail. A membrane is not interchangeable with any other membrane. Its behavior depends on which phospholipids are present, which fatty acids occupy those phospholipids, how much cholesterol is present, how sphingolipids are distributed, how ordered or disordered the surface becomes, and how vulnerable the structure is to oxidation or mechanical disruption. Those factors shape permeability, thickness, flexibility, curvature, electrical behavior, receptor clustering, and signaling fidelity. A membrane that is too rigid creates one kind of problem. A membrane that is too unstable or oxidatively damaged creates another. A membrane overloaded with poorly protected polyunsaturated material may allow high signaling flexibility while also becoming chemically fragile. A membrane built with greater structural stability may preserve gradients and protein behavior more reliably but alter mobility in other ways. Biology is constantly solving this material balancing act. The health of the system depends on whether that balance remains coherent across tissues and over time.

That is why membranes sit underneath so many processes that are usually discussed separately. Neural firing depends on membrane excitability and ion channel behavior. Hormone signaling depends on receptor function within specific membrane environments. Immune activation depends on membrane reorganization, receptor assembly, vesicle trafficking, and later the release of lipid-derived mediators. Barrier tissues depend on membrane integrity plus the protein structures anchored to them. Mitochondrial output depends on the ability of membranes to maintain proton separation and organize respiratory complexes. Even mechanical behavior at the tissue level depends partly on whether cell membranes and associated lipid structures can absorb stress without destabilizing the signaling systems built into them. The body looks like many systems from the outside, but at depth those systems are repeatedly operating through variations of the same membrane logic.

This also explains why biological breakdown often begins long before conventional disease categories become obvious. Membranes can lose quality gradually. They can become more oxidized, less stable, more compositionally distorted, less able to support receptor precision, less effective at holding gradients, and more likely to amplify inflammatory noise. The early signs may appear disconnected. A person notices unstable energy, poorer recovery, more reactivity to food or stress, changes in mood, reduced exercise tolerance, worsening metabolic control, or a greater tendency toward chronic irritation in tissues. These do not always look like membrane problems because the membrane is not visible in ordinary medical language. But much of what the person is experiencing may be the downstream behavior of surfaces that no longer organize biology cleanly. The system has not lost all function. It has lost structural precision.

Seen from this angle, the membrane is where structure and signaling become inseparable. It is the place where matter becomes information-bearing. A receptor does not just detect a hormone because the hormone exists. It detects it in a certain membrane state, with a certain lipid neighborhood, under a certain curvature and cholesterol distribution, with certain probabilities of clustering and internalization. An inflammatory enzyme does not merely act because the gene for that enzyme is expressed. It acts because the membrane provides the substrate access and physical conditions needed for action. A mitochondrion does not merely burn fuel because fuel is present. It produces energy because membrane architecture permits organized electron flow. Function is therefore not suspended above structure. Function is the behavior of structure under conditions.

For that reason, any serious discussion of health has to begin lower than symptoms, lower than blood markers, and lower than even many familiar biochemical pathways. It has to begin at the level of the material surfaces that make organized life possible. Membranes are the foundation because they are the condition for compartmentalization, signaling, energy conversion, selective exchange, and biological identity itself. Once that is understood, the rest of physiology starts to align. Nutrients stop looking like isolated chemicals and start looking like materials that alter surfaces. Chronic disease stops looking like a list of unrelated malfunctions and starts looking more like the accumulated consequences of structural distortion. And omega-3, which is so often discussed as a supplement with benefits, can finally be placed where it belongs: inside the membrane story, where biology actually begins.

Compartmentalization and Control

Life depends on separation. Not symbolic separation, but physical separation that allows different chemical conditions to exist at the same time inside the same organism. A living body cannot function as one open fluid space where everything mixes freely. If that happened, gradients would collapse, reactions would interfere with one another, signaling would lose direction, and the distinction between useful chemistry and destructive chemistry would disappear. Compartmentalization is the solution to that problem. It allows the body to divide itself into controlled zones, each with its own composition, pressure, charge distribution, substrate concentration, and functional purpose. The membrane is what makes that division real. Once a membrane defines a compartment, biology gains the ability to control what enters, what leaves, what accumulates, what reacts, and what remains excluded. That is the beginning of regulation in the most literal sense. Control is not first a matter of hormones, genes, or feedback loops. It is first a matter of whether the system can hold separate spaces long enough for those higher forms of control to even exist.

The cell itself is the first major example. It maintains an internal environment that is chemically different from the fluid surrounding it, and that difference is not incidental. Intracellular potassium remains high while sodium is kept relatively low. Calcium is held under tight restriction because even small increases can trigger powerful downstream effects. pH is buffered within narrow ranges because enzyme systems depend on local chemical stability. Nutrients are brought in selectively, waste is moved out selectively, and signaling molecules are either admitted, excluded, degraded, recycled, or transported according to need. None of this happens in an open system. It depends on membranes that can preserve concentration differences against the constant tendency of molecules to diffuse toward equilibrium. In practical terms, the membrane allows the cell to say no. It can refuse indiscriminate entry. It can prevent the loss of critical molecules. It can control timing. It can turn transport into an active decision rather than a passive leak.

Inside the cell, the same logic becomes more elaborate. The body does not place all chemistry into one intracellular pool and hope that specificity will emerge from molecular goodwill. It builds internal compartments because precision requires separation. The nucleus isolates the genome from the cytoplasmic environment while still allowing tightly regulated communication through nuclear pores. The mitochondrion creates two membrane-defined spaces so electron transport can build a proton gradient across the inner membrane and convert that gradient into ATP. Lysosomes contain acidic degradative chemistry that would be destructive if released without control. Peroxisomes handle oxidative reactions that need their own boundary conditions. The endoplasmic reticulum organizes protein synthesis, folding, and lipid handling within its own membrane network. Vesicles move cargo in enclosed form because transport without containment would create chemical disorder. Compartmentalization therefore does not just make biology tidy. It prevents incompatibility. It allows one reaction to occur intensely in one place without corrupting the conditions needed somewhere else.

This creates a deeper definition of control than the word usually carries. In ordinary language, control sounds like command from above, as if the body is centrally managed by regulatory molecules issuing instructions down a chain. Biology does use layered signaling, but that signaling only works because compartments constrain possibility. A hormone may circulate systemically, but its effect still depends on whether the target tissue can receive it, buffer it, amplify it, or terminate it within the architecture of its compartments. A calcium signal can activate contraction, secretion, or transcription depending on where calcium rises, how fast it rises, how long it remains elevated, and which local proteins are present to interpret it. A reactive oxygen species can serve as a controlled signal in one compartment and become damaging chemistry in another. Control is therefore never just about the presence of a molecule. It is about where that molecule exists, where it is prevented from existing, and how the surrounding boundary structure limits its reach.

This is why loss of compartmental integrity produces disproportionate consequences. When a barrier fails, chemistry that was supposed to remain local spreads into spaces that were not built to handle it. When mitochondrial membranes lose integrity, proton gradients weaken, ATP production becomes less efficient, and electron leakage can rise. When lysosomal contents escape, degradative processes begin damaging the wrong targets. When intestinal barrier function deteriorates, microbial fragments, incompletely processed food components, and inflammatory stimuli gain greater access to immune surfaces beneath the epithelial layer. When vascular or tissue barriers become more permeable, fluid shifts, immune traffic, and signaling noise increase. These are not merely examples of damage occurring in isolated places. They are examples of lost control through failed boundaries. Once compartmentalization weakens, the system loses the ability to keep processes in their proper zones, and biological behavior becomes less selective, more expensive, and more chaotic.

The nervous system offers one of the clearest demonstrations of this principle. Neurons rely on membrane-defined compartments to maintain resting potential, generate action potentials, release neurotransmitters at synapses, and recover after signaling events. The signal only works because ions are separated, channels open in a controlled sequence, and neurotransmitter release occurs into a narrow synaptic space rather than into general tissue fluid. The brain as a whole depends on larger compartmental controls as well, including the blood-brain barrier, specialized extracellular environments, and glial regulation of local chemistry. Remove those layers of separation and neural precision degrades quickly. The same is true in the immune system, where discrimination depends on controlling where antigens are encountered, where inflammatory mediators are generated, where immune cells traffic, and when damaged material is cleared without spilling its contents across surrounding tissue. The body maintains intelligence through boundaries. Without boundaries, information turns into noise.

Lipid structure sits underneath all of this because membranes are the physical basis of compartmentalization. Their composition determines how effectively a boundary can hold gradients, resist uncontrolled permeability, support transport proteins, recover from stress, and preserve signaling precision under load. A membrane that is compositionally weak, excessively oxidized, overly permeable, or mechanically unstable may still exist, but it does not provide the same level of control. It allows more leakage, more misfiring, more unintended molecular contact, and more distortion of timing. A stable membrane does the opposite. It sharpens distinction between compartments. It supports selective transport instead of indiscriminate movement. It preserves the conditions needed for high-resolution biological behavior. This is one reason lipid quality matters so much beyond the crude language of energy intake. The body is not just fed by fats. It is governed through structures partly made from them.

Compartmentalization also explains why chronic dysfunction often feels diffuse before it becomes diagnosable. Control rarely disappears all at once. More often it erodes gradually. Barriers become slightly more permissive. Membranes become slightly less reliable. Signaling molecules persist a little longer in places where they should have been cleared. Oxidative reactions reach a little further than they should. Immune recognition becomes slightly less selective. Energy production becomes slightly less contained. Early on, this does not look like one dramatic pathology. It looks like accumulated imprecision. The person becomes less resilient, less stable, less capable of clean transitions between rest and stress, activation and recovery, feeding and fasting, challenge and repair. The compartments are still present, but the quality of control they provide has declined.

Seen clearly, compartmentalization is not a side feature of biology. It is what allows control to exist in the first place. The body does not regulate by floating commands through undifferentiated chemistry. It regulates by building spaces, protecting those spaces, and using those spaces to determine what kind of reactions are possible and where. Once that framework is established, signaling becomes meaningful, energy conversion becomes efficient, immune defense becomes discriminating, and tissue behavior becomes coordinated instead of random. This is why membrane integrity and lipid architecture deserve such central attention. They are not one topic among many. They are part of the physical basis by which the body holds order against collapse.

Lipids as Structure, Not Just Fuel

One of the most limiting ideas in modern nutrition is the habit of treating fat primarily as stored energy. In that framework, lipids matter because they contain calories, slow digestion, influence appetite, and can be burned when glucose is not immediately available. All of that is true, but it describes only one layer of lipid biology, and not the deepest one. The more foundational role of lipids is structural. They are part of the material from which the body builds itself. They form membranes, define compartment boundaries, shape organelle behavior, influence tissue stability, and create the physical environment in which proteins, receptors, enzymes, and transport systems must operate. When lipids are viewed only as fuel, the body gets interpreted like an engine that occasionally uses fat for combustion. When lipids are viewed structurally, the body looks different. It becomes a built system whose performance depends on the quality, balance, and durability of the materials used to construct its surfaces.

This matters because the body does not merely use lipids after they are eaten. It incorporates them. Fatty acids are esterified into phospholipids, packed into membranes, stored in droplets, transported in lipoproteins, converted into signaling molecules, and positioned within tissues according to ongoing metabolic need. Once incorporated, they change the behavior of the structure they enter. A membrane containing different lipid species does not just look different on a chemistry chart. It behaves differently under stress, responds differently to signals, and supports different patterns of receptor movement, ion transfer, permeability, and enzyme activity. That means dietary fat is not simply entering a furnace. It is contributing to the construction, repair, and remodeling of biological matter. This is one reason why the same calorie intake can produce very different physiological outcomes depending on what kinds of lipids are repeatedly being supplied and what broader metabolic conditions those lipids enter.

The structural role of lipids begins with the membrane, but it does not stop there. Lipids determine how tightly a membrane packs, how much lateral movement occurs within it, how vulnerable it is to oxidation, how easily it bends to form vesicles, how stable it remains under mechanical stress, and how effectively it can host proteins that need a certain physical environment in order to function well. Cholesterol contributes to membrane order and local stiffness. Saturated fatty acids tend to support tighter packing and greater structural stability. Monounsaturated fats can support flexibility while maintaining relative resilience. Polyunsaturated fats increase fluidity and expand signaling potential, but they also introduce greater chemical fragility because their double bonds are more susceptible to oxidation. None of these characteristics are abstract. They alter how real tissues behave. A neuron, an immune cell, an intestinal epithelial cell, and a hepatocyte all inherit part of their operating behavior from the lipid composition of the surfaces through which they function.

This changes the way energy itself should be understood. The body certainly oxidizes lipids for ATP production, especially in tissues adapted for high rates of fat use such as skeletal muscle, cardiac muscle, and liver under appropriate conditions. But even here, structure remains upstream. Fat cannot be converted into energy efficiently unless mitochondria are physically capable of doing the work. That requires intact mitochondrial membranes, preserved cristae architecture, controlled proton impermeability, and lipid environments that stabilize respiratory complexes rather than destabilize them. The body does not extract energy from fat in a structural vacuum. It extracts energy through lipid-built organelles whose own function depends on lipid integrity. In other words, lipids are involved on both sides of the equation. They serve as potential fuel, but they also help determine whether the machinery that burns fuel can operate cleanly. The old picture of fat as input and mitochondria as passive burners misses that the machinery itself is partly made from lipid-dependent architecture.

The immune system reveals the same principle in another form. Lipids do not only sit in immune cell membranes as inert background material. They help organize receptor clusters, shape the immunological synapse, influence membrane trafficking during activation, and provide the substrate for inflammatory and pro-resolving mediator synthesis. Arachidonic acid, EPA, and DHA are not just nutrients floating in plasma with separate brand identities. They are structural components that can later be mobilized into signaling cascades when phospholipase activity releases them from membrane phospholipids. This means that what appears during inflammation is partly determined by what has already been built into tissue. The inflammatory output of the body is not generated from nothing at the moment of stress. It emerges from stored material. The membrane is acting as both structure and reservoir. That is why long-term lipid intake shapes immune behavior over time even when no obvious acute symptom is present.

The nervous system depends especially heavily on this structure-first view. Neural tissue is dense with lipid material because signal transmission, synaptic vesicle release, membrane excitability, and insulation all require surfaces with specific physical properties. Myelin is lipid-rich because rapid conduction depends on electrical separation. Synaptic membranes require precise composition because neurotransmission depends on curvature, vesicle fusion, receptor organization, and rapid membrane recycling. Brain lipids are not there as emergency calories stored near neurons for convenience. They are part of what allows neurons to behave like neurons. When lipid composition shifts unfavorably, the effect is not limited to energy supply. It can alter signaling stability, membrane excitability, inflammatory sensitivity, and the quality of neural communication itself. That is why the conversation around lipids and brain health becomes shallow when it is reduced to whether a fat "feeds the brain." The brain is partly built from lipid architecture, and its behavior follows the quality of that architecture.

This structural lens also clarifies why some fats can support stability while others can increase volatility when the system is not properly protected. A highly unsaturated lipid may contribute useful fluidity and signaling potential, but if oxidative defense is poor, if membrane repair is inadequate, or if inflammatory pressure is already high, that same lipid can become part of an unstable surface that is easily damaged and then converted into reactive byproducts. On the other side, more saturated structures may improve durability and lower susceptibility to peroxidation, but excessive rigidity in the wrong context can also impair certain forms of membrane behavior. Biology is never solved by slogans. The real question is what kind of structure a given lipid pattern creates across a real tissue under real metabolic conditions. This is why the phrase healthy fats often fails to explain anything meaningful. Lipid value depends on role, proportion, tissue context, oxidative environment, and the structural state of the organism already receiving it.

Once lipids are understood as structure, the timeline of nutritional change also becomes easier to interpret. Structural remodeling is slower than pharmacologic stimulation. A membrane does not instantly transform because one meal contained more omega-3 or less seed oil. Tissue composition changes over repeated exposure, selective incorporation, turnover, oxidation, repair, and replacement. That is one reason people often misunderstand fat-based interventions. They expect a signaling molecule result from what is actually a remodeling process. Structural inputs work by changing the material conditions of the system over time. Membrane composition gradually shifts. Receptor behavior gradually shifts with it. Inflammatory substrate availability gradually shifts. Mitochondrial resilience, barrier behavior, and signal fidelity can then begin to move in new directions. This is not the pace of a stimulant or a pain reliever. It is the pace of construction.

For that reason, lipids should be thought of less as optional dietary macros and more as ongoing building inputs that happen to carry energy. That order

matters. Their caloric value is real, but it is secondary to the deeper fact that they enter tissues and influence what those tissues are physically like. The body is not a furnace wrapped in flesh. It is a layered, compartmentalized structure whose surfaces determine much of its behavior. Lipids participate directly in that construction. They help define whether membranes are stable or fragile, whether signals are clean or distorted, whether inflammation can resolve or only persist, whether mitochondria can hold gradients, and whether tissues can preserve order under stress. Once that becomes the frame, the discussion of omega-3, omega-6, saturated fat, phospholipids, cholesterol, and membrane remodeling stops being a side conversation about dietary preference.
It becomes a conversation about the materials from which biological performance is built.

Chapter 2

Membranes as Decision-Making Surfaces

The membrane is usually introduced as a boundary, and that description is correct as far as it goes, but it is still too passive to explain what membranes actually do. A membrane does not merely separate inside from outside. It interprets contact. It determines whether a molecule will be ignored, transported, resisted, internalized, amplified into a signal, or converted into a larger change in cellular behavior. In that sense, the membrane functions less like a wall and more like a decision surface. It is the place where the cell encounters the world and decides what that encounter means. Every tissue in the body depends on this process. Nutrients arrive, hormones circulate, inflammatory signals appear, microbes or microbial fragments make contact, mechanical force distorts the surface, temperature changes alter membrane behavior, electrical gradients shift, and the cell must continuously determine whether these inputs represent fuel, threat, instruction, noise, or damage. Those determinations are not made in abstraction. They are made through the physical properties and molecular organization of the membrane itself.

This is why membrane biology belongs at the center of physiology rather than at its edge. The cell does not first understand a signal and then pass that signal through the membrane as a delivery route. The membrane is part of the interpretive mechanism. A receptor embedded in a membrane does not respond only because a ligand binds to it. It responds within a local field defined by lipid composition, cholesterol content, membrane thickness, surface charge, curvature, oxidative state, and the presence or absence of neighboring proteins. That local field changes the probability of receptor clustering, the stability of active conformations, the speed of internalization, the access of kinases and phosphatases, and the likelihood that a brief external event becomes a sustained intracellular response. What looks from the outside like a simple on-off signal is usually the end result of many smaller physical decisions built into the surface architecture. The membrane does not think in the psychological sense, but it continuously sorts inputs into biological consequences.

This decision-making role becomes clearer once signaling is understood as a spatial event rather than a purely chemical one. Molecules do not act in empty space. They collide within structured environments. Receptors are not scattered randomly across a featureless sheet. They occupy domains, enter clusters, separate from other proteins, move into ordered regions, leave those regions, bind adaptors, and participate in transient signaling assemblies whose formation depends on membrane conditions. A hormone signal can be strong in one membrane context and weak in another even when hormone concentration remains the same. An inflammatory trigger can be amplified or dampened depending on how membrane lipids shape receptor behavior and downstream enzyme access. A growth signal can persist too long if the surface organization that normally restrains it has been altered. These are not minor effects. They are part of how the cell decides what kind of state it is in and what it should do next.

The concept of the membrane as a decision surface also explains why lipids influence behavior far beyond their caloric value. A change in membrane composition is not just a biochemical substitution. It is a change in interpretive architecture. Alter the balance of saturated, monounsaturated, and polyunsaturated fatty acids within phospholipids, and you alter the packing characteristics of the membrane. Alter packing, and you alter receptor mobility, microdomain formation, membrane permeability, mechanical resilience, and enzyme-substrate interactions. Change cholesterol distribution, and ordered regions may become more or less stable. Increase oxidative damage, and the membrane may become more disorganized, more permeable, and less capable of hosting precise signaling events. The cell then begins making different decisions from the same external world because the surface through which it reads that world has changed. This is one of the deepest reasons that nutrition, inflammation, oxidative stress, endocrine signaling, and chronic disease cannot be understood as separate conversations. They converge at the membrane.

The immune system makes this especially obvious. An immune cell does not merely possess receptors for threat. It has to organize those receptors into functional patterns on the membrane surface, distinguish weak noise from true danger, assemble signaling complexes, change shape, move, engulf, secrete, and later deactivate or resolve. Every one of those steps depends on membrane behavior. If the membrane becomes compositionally distorted, oxidatively damaged, or overloaded with unstable signaling substrate, immune interpretation changes. Threat may be recognized too aggressively, too diffusely, or for too long. Activation may occur readily while resolution remains incomplete. The cell may enter inflammatory states faster than it can leave them. This is not because immune cells have suddenly forgotten their purpose. It is because the surface through which they make decisions no longer supports clean discrimination. A body can therefore become chronically inflamed not only because inflammatory signals exist, but because its decision-making surfaces have become less precise.

The nervous system depends on the same principle under different constraints. Neurons and glial cells must handle electrical signaling, receptor trafficking, synaptic vesicle fusion, local inflammatory surveillance, and rapid adaptation to incoming information. These processes require membranes that can support highly specific patterns of excitability and communication. A synaptic membrane must decide whether a neurotransmitter pulse should trigger a strong postsynaptic response, a weak one, a temporary change in receptor density, or a longer-term plastic adaptation. That decision is not made by neurotransmitter concentration alone. It depends on receptor state, membrane composition, channel behavior, scaffold stability, and local lipid organization. When membranes are altered, the nervous system may not fail dramatically at first. Instead it becomes noisier, more reactive, less stable, or less efficient. Precision declines before catastrophe appears. The decision surface is still operating, but it is making lower-quality decisions because its structure has changed.

This framework also clarifies why chronic dysfunction often presents as dysregulation rather than simple deficiency. A person may have enough hormones in circulation yet still show poor response. They may have immune activity that will not turn off, appetite signals that do not match energy state, stress responses that remain exaggerated after the stressor has passed, or inflammatory chemistry that persists long after the original insult. In many cases the problem is framed in terms of too much or too little of a signaling molecule. Sometimes that is true. But often the more foundational issue is that the membrane surface interpreting the signal has become distorted. The system is not merely lacking input. It is misreading input. Decision quality has degraded at the interface layer. That leads to amplification where restraint was needed, resistance where responsiveness was needed, leakage where compartmental control was needed, and persistence where termination was needed.

Once membranes are understood as decision-making surfaces, the subject of omega-3 expands naturally into a much larger argument. Omega-3 fatty acids are not interesting only because they can become anti-inflammatory metabolites or support a desirable ratio on paper. They matter because they enter the membrane and help shape the physical conditions under which cellular decisions are made. They influence substrate availability for future mediator synthesis, but they also alter membrane behavior before those mediators are ever produced. They can change how receptors cluster, how signals propagate, how inflammatory responses escalate, and whether resolution pathways have access to the structural material required to function. This does not mean omega-3 acts alone or solves everything. It means omega-3 belongs to the architecture of interpretation. It helps determine what kind of surface the cell is using to read its environment.

The deeper message of this chapter is that biology does not decide through disembodied information. It decides through matter arranged into responsive surfaces. The membrane is where chemistry becomes meaning for the cell. It is where contact becomes instruction, where instruction becomes activation or restraint, and where long-term structural inputs shape short-term behavior. Once that is seen clearly, many scattered topics begin to align. Receptor sensitivity, inflammation, insulin resistance, neurotransmission, immune tolerance, endothelial function, barrier integrity, and recovery capacity all begin to look less like isolated failures and more like different expressions of how well the body's decision-making surfaces are built. That is the level at which the lipid story becomes coherent, and it is the level required for understanding why membrane composition is never just background material. It is part of how the body decides what to do next.

The Cell Membrane as an Interface

The cell membrane is often described as a border, but border is too static a word for what it actually is. A true biological membrane is an interface. It is the active surface where the cell meets everything it does not fully control and must therefore evaluate, manage, or transform. Nutrients arrive at this surface. Hormones arrive at this surface. Mechanical stress reaches this surface. Immune signals, microbial fragments, toxins, electrical changes, osmotic shifts, and inflammatory mediators all reach this surface. The cell membrane is the first place where outside conditions become intracellular consequences. It does not merely separate two environments. It governs the terms of contact between them. That is what makes it an interface rather than a wrapper. The membrane allows the cell to remain distinct from its environment while still exchanging matter and information with it in a controlled way. Without that interface, the cell could neither preserve its identity nor participate in a larger organism.

This interface function depends on more than the existence of a lipid bilayer. It depends on the membrane being built as a selective and responsive surface. Embedded within it are receptors, ion channels, transporters, docking proteins, adhesion molecules, enzymes, and structural anchors, all positioned inside a material environment that affects how they behave. A receptor only matters if the membrane can hold it in the right orientation, allow it to move when movement is required, cluster it when clustering is required, and connect it to intracellular signaling machinery once binding occurs. A transporter only works if the membrane can preserve the gradient that gives transport meaning. An ion channel only matters if the membrane can maintain the separation of charge and concentration that makes opening and closing consequential. The membrane therefore does not simply host molecular tools. It creates the conditions that make those tools usable.

Because it is an interface, the membrane has to solve two problems at once. It has to defend the cell from indiscriminate mixing with the outside world, and it has to allow carefully selected exchange with that same world. If it becomes too permissive, the cell loses control over ions, water, metabolites, and signaling exposure. If it becomes too rigid or poorly responsive, transport becomes inefficient, signaling becomes blunt, and adaptation slows. The membrane has to remain stable without becoming inert. It has to remain dynamic without becoming leaky. That balance is one of the most important material challenges in biology, and lipid composition sits near the center of it. The kinds of fatty acids built into membrane phospholipids, the local cholesterol content, the presence of sphingolipids, the degree of oxidative injury, and the mechanical demands placed on the tissue all influence how well that interface performs. What the membrane is made from changes how it negotiates the outside world.

This is why the membrane is not just a line between inside and outside but a site of interpretation. The same external signal can produce different cellular outcomes depending on membrane state. A hormone may bind its receptor, but the intensity, duration, and downstream quality of that response depend partly on how the receptor is positioned within the membrane, what nearby lipids stabilize or destabilize it, and whether the surrounding surface supports clean signal transfer or introduces noise. The same nutrient may be absorbed efficiently in one membrane condition and poorly in another. The same inflammatory trigger may produce an exaggerated response in a disordered membrane and a more proportionate response in a stable one. The membrane does not think, but it determines how much meaning an external event is allowed to carry. That is why it behaves like an interface in the deepest sense. It is the point where contact is translated into consequence.

This becomes even clearer when the membrane is viewed as a layered communication surface rather than a simple barrier. On its outer face, it presents receptors and adhesion structures to the extracellular environment. Within the bilayer, it organizes proteins in space, alters their mobility, and creates microdomains where certain interactions are more likely to occur. On its inner face, it anchors signaling machinery to the cytoskeleton and intracellular pathways that will execute the result of the encounter. An event at the outer surface therefore does not stay at the outer surface. It propagates through the membrane into the cell's internal architecture. A binding event can alter gene expression. A mechanical deformation can change ion flow. A change in membrane composition can alter endocytosis, exocytosis, motility, or immune recognition. The membrane is a translation layer between external conditions and internal action.

This interface role is especially important in tissues that live under constant environmental exposure. Intestinal epithelial cells face food components, microbial products, bile acids, enzymes, and immune surveillance signals all at once. Their membranes must allow nutrient absorption while resisting uncontrolled entry of harmful material. Endothelial cells lining blood vessels must respond to circulating molecules, shear stress, immune signals, and redox changes while preserving vascular integrity. Immune cells must use their membranes to detect threat, distinguish self from non-self, form contact zones with target cells, and later disengage when the job is done. Neurons must receive neurotransmitters, maintain electrical gradients, and recycle signaling machinery at high speed without losing stability. In each case, the membrane is not an accessory to function. It is where function begins, because it is where exchange with the world is structured rather than random.

This also explains why changes in membrane composition can reshape physiology so broadly. When the interface changes, the quality of contact changes. If the membrane becomes more oxidized, permeability can shift and receptor behavior can degrade. If the lipid environment becomes less stable, signaling complexes may assemble less cleanly or disassemble improperly. If the membrane becomes overloaded with substrates that favor inflammatory mediator release under stress, immune signaling can become more easily amplified. If the membrane loses structural resilience, cells may become more vulnerable to mechanical or oxidative injury. These changes do not stay confined to one biochemical pathway because the membrane is upstream of many pathways at once. It is the platform through which multiple systems encounter their inputs. A degraded interface produces degraded interpretation across the organism.

For that reason, the cell membrane should be understood as one of the body's primary control surfaces. It decides what gets in, what stays out, what gets sensed, what gets ignored, what gets transported, what gets stored, and what gets turned into action. It is not doing this alone, and it is not doing it consciously, but it is doing it materially. Its composition, organization, and stability determine how precisely the cell can engage with its environment without being overwhelmed by it. Once that is understood, the importance of lipid architecture becomes much harder to ignore. Lipids are not merely passive ingredients in the membrane. They shape the interface itself, and by shaping the interface, they help shape the behavior of the cell, the tissue, and eventually the organism built from them.

Receptors, Fluidity, and Signal Interpretation

A receptor is often described as if it were a fixed lock waiting for the right key, but that image removes the receptor from the material surface that gives it meaning. Receptors do not float in empty space. They are embedded in membranes, and that embedding changes how they behave before any ligand ever arrives. The membrane affects receptor orientation, movement, clustering, conformational flexibility, access to signaling partners, and the rate at which activated receptors are internalized or recycled. This means signal interpretation begins before binding. The receptor is already being conditioned by the physical state of the membrane surrounding it. A hormone, neurotransmitter, cytokine, or growth factor may be present in circulation, but the effect of that signal still depends on whether the membrane is able to host a receptor in a way that preserves precision instead of noise.

Fluidity sits near the center of this problem because membranes have to remain mobile enough to support signaling while stable enough to preserve structure. A membrane that is too rigid can restrict receptor movement, reduce the ability of receptors to cluster into active complexes, impair vesicle fusion, and interfere with conformational changes required for signal transfer. A membrane that is too disordered can create a different problem. Receptors may move excessively, signaling complexes may assemble too loosely or too unpredictably, permeability may rise, and the surface can become more vulnerable to oxidative injury and interpretive instability. Biology therefore does not aim for maximum fluidity or minimum fluidity. It aims for usable fluidity within a stable structural framework. The membrane has to allow motion without becoming incoherent. It has to permit adaptation without losing control of the surface on which that adaptation occurs.

Receptors are highly sensitive to that balance because their function is not only chemical but spatial. Many receptors need to cluster after binding in order to amplify a signal. Others need to be segregated from inhibitory proteins before activation can proceed. Some require movement into cholesterol-rich or sphingolipid-rich membrane microdomains where the local environment supports certain protein-protein interactions. Some depend on rapid endocytosis after activation so the signal can be terminated or redirected. All of this is influenced by the material state of the membrane. The same receptor can generate a different biological response in two cells not because the receptor itself is genetically different, but because the lipid environment alters how that receptor behaves as part of a surface system. Signal interpretation is therefore partly a matter of membrane mechanics. The cell is not only asking whether a ligand bound. It is also determining what that binding event should be allowed to become.

This is one reason membrane composition has such broad physiological consequences. Saturated fatty acids tend to promote tighter packing and structural firmness. Monounsaturated fats can preserve flexibility while maintaining relatively good stability. Polyunsaturated fats increase membrane mobility and can support dynamic signaling behavior, but they also introduce more chemical fragility because their double bonds are more easily oxidized. Cholesterol adds another layer by buffering membrane behavior, preventing excessive disorder in some contexts while preventing excessive rigidity in others. Sphingolipids contribute to ordered domains that help organize receptor activity and signal sorting. The membrane is therefore not simply more fluid or less fluid. It contains regions with different physical properties, and receptors behave differently depending on where they sit within that landscape. Signal quality emerges from the organization of this material terrain.

The consequences of altered fluidity become obvious in endocrine and metabolic signaling. A cell may be exposed to insulin, thyroid hormone, cortisol, leptin, or other circulating messengers, yet still respond poorly if receptor behavior at the membrane has become distorted. This is often framed solely as receptor resistance or downstream signaling failure, but the membrane layer is frequently underappreciated. If receptors cannot cluster correctly, if local lipid domains are disorganized, if oxidative injury has altered the surrounding phospholipids, or if membrane turnover has produced a surface that no longer supports clean conformational change, the signal can be weakened, prolonged incorrectly, or interpreted with reduced fidelity. The body then behaves as though it has insufficient signaling even when the messenger itself is present. In that case the problem is not absence of instruction. It is degraded interpretation at the surface.

The immune system depends on this same principle in a more dynamic setting. Immune receptors have to discriminate between background noise and meaningful threat. They often do this through threshold behavior, which depends on receptor density, clustering, membrane microdomain organization, and the speed with which signaling assemblies form and dissolve. A membrane that is compositionally unstable or excessively oxidized can lower the quality of that discrimination. Threat detection may become overactive, sustained too long, or poorly resolved. The cell may activate too easily and terminate too slowly. This is one pathway by which structural membrane problems become chronic inflammatory behavior. The immune cell is still receiving signals, but the surface through which it interprets those signals has become less reliable. A small input can begin to produce a larger and more persistent response than the original event justified.

Neural signaling is equally dependent on membrane fluidity and receptor interpretation. Neurotransmitter receptors, ion channels, synaptic docking proteins, and vesicle release machinery all operate within membranes that must maintain fast dynamics without sacrificing precision. If fluidity drops too low, receptor mobility and vesicle fusion can become impaired. If disorder rises too high, electrical stability and signaling precision can begin to deteriorate. This does not always produce immediate failure. More often it produces noise. Synaptic timing becomes less exact. Recovery from signaling becomes less efficient. Excitability shifts. Inflammatory sensitivity in neural tissue may rise. The person experiences the downstream behavior as changes in mood, attention, resilience, sensitivity, or cognitive sharpness, but underneath those effects is a membrane-level problem of signal interpretation being carried out on altered surfaces.

This also clarifies why omega-3 cannot be understood simply as a nutrient that turns inflammation up or down. EPA and DHA enter phospholipids and change membrane properties over time. That changes substrate availability for future signaling molecules, but it also changes the physical environment in which receptors and channels operate. In some tissues this can improve flexibility, receptor behavior, or signal transduction. In other contexts, especially when oxidative protection is weak or membrane instability is already high, increasing highly unsaturated lipids without structural support may introduce vulnerability as well. The issue is never just whether a fatty acid is good in isolation. The issue is what kind of interpretive surface it helps build.

Signal interpretation is only as good as the membrane through which the signal is being read.

Receptors, fluidity, and signal interpretation therefore belong to the same system. A receptor is not a detached sensor. It is a protein embedded in matter, and that matter changes the meaning of the signal it receives. Fluidity is not a cosmetic feature of the membrane. It is part of what determines whether receptors can move, cluster, change shape, terminate signals, and communicate with intracellular machinery at the right intensity and duration. When this relationship is stable, the cell reads its environment with high precision. When it is distorted, the same world begins to produce worse decisions. Hormones can be present but poorly felt. Immune triggers can be exaggerated. Neurotransmitters can become noisier. The membrane is not just where signals arrive. It is part of how signals become biologically real.

How Membrane Composition Alters Reality

The body does not experience the world directly. It experiences the world through surfaces. Every nutrient, hormone, cytokine, neurotransmitter, mechanical force, temperature shift, microbial fragment, and oxidative stressor reaches the cell only by first encountering a membrane. That means the cell's version of reality is always filtered through composition. The membrane is not a neutral window. It is an active material layer that changes what can be sensed, how strongly it can be sensed, how long the signal persists, and whether the signal is translated into useful action or into distortion. Change the composition of the membrane and the world the cell lives in changes with it, even if the external environment remains the same. Two cells exposed to the same molecule are not necessarily living in the same biological reality if their membranes are built differently. They will not read the same input the same way, because the input is being processed through different physical conditions.

This is one of the most important reasons composition cannot be treated as a minor biochemical detail. A membrane enriched in more stable lipid species behaves differently from one enriched in highly unsaturated, oxidation-prone material. A membrane with coherent cholesterol distribution behaves differently from one in which ordered domains are unstable or poorly maintained. A membrane with adequate phospholipid turnover and structural repair behaves differently from one that has accumulated damaged lipids faster than they can be removed. These differences alter permeability, charge behavior, thickness, flexibility, protein mobility, vesicle formation, and the probability that receptors and enzymes will encounter the right partners at the right time. The cell then begins drawing different conclusions from the same external event. A signal that should have been brief may linger. A stimulus that should have remained local may spread. A threat that should have been resolved may stay active because the surface conditions favor escalation more than closure. Reality, at the cellular level, is not just what arrives. It is what the membrane allows arrival to become.

This helps explain why membrane composition alters not only signaling intensity but signaling meaning. A hormone does not simply carry a message in pure form from the bloodstream into the cell. It meets a receptor embedded in a specific lipid environment, and that environment changes whether the receptor is properly folded, how easily it clusters, whether it enters an ordered membrane region, how effectively it couples to downstream proteins, and how rapidly the signal is terminated or internalized. The same hormone concentration can therefore produce different physiological outcomes depending on membrane state. The same principle applies to immune recognition. A receptor meant to detect danger may become oversensitive in a disordered membrane, less selective in an oxidized membrane, or unable to terminate correctly in a membrane that cannot reorganize cleanly once activation has occurred. What the cell interprets as danger, safety, abundance, scarcity, or injury is partly determined by the composition of the surface doing the interpretation.

This is why chronic dysfunction often feels like the body has started misreading reality. A person becomes unusually reactive to food, stress, exertion, temperature, or inflammation. Hormonal signals seem present but ineffective. Appetite cues no longer match energy state. Immune activity activates too easily and turns off too slowly. Neural signaling becomes more erratic, less stable, or more easily overstimulated. These are usually described as separate forms of dysregulation, but many of them can be understood more clearly as interpretive problems emerging from altered membrane composition. The world reaching the body has not necessarily changed in proportion to the reaction. The body's surface architecture has changed, and with it the threshold, fidelity, and timing of biological response. In practical terms, the organism begins living in a noisier version of reality because its interfaces are no longer filtering and translating information with the same precision.

The physical properties of different lipids are central to this effect. Saturated fatty acids tend to support tighter packing, lower permeability, and greater resistance to oxidative distortion, which can increase structural stability but also reduce mobility if present without balance. Monounsaturated fats often preserve fluid behavior while maintaining good resilience. Polyunsaturated fats expand flexibility and signaling range, but their double bonds increase susceptibility to peroxidation, which means they can enrich function under protected conditions and increase fragility under unprotected ones. Cholesterol acts as a structural buffer and organizer, modifying disorder in one region while preserving fluidity in another. Sphingolipids help create ordered membrane microdomains that shape receptor localization and signal sorting. None of these features are abstract biochemical trivia. They are the physical basis of interpretation. They determine whether the membrane behaves like a stable control surface or a chemically unstable field that distorts the signals passing through it.

This is especially important because membrane composition is not static. It is continuously remodeled by diet, endogenous lipid metabolism, oxidative stress, inflammation, hormonal state, mitochondrial function, lipoprotein transport, phospholipid turnover, and tissue-specific demands. A person is not carrying one fixed membrane identity throughout life. Their surfaces are being rebuilt in real time, sometimes gradually and sometimes under heavy metabolic pressure. This means reality at the cellular level is also moving. A tissue exposed to repeated oxidative injury may begin interpreting routine inputs as more threatening because its membrane environment has become easier to destabilize. A tissue repeatedly supplied with unstable lipids but insufficient antioxidant and repair support may develop high signaling volatility without durable control. Another tissue may become excessively rigid, less adaptive, and less capable of dynamic response. These are not merely changes in composition. They are changes in the rules by which the cell reads the world.

The nervous system makes this especially clear. A neuron depends on membrane composition for excitability, receptor behavior, synaptic vesicle cycling, and recovery after stimulation. Change that composition and sensory thresholds change, mood regulation changes, attention changes, signal-to-noise ratio changes, and inflammatory sensitivity within neural tissue can change as well. The person experiences this as a psychological or cognitive shift, but part of what has changed is the membrane-level reality through which neural signals are being interpreted. The immune system follows the same logic through a different expression. Membrane composition changes how aggressively receptors assemble, how easily inflammatory cascades begin, how lipid mediator substrates are stored and released, and whether resolution can be organized once the initial response should end. The immune cell is not just fighting the world. It is reading the world through its own surface material, and when that material changes, its definition of threat changes with it.

This is the level at which omega-3 becomes meaningful in a deeper way. Omega-3 fatty acids do not simply add a beneficial compound to the bloodstream. They alter membrane composition over time, and by altering membrane composition they alter what kind of world the cell is inhabiting. They change the reservoir from which signaling molecules can later be generated, but they also change receptor environment, membrane curvature behavior, surface flexibility, and the probabilities of certain signaling events occurring. That does not make omega-3 universally corrective in every context. A highly unsaturated membrane that lacks oxidative protection can become vulnerable even while gaining signaling flexibility. A tissue overloaded with inflammatory competition may incorporate omega-3 without fully expressing its benefits. A person may require broader structural correction, not just one substrate change. But the principle remains the same. When membrane composition changes, reality changes for the cell.

Seen clearly, this is one of the most important unifying ideas in biology. Cells do not respond to the world as detached processors of clean information. They respond through material surfaces that decide what counts as a signal, what counts as noise, what crosses the threshold for activation, and whether activation can later be resolved. Membrane composition therefore alters behavior at every level above it. It changes immune tone, hormonal sensitivity, neurotransmission, barrier control, mitochondrial efficiency, and stress tolerance because all of those processes depend on how the cell interprets contact. The membrane is the lens, and lipid composition changes the lens. Once that is understood, many forms of chronic dysfunction stop looking mysterious. The system is not always failing because the world is too hostile. Sometimes it is failing because the surface through which the world is being read has been rebuilt into something less precise, less stable, and less capable of telling the difference between signal and distortion.

Lipid Structure Determines Cellular Behavior

Cells do not behave according to genes alone, and they do not behave according to signaling molecules alone. They behave through the material conditions in which genes are expressed and signals are interpreted. Lipid structure is one of the deepest of those conditions. It determines the quality of the membrane, the stability of compartments, the movement of receptors, the organization of microdomains, the permeability of surfaces, the vulnerability of those surfaces to oxidation, and the availability of stored fatty acid substrates that can later be turned into signaling molecules. Because of that, lipid structure does not merely support cellular behavior from the background. It helps generate it. Change the lipid architecture of a cell and you change what that cell can sense, how precisely it can respond, how strongly it reacts, how long it stays activated, and how well it returns to baseline once the event has passed.

This becomes easiest to see when the membrane is treated as part of the decision system rather than as passive packaging. A receptor embedded in a well-built membrane behaves differently from the same receptor embedded in a membrane that is disordered, oxidized, overly permeable, or compositionally unstable. In one setting, ligand binding may lead to clean clustering, efficient downstream coupling, appropriate amplification, and timely signal termination. In another, the receptor may cluster poorly, over-cluster, couple weakly, internalize incorrectly, or remain active longer than it should. The difference is not necessarily in the receptor protein itself. The difference is in the surface that holds it. The cell then behaves differently because its interpretive machinery is being run through a different physical environment. What appears from the outside as altered sensitivity, resistance, hyperreactivity, or dysregulation is often the behavioral expression of altered lipid structure.

The same principle governs ion channels and transporters. Cellular excitability, nutrient uptake, waste export, osmotic control, calcium signaling, and electrochemical gradient maintenance all depend on proteins that must operate inside membranes with usable physical properties. If the lipid environment becomes too rigid, channel gating and transporter cycling may become mechanically impaired. If the membrane becomes too disordered or oxidatively damaged, permeability can rise in unwanted ways and charge separation can become harder to maintain cleanly. That means even basic cellular timing changes when lipid structure changes. The cell may depolarize more easily, recover more slowly, leak ions more readily, import substrates less selectively, or lose gradient-dependent control over its own chemistry. Behavior at that point is no longer being determined simply by which proteins are present. It is being determined by whether the membrane gives those proteins a stable platform on which to work.

Lipid structure also determines behavior by shaping how the cell handles stress. A membrane built from highly oxidation-prone material behaves differently under inflammatory pressure than a membrane built from more stable material. Once reactive oxygen species rise, peroxidation can spread through vulnerable lipids, altering membrane integrity, damaging local proteins, changing permeability, and generating reactive breakdown products that further distort signaling. A cell with structurally resilient membranes can absorb a greater degree of metabolic or inflammatory stress before its behavior becomes chaotic. A cell with fragile membranes begins misfiring earlier. It becomes easier to activate, harder to stabilize, and slower to recover. This is why the same inflammatory load or oxidative burden can produce very different outcomes in different tissues or different people. Stress does not act on blank surfaces. It acts on built material, and the structure of that material determines how the cell behaves under pressure.

Immune behavior is heavily shaped by this logic. Immune cells depend on membrane structure to assemble receptors, form immunological synapses, engulf targets, release signaling molecules, migrate through tissue, and later shift from activation to resolution. The ability to recognize a threat is only one part of the problem. The cell also has to regulate the magnitude and duration of the response. If membrane composition favors unstable signaling, inflammatory cascades can begin too easily and terminate too poorly. If lipid substrate pools are skewed toward mediators that intensify inflammation more readily than they support its resolution, immune behavior shifts further in that direction. The immune system then appears overreactive or chronically activated, but underneath that pattern is a structural issue. The cell is behaving according to the materials built into its surface and stored within its membranes. Inflammation is not being generated from nothing. It is being generated from architecture.

Neural behavior follows the same rule through a different kind of membrane demand. Neurons require tightly controlled excitability, rapid vesicle fusion, receptor trafficking, synaptic plasticity, and membrane recovery after repeated firing. All of that depends on lipid structure. A membrane that is too rigid may slow receptor movement and vesicle dynamics. A membrane that is too unstable may increase noise, alter ion channel behavior, and reduce signaling precision. The result may not be immediate neurological failure. More often it is altered behavior at the system level: greater irritability, poorer signal-to-noise ratio, reduced resilience, unstable mood, diminished focus, altered sensory thresholds, or impaired recovery from stimulation. These effects are often described in purely chemical or psychological language, but the chemistry is still being executed through membranes. The neuron behaves the way its surface allows it to behave.

Mitochondrial behavior is equally dependent on lipid structure, and this is often missed because metabolism is usually described in terms of fuel supply rather than machine integrity. The mitochondrion does not produce ATP simply because fatty acids, glucose, or other substrates are present. It produces ATP because its inner membrane can organize the electron transport chain, hold a proton gradient, maintain cristae structure, and prevent excessive proton leak. Cardiolipin and other membrane components play direct roles in stabilizing respiratory complexes and preserving the architecture required for oxidative phosphorylation. If mitochondrial lipid structure degrades, behavior changes. Electron transfer becomes less efficient. Reactive oxygen species may rise. ATP production becomes more expensive. Stress signaling increases. The cell then behaves like it is underpowered, inflamed, or metabolically inflexible because the membrane architecture of its energy system no longer supports clean output. Fuel alone cannot fix that. The behavior is being determined by structure.

This is also why lipid structure creates long time-horizon effects that are often misunderstood. The body remodels membranes gradually through repeated dietary exposure, endogenous synthesis, lipoprotein transport, oxidative damage, repair, and phospholipid turnover. Cellular behavior therefore shifts over time as structure shifts. A person does not wake up one day with a completely different signaling system because of a single meal. But repeated incorporation of certain lipids, repeated exposure to oxidative stress, repeated inflammatory activation, and repeated failure of repair can slowly rebuild tissues into different behavioral states. Receptors may become less precise. Immune cells may become more triggerable. Mitochondria may become less efficient. Barriers may become more permissive. Neural tissue may become more reactive. What looks like a collection of unrelated chronic problems is often the accumulated behavioral output of slowly remodeled lipid architecture.

This is the deeper reason omega-3, omega-6, saturated fat, cholesterol, phospholipids, and membrane turnover matter. They are not simply nutrients or risk factors floating above the body as abstract variables. They become part of the surfaces through which behavior emerges. Omega-3 can alter membrane flexibility, receptor environment, and the substrate pool for pro-resolving mediators. Arachidonic acid can provide substrate for potent inflammatory signaling. Saturated structures can increase stability and reduce oxidative fragility, though excessive rigidity in the wrong context can create different limitations. Cholesterol can organize and buffer membrane behavior. The point is not that one class of lipid always determines outcome in isolation. The point is that cellular behavior is built from the combined structural consequences of the lipid environment. The cell behaves according to what it is made from.

Once this is understood, many physiological contradictions become easier to interpret. A signal can be present but not produce the expected effect because the membrane cannot read it well. A tissue can look inflamed not only because inflammatory triggers exist, but because its structural state amplifies those triggers and prevents clean resolution. A mitochondrion can have access to fuel and still generate poor energy because the membrane architecture required for conversion is degraded. A person can feel unstable across many systems at once because the surfaces governing those systems have been remodeled into a less coherent state. Lipid structure determines cellular behavior because behavior is not separate from structure. It is structure in motion, structure under stress, structure interpreting input, and structure deciding what the cell can become from one moment to the next.

Chapter 3

The Three Roles of Lipids

Lipids are usually discussed in fragments. In one context they are described as fuel. In another they are described as membrane material. In another they appear as precursors for hormones, inflammatory mediators, or signaling molecules. Each of those descriptions is true, but the separation has created confusion because it encourages people to think these are different stories rather than different expressions of the same biological reality. The same lipid that becomes part of a membrane can later be mobilized under stress. The same fat that serves as stored energy can alter signaling indirectly by changing insulin dynamics, mitochondrial load, or substrate competition. The same fatty acid incorporated into phospholipids can later be released and converted into eicosanoids, resolvins, protectins, or other signaling molecules that change immune behavior, vascular tone, and tissue repair. Lipids do not live in one category at a time. They move between structural, energetic, and signaling roles depending on tissue state, metabolic context, and the needs of the organism. That is why they sit so close to the center of physiology. They are not one nutrient class among many. They are one of the body's major multi-role material systems.

The first role of lipids is structural, and this is the most foundational because it sits underneath the other two. Lipids build membranes. They create the boundary conditions required for compartmentalization, gradient control, receptor function, vesicle trafficking, barrier integrity, organelle identity, and cellular decision-making. Without lipid structure, there is no meaningful inside and outside, no mitochondrial membrane capable of oxidative phosphorylation, no synaptic membrane capable of rapid neurotransmission, and no epithelial surface capable of regulating absorption without losing barrier control. Structural lipids do not merely hold the body together in the crude mechanical sense. They create the surfaces through which biological order is maintained. Their saturation level, fatty acid composition, cholesterol interaction, oxidative stability, and distribution within phospholipids all change how the membrane behaves. That means structural lipids determine not just what the body is made of, but how its interfaces perform under normal conditions and under stress.

The second role of lipids is energetic. This is the role most people know, but it is often explained too simplistically. Lipids are energy-dense molecules, and many tissues are adapted to oxidize fatty acids efficiently under the right metabolic conditions. Triglycerides store large amounts of chemical energy in a compact, water-sparing form. During fasting, sustained exercise, carbohydrate restriction, or ordinary background metabolism in certain tissues, fatty acids can be mobilized from adipose tissue, transported into cells, activated, shuttled into mitochondria, and oxidized to generate acetyl-CoA, reducing equivalents, and eventually ATP. That energetic function matters enormously, but even here the structural story remains upstream. Lipids can only serve as efficient fuel if the machinery that processes them is intact. Mitochondria must have functional membranes. Carnitine-dependent transport must work. Electron transport complexes must remain organized. The cell must be able to handle beta-oxidation products without creating excessive oxidative stress or redox imbalance. So even the energetic role of lipids cannot be separated from structure. The body does not simply burn fat. It uses structurally organized systems to convert certain lipids into usable energy under defined physiological conditions.

The third role of lipids is signaling, and this is where much of their complexity becomes visible. Lipids are not silent materials. They act as precursors, cofactors, organizers, and direct participants in communication. Membrane-derived fatty acids can be released and converted into eicosanoids, leukotrienes, prostaglandins, thromboxanes, lipoxins, resolvins, protectins, maresins, and many other mediator classes that influence inflammation, vascular behavior, platelet activity, immune recruitment, pain signaling, and tissue resolution. Cholesterol serves as the backbone for steroid hormone synthesis, making lipid biology central to endocrine regulation. Phosphoinositides and related membrane lipids participate directly in intracellular signaling cascades. Diacylglycerol and ceramides influence kinase activity, apoptosis, insulin signaling, and stress responses. Lipid rafts and membrane microdomains help determine which receptors encounter which partners and how strongly downstream pathways are activated. In other words, lipids do not simply carry signals after other systems have spoken. They are part of the language of the body itself.

These three roles are not parallel tracks. They constantly overlap. A membrane phospholipid is structural until phospholipase activity releases one of its fatty acids for signaling. A stored triglyceride is energetic until its mobilization changes the hormonal and inflammatory environment of the body. A signaling lipid can alter gene expression and thereby reshape future structural composition. The body is continuously converting lipids from one role into another. That conversion is part of metabolic intelligence. It allows stored matter to become energy during demand, structural material to become inflammatory substrate during threat, and signaling molecules to drive reconstruction after damage. But it also means that lipid imbalance rarely stays confined to one domain. A problem that begins as poor membrane composition can later appear as signaling distortion. A problem that begins as disordered fuel handling can eventually change membrane turnover and inflammatory behavior. A person may think they have separate issues involving energy, inflammation, and tissue fragility when in fact all three are expressions of disrupted lipid role integration.

This integration is especially important in chronic disease. A body built from unstable membrane lipids may interpret signals poorly, leak gradients more readily, and become easier to activate under stress. If that same body also stores and mobilizes fat in a metabolically dysregulated way, energetic instability increases. If the stored and structural lipid pools are also biased toward pro-inflammatory signaling outputs, the organism does not just have an inflammation problem or an energy problem or a structural problem. It has a lipid coordination problem. The three roles are no longer cooperating. Structure becomes fragile, fuel handling becomes inefficient, and signaling becomes distorted. The result is the familiar pattern of chronic modern dysfunction: unstable energy, exaggerated inflammatory behavior, poor recovery, barrier weakness, endocrine inconsistency, vascular stress, neural irritability, and difficulty returning cleanly to baseline once a challenge has passed.

This is why any serious discussion of omega-3 must be placed inside all three roles at once. Omega-3 fatty acids are structural because they enter phospholipids and alter membrane composition. They are signaling-relevant because EPA and DHA provide substrate for specialized mediator families involved in inflammatory resolution. They are also energetically relevant, though less central in this regard than some other fats, because their presence influences whole-system substrate balance, membrane-dependent mitochondrial performance, and the broader metabolic environment in which energy conversion occurs. Yet omega-3 never acts alone. Its effects depend on the surrounding lipid landscape. A membrane already destabilized by oxidative burden may not benefit from additional highly unsaturated material unless protective systems improve at the same time. A body overloaded with competing omega-6-derived signaling may not express the full benefits of omega-3 incorporation until that broader balance changes. A person with poor mitochondrial structure may not experience better energy simply because fatty acid composition shifts. The three roles always remain entangled.

The same logic applies to saturated fats, monounsaturated fats, phospholipids, cholesterol, and tissue-specific lipid distributions. Saturated fats tend to support structural stability and lower oxidative fragility, but their effects depend on proportion and context. Monounsaturated fats often provide a useful balance between flexibility and resilience. Cholesterol is not simply a cardiovascular talking point. It is a membrane organizer and hormone precursor. Phospholipids are not merely dietary trivia. They are the architecture of cell surfaces and organelle boundaries. Arachidonic acid is not merely inflammatory. It is a normal signaling substrate whose timing and magnitude matter. DHA is not merely brain food. It is part of the material environment of neural membranes. The mistake is to isolate one lipid and ask whether it is good or bad as though biology worked by moral categories. The better question is what role that lipid is serving, in what tissue, under what conditions, and how its presence alters the coordination between structure, fuel use, and signaling.

Once lipids are understood in these three roles, many confusions in nutrition and medicine begin to clear. Fat is no longer just a calorie category. Inflammation is no longer just a matter of immune molecules floating in blood. Energy is no longer just a question of eating enough or restricting enough. The body starts to look more coherent because lipids are being seen at the level where they actually operate. They build the surfaces. They store and release fuel. They generate and organize signals. When these roles are aligned, the organism gains stability, efficient energy handling, and cleaner control over inflammatory timing and tissue behavior. When they are misaligned, the same organism begins to fragment into the separate disease categories people usually encounter. The categories are real at the clinical level, but underneath them is one recurring problem: the body is trying to govern itself through lipid systems whose structural, energetic, and signaling functions no longer fit together cleanly.

The purpose of this chapter is not just to define three lipid roles as an academic exercise. It is to establish a framework for the rest of the book. From here forward, whenever a lipid appears in the discussion, the real question will be which role is being emphasized and which other roles are being indirectly altered at the same time. A fatty acid entering a membrane is never only structural. A signaling mediator released during inflammation is never unrelated to the membrane it came from. A fuel substrate entering mitochondria is never separate from the membrane conditions that determine how well that oxidation can proceed. The body uses lipids because lipids can become matter, energy, and instruction without leaving the same biological language. That is their power. It is also why misunderstanding them has produced so much confusion in modern health thinking.

Structural Lipids

Structural lipids are the lipids the body uses to build itself. That statement sounds simple, but it has consequences that reach through nearly every level of physiology. A structural lipid is not defined by whether it can be burned for energy or turned into a signaling molecule later. It is defined by the fact that it becomes part of the physical architecture of the cell. It enters membranes, contributes to organelle boundaries, affects barrier integrity, shapes the local environment around proteins, and helps determine whether cellular surfaces remain stable, flexible, selective, and responsive under stress. Structural lipids therefore do not sit at the edge of biology as passive material. They help create the surfaces through which biology is allowed to happen. When their composition is coherent, cells maintain cleaner signaling, stronger compartment control, better gradient stability, and more reliable tissue behavior. When their composition is poor, function becomes less precise long before obvious structural failure appears.

The most important structural lipids in the body are phospholipids, sphingolipids, cholesterol, and the fatty acids esterified into those larger membrane components. Phospholipids form the basic bilayer architecture because their water-attracting head groups and water-avoiding fatty acid tails allow them to self-organize into membranes. That self-assembly gives biology one of its most powerful material tools: a boundary that can hold difference across two sides while still allowing regulated exchange. But phospholipids are not all the same. Their head groups differ, their fatty acid chains differ, and the position of those chains within the molecule affects curvature, packing, charge behavior, and local protein interaction. Phosphatidylcholine, phosphatidylethanolamine, phosphatidylserine, phosphatidylinositol, cardiolipin, and other membrane phospholipids each contribute different physical and signaling properties depending on tissue and compartment. The membrane is never just made of generic fat. It is built from specific lipids arranged into specific environments.

Cholesterol belongs inside this structural discussion because it is one of the major organizers of membrane behavior. It inserts itself between phospholipids and changes how they pack. In some contexts it reduces excessive membrane fluidity. In others it prevents phospholipids from packing too tightly. It stabilizes certain membrane regions, helps form ordered microdomains, changes permeability, and influences the movement and clustering of receptors and other membrane proteins. Cholesterol is often discussed only in relation to blood transport or cardiovascular risk, but inside tissues it plays a more basic role. It is part of the architecture that determines whether a membrane behaves like a reliable control surface or a surface that becomes too disordered, too permeable, or too unstable under pressure. A membrane without sufficient structural organization cannot interpret signals cleanly, and cholesterol is one of the molecules that helps maintain that organization.

Sphingolipids add another layer of structure that is often overlooked. They contribute to membrane order, support the formation of microdomains, and are especially important in tissues that require durable signaling surfaces, including neural tissue. Sphingomyelin, glycosphingolipids, and related molecules help create more ordered regions within membranes that can sort proteins, cluster receptors, and alter how signals are initiated and contained. In myelin, these structural lipids become especially important because rapid conduction depends on a stable lipid-rich insulating architecture. In immune and epithelial tissues, they participate in surface identity and signal organization. Like other structural lipids, sphingolipids are not inert building blocks. Their presence changes how the membrane behaves as a living interface.

The fatty acid composition attached to structural lipids matters just as much as the lipid class itself. A phospholipid carrying saturated fatty acids will pack differently from one carrying monounsaturated or polyunsaturated fatty acids. Saturated chains generally produce tighter packing and greater resistance to oxidative disruption. Monounsaturated chains often allow a useful balance between movement and durability. Polyunsaturated chains increase flexibility and can support dynamic membrane behavior, but their multiple double bonds also increase susceptibility to peroxidation. This means structure is never just about having enough membrane material. It is about what kind of membrane material has been built. A cell surface enriched in highly unsaturated lipids may become more flexible and signaling-capable, but if the oxidative environment is poor, that same surface may become chemically fragile and easier to damage under inflammatory stress. The structural value of a lipid cannot be separated from the physical demands placed on the tissue receiving it.

This is why structural lipids determine so much more than the appearance of a membrane on a diagram. They influence receptor behavior, transporter efficiency, vesicle fusion, membrane curvature, mechanical resilience, permeability, ion leakage, and the ability of the cell to preserve gradients across time. A membrane must be stable enough to resist collapse into indiscriminate mixing, but dynamic enough to allow transport, signaling, and adaptation. Structural lipids create that balance. They decide whether a receptor can cluster correctly, whether a channel sits in the right physical environment, whether an immune synapse forms cleanly, whether mitochondrial membranes hold proton gradients efficiently, and whether barrier tissues can remain selectively permeable rather than diffusely leaky. In this sense, structural lipids are not merely construction material. They are performance material.

The importance of structural lipids becomes even clearer when tissues are compared. Neural tissue depends on specialized membrane composition because excitability, synaptic transmission, myelination, and long-range stability all require finely tuned lipid surfaces. Mitochondria depend on structurally specific lipids such as cardiolipin to preserve cristae architecture and maintain respiratory complex organization. The intestinal lining depends on membrane integrity and lipid-supported junctional organization to preserve barrier control while still permitting absorption. Immune cells depend on surface structure to assemble receptors, reorganize their membranes during activation, and later shift into resolution states. Endothelial cells depend on membrane composition to regulate vascular tone, signal perception, and permeability. Each tissue uses structural lipids according to its own demands, but the rule remains the same. What the membrane is made from changes what the tissue can do.

Structural lipids also create long memory inside the body. Once incorporated into membranes, they do not behave like fleeting signals that vanish in minutes or hours. They become part of tissue architecture until turnover, damage, remodeling, or replacement changes them. That means diet, endogenous synthesis, stress exposure, oxidative burden, inflammation, and repair capacity all gradually shape structural identity over time. A person is not just eating fat in the short-term metabolic sense. They are contributing to the material pool from which future membranes will be built and rebuilt. This is one reason structural dysfunction often develops slowly. The tissue is being remodeled over months and years, and the consequences appear first as altered behavior before they appear as visible damage. Recovery also follows this slower logic. Rebuilding structural lipid architecture is more like reconstruction than stimulation. It requires time, repeated material input, and a physiological environment that allows new structure to persist.

This is also the level at which omega-3 becomes biologically meaningful beyond marketing language. EPA and DHA matter partly because they are structural lipids once incorporated into phospholipids. They change membrane characteristics, alter substrate pools for future signaling, and modify the environment in which receptors, channels, and enzymes operate. But they are only one part of structural lipid biology. Cholesterol, sphingolipids, saturated fatty acids, monounsaturated fatty acids, phospholipid head groups, and tissue-specific remodeling systems all influence the final surface behavior of the membrane. That is why no single lipid should be treated as the whole story. A membrane is a composite structure. Its behavior emerges from the relationships among its parts, not from the presence of one favored nutrient in isolation.

Understanding structural lipids correctly changes the entire nutritional and physiological frame. The body is no longer seen as a machine that runs on fuel and occasionally uses fat for secondary tasks. It becomes a built system that must continuously maintain its surfaces. Structural lipids are part of how that maintenance happens. They determine whether boundaries hold, whether signals are interpreted with precision, whether energy-producing compartments remain intact, whether immune behavior stays discriminating, and whether tissues can absorb stress without losing coherence. They do not merely support life from the background. They are part of the material basis of order. Without them, biology does not simply become inefficient. It becomes less able to remain itself.

Energetic Lipids

Energetic lipids are the lipids the body uses as concentrated fuel, but even that description needs to be tightened because it is often interpreted too casually. The body does not simply burn fat in a generic sense. It stores specific lipid forms, mobilizes them under defined hormonal conditions, transports them through tightly controlled systems, activates them enzymatically, and then channels them into mitochondria or related oxidative pathways where their chemical energy can be extracted in a stepwise manner. This makes energetic lipids more than passive reserves. They are part of a controlled fuel architecture. Their value lies not only in the amount of energy they contain, but in the way they allow the body to store large amounts of usable fuel without carrying it in a hydrated, bulky, chemically disruptive form. Triglycerides solve a physical problem for the organism. They permit dense energy storage that does not destabilize cellular water balance, and that storage gives the body metabolic range across fasting, exercise, illness, overnight repair, and ordinary day-to-day intervals between meals.

The major energetic lipids are triglycerides, which consist of three fatty acids esterified to a glycerol backbone. In adipose tissue, triglycerides function as the primary long-term energy reserve. In food, triglycerides also serve as a major incoming lipid form that must be digested, absorbed, repackaged, transported, and either oxidized or stored. Their central role in energy biology comes from the fatty acids they carry. These fatty acids contain long hydrocarbon chains rich in reduced carbon-hydrogen bonds, which makes them chemically valuable as oxidative substrate. When the body mobilizes stored triglyceride, lipolysis releases fatty acids that travel through circulation, usually bound to albumin, until they are taken up by tissues capable of using them. Once inside the cell, those fatty acids are activated to acyl-CoA derivatives and, for long-chain species, usually transported into mitochondria through the carnitine shuttle. There they undergo beta-oxidation, generating acetyl-CoA, NADH, and FADH2, which feed into the citric acid cycle and electron transport chain. The energy potential of fat is therefore real, but it is accessed through layered control rather than through simple combustion.

This control matters because energetic lipids are not meant to be burned indiscriminately. Their use depends on metabolic context. In the fed state, especially when insulin is elevated, fat storage is favored and lipolysis is suppressed. In fasting, lower insulin and higher counterregulatory signals such as glucagon, catecholamines, and in some contexts cortisol, increase triglyceride breakdown and fatty acid mobilization. During prolonged low-intensity exercise, fatty acid oxidation contributes substantially to ATP production. During carbohydrate restriction or longer fasting states, hepatic fatty acid oxidation rises and ketogenesis can begin converting acetyl-CoA into ketone bodies that distribute energy more widely, especially to tissues like the brain during adaptation. Energetic lipids are therefore governed by timing, hormonal state, tissue demand, oxygen availability, mitochondrial capacity, and redox handling. The body does not just ask whether fat is available. It asks whether present conditions allow fat to be used efficiently without destabilizing other layers of metabolism.

This is one reason the phrase fat burning is often too crude to explain what is actually happening. Oxidizing fatty acids efficiently requires intact cellular machinery. Mitochondria need structurally sound membranes, organized respiratory complexes, adequate oxygen delivery, appropriate cofactor status, and sufficient redox balance to handle electron flow cleanly. If mitochondrial function is impaired, fatty acid delivery alone does not guarantee efficient energy production. In that case, energetic lipids may be abundant while usable energy remains poor. The problem is no longer substrate scarcity. The problem is conversion quality. A person may store fat well, mobilize fat poorly, transport fat adequately but oxidize it inefficiently, or generate excessive incomplete oxidation products when mitochondrial throughput cannot keep pace. This makes energetic lipids inseparable from the structural theme established earlier in the book. Fuel only matters if the machine using the fuel retains the architecture required to process it.

Energetic lipids also influence stability in ways that glucose-based discussions often obscure. Fatty acid oxidation generally supports slower, steadier ATP production than rapid glycolytic flux, especially in tissues designed for sustained oxidative work. Cardiac muscle, resting skeletal muscle, and liver rely heavily on lipid oxidation under many normal conditions because fat provides a large and durable energy stream. This can create metabolic steadiness when mitochondrial function, oxygen delivery, and hormonal coordination are intact. But energetic stability is never just a property of the fuel itself. It depends on whether fatty acid mobilization is proportionate, whether insulin and glucagon timing remain coherent, whether the person can transition between substrates without excessive friction, and whether tissues are receiving a lipid supply they can actually oxidize instead of merely store. Fat is often described as a stable fuel, and it can be, but only inside a system built to access it properly.

The energetic role of lipids also intersects with stress physiology. During acute stress, catecholamines increase lipolysis, releasing fatty acids into circulation to provide fuel for tissues facing higher demand. During prolonged stress, however, energetic lipid use can become distorted. Excessive fatty acid flux into tissues that cannot oxidize efficiently may increase lipid intermediates, redox strain, and inflammatory stress. The same substrate that supports resilience in one metabolic context can contribute to dysfunction in another if flux exceeds processing capacity. This is one reason lipid metabolism cannot be reduced to simple praise of fat oxidation. The question is not only whether the body can mobilize fat, but whether it can match mobilization to oxidation without creating spillover, incomplete combustion, or signaling disruption. Energetic lipids support the organism when fuel release, transport, mitochondrial handling, and tissue demand remain coordinated. They become destabilizing when those layers separate.

This coordination is especially important in the liver, which acts as a major traffic hub for energetic lipid handling. The liver takes up fatty acids, oxidizes them, re-esterifies them, packages them into lipoproteins, and under certain conditions converts part of their acetyl-CoA load into ketone bodies. When hepatic handling remains coherent, lipids can be directed toward energy production or export according to need. When it becomes overloaded, especially in the presence of excessive nutrient flux, insulin dysregulation, mitochondrial strain, or chronic inflammatory stress, the liver may accumulate triglycerides and lose the clean balance between oxidation, storage, and export. This is not simply a problem of too much fat. It is a problem of energetic lipid traffic losing control. Storage begins to outpace use, or delivery begins to outpace processing, and the liver shifts from being an adaptive fuel coordinator to being a bottleneck.

Energetic lipids also differ from structural lipids in their time behavior. Structural lipids become part of tissue architecture and influence performance over longer remodeling windows. Energetic lipids are more immediately mobilizable. They exist partly to be called upon during need. Yet even here the distinction is not absolute. A triglyceride reserve can alter systemic signaling through adipokines, lipolytic flux, and substrate competition. A fatty acid released for fuel can later influence inflammatory pathways or membrane remodeling indirectly. A tissue chronically exposed to high energetic lipid turnover may gradually change its structure in response. The body does not maintain a perfect wall between lipid roles. It maintains shifting priority. Energetic lipids are the lipid pool most immediately available for oxidation, but they remain connected to the signaling and structural consequences of how they are stored and used.

This is where common misunderstandings about dietary fat and metabolic health usually begin. People often assume that consuming fat directly means becoming better at using fat. That is not automatically true. Efficient use of energetic lipids depends on digestive capacity, bile flow, lipase activity, intestinal absorption, chylomicron transport, lipoprotein handling, mitochondrial density, carnitine availability, redox balance, endocrine context, and tissue-level oxidative demand. A person can eat more fat and still fail to oxidize it well if the system required to handle it is underbuilt or metabolically inflexible. On the other side, a person with good mitochondrial function and well-regulated lipid metabolism may derive remarkable stability from energetic lipids because the system can mobilize, transport, and oxidize them with relatively low volatility. The difference is not ideological. It is architectural.

Seen clearly, energetic lipids are not just calories stored in fat tissue or calories consumed in food. They are part of the body's time-management system for energy. They allow energy collected during abundance to remain available during scarcity. They allow tissues to perform long-duration work without constant dependence on immediate carbohydrate intake. They support fasting survival, nighttime metabolism, physical endurance, and background cellular maintenance. But their usefulness always depends on structural integrity and signaling coordination. The body has to know when to release them, where to send them, how quickly to oxidize them, and when to stop. That is why energetic lipids cannot be understood in isolation from membranes, hormones, and mitochondrial architecture. They are the fuel role of lipid biology, but they are still being governed by the same larger principle running through this book: biological performance emerges from organized structure, and even fuel only becomes useful when the system using it is built well enough to stay in control.

Signaling Lipids

Signaling lipids are the lipids that carry instruction, timing, and state information inside the body. They do not just sit in tissues as structural matter and they do not just wait to be oxidized as fuel. They participate directly in communication. Some act as precursors that are released from membranes and rapidly converted into local mediators. Some function as membrane-organizing lipids that change which receptors can interact and how strongly signals are amplified. Some serve as intracellular second messengers that alter kinase activity, calcium handling, gene transcription, vesicle movement, apoptosis, or metabolic direction. Others provide the molecular backbone for steroid hormones that coordinate physiology across entire organs and tissues. When signaling lipids are understood properly, it becomes obvious that lipids are not just supporting communication from the edges. They are part of the language the body uses to decide what state it is in and what state it should enter next.

One of the clearest examples is the release of fatty acids from membrane phospholipids during stress, injury, immune activation, or normal signaling events. A membrane is not just a surface. It is also a stored signaling reservoir. Phospholipase enzymes can liberate arachidonic acid, EPA, DHA, and other fatty acids from phospholipid positions, and once released, those substrates enter enzymatic pathways that generate prostaglandins, thromboxanes, leukotrienes, lipoxins, resolvins, protectins, maresins, and related mediators. These molecules do not merely announce that something has happened. They shape the character of the response. They influence vascular tone, platelet behavior, immune cell recruitment, pain sensitivity, fever generation, vascular permeability, phagocytosis, debris clearance, tissue repair, and the active termination of inflammation. That means the signaling output of the body is partly determined by what has already been built into its membranes. The body does not invent inflammatory language at the moment of crisis. It draws from stored lipid material and converts that material into instruction.

This gives signaling lipids a distinctive kind of biological power. A protein signal often depends on prior gene expression, translation, folding, trafficking, and release. Lipid signaling can move faster because much of the substrate is already present in the membrane waiting to be mobilized. The membrane therefore functions as a preloaded signaling platform. Once a trigger reaches threshold, the cell can rapidly generate potent local messages without first synthesizing every component from scratch. That speed is useful in immunity, hemostasis, tissue injury, and many forms of stress adaptation, but it also creates risk. If the stored lipid substrate pool is compositionally biased toward signaling patterns that intensify activation more readily than they support closure, the cell may enter inflammatory states with far greater ease than it exits them. Signaling lipids therefore do not just help explain why inflammation happens. They help explain why inflammation takes the specific shape it takes and why that shape may become persistent in some organisms and not in others.

Arachidonic acid is central to this discussion because it is one of the major membrane-derived substrates for eicosanoid synthesis. Once released, it can be converted into prostaglandins, thromboxanes, leukotrienes, and other mediator families that influence vasodilation, vasoconstriction, platelet aggregation, vascular leakage, leukocyte trafficking, smooth muscle behavior, pain generation, and multiple layers of immune activation. Arachidonic acid is not inherently pathological. It is a normal and necessary signaling substrate. The problem begins when its mobilization is excessive, poorly contained, or insufficiently followed by resolution chemistry. In that context, the body remains biased toward initiation. The signaling system becomes good at starting defense and poor at finishing it. EPA and DHA matter partly because they change this signaling terrain. They can compete for enzymatic access, alter mediator output, and provide substrate for specialized pro-resolving mediators that help terminate inflammatory activity, restore tissue order, and shift the body from escalation toward completion. This is one of the deepest reasons omega-3 belongs in a signaling chapter rather than being confined to a supplement chapter.

Signaling lipids are not limited to inflammatory mediators released into the extracellular environment. Many operate inside the membrane itself or on the cytoplasmic side of it as part of intracellular instruction systems.

Phosphoinositides help determine membrane identity, vesicle trafficking, cytoskeletal behavior, and signal relay through pathways that influence growth, metabolism, migration, and survival. Diacylglycerol functions as a second messenger that activates protein kinase C and related pathways, altering cell activation states, secretion patterns, proliferation signals, and stress responses. Ceramides participate in stress signaling, apoptosis, insulin signaling interference, membrane domain formation, and inflammatory amplification under certain conditions. Sphingosine-1-phosphate helps regulate vascular integrity, immune cell trafficking, lymphocyte movement, and survival signaling. In each case, the lipid is not just a passive membrane component. It is participating directly in cellular logic. It changes what the cell does next.

Cholesterol also belongs here, not only because of its membrane-organizing role but because it is the raw material for steroid hormone synthesis. Cortisol, aldosterone, testosterone, estradiol, progesterone, and other steroid hormones all emerge from cholesterol metabolism. That places lipid biology inside endocrine command. Steroid hormones alter metabolism, mineral balance, reproduction, immune tone, circadian timing, tissue growth, stress response, and long-term adaptation. The body therefore uses lipids not only for local signaling events at the membrane surface but also for long-distance hormonal coordination across the entire organism. A change in lipid handling can alter endocrine capacity. A change in endocrine state can alter lipid storage, membrane remodeling, inflammatory behavior, and energetic flux. These are not separate systems. They are linked through lipid-based signaling architecture.

The membrane's physical organization also creates signaling effects before any lipid mediator is enzymatically released. Certain lipids help form ordered microdomains that concentrate or exclude specific receptors and signaling proteins. That means lipid arrangement determines who can talk to whom at the surface. A receptor placed into one membrane neighborhood may activate strongly because the local partners needed for amplification are present. The same receptor in a different lipid neighborhood may remain quiet, terminate quickly, or fail to couple efficiently. This is signaling by architecture. The membrane is not just storing future mediators. It is already shaping current signal quality by controlling protein geography. In that sense, signaling lipids act both chemically and spatially. They generate messages, and they organize the surfaces across which those messages can be interpreted.

This dual role helps explain why signaling lipids can produce both adaptation and pathology. Under controlled conditions, they allow fast local coordination, tissue repair, immune defense, vascular responsiveness, endocrine regulation, and organized recovery after stress. Under distorted conditions, they can drive chronic inflammation, pain persistence, thrombosis risk, endothelial dysfunction, metabolic rigidity, immune overactivation, and failure of resolution. The difference is rarely the existence of signaling lipids themselves. The difference is proportion, timing, substrate balance, membrane state, oxidative load, enzymatic control, and whether the organism can transition from activation to completion without getting trapped in the middle. Signaling lipids are powerful because they are embedded in the structure of the body. They are close to the point of action, and they can move the system quickly. That same closeness is why lipid imbalance can have such broad effects.

This is also why signaling lipids create memory inside tissues. A membrane enriched over time with certain fatty acid patterns becomes a reservoir for future signaling outcomes. A tissue repeatedly exposed to oxidative stress or inflammatory pressure may shift not only its acute mediator production but also the composition of the membrane from which later mediators will be drawn. The next response is therefore shaped by the history of previous structure. A cell that has been rebuilt under chronic inflammatory conditions may become easier to activate because its membranes now contain a substrate mix and signaling organization that favor faster escalation. Another cell supported toward better membrane remodeling and better resolution chemistry may begin responding with greater proportionality. The tissue is not merely reacting in the present. It is reacting through stored structural history.

Seen clearly, signaling lipids are the reason lipids cannot be reduced to calories or even to membrane material alone. They are part of the body's operational language. They tell blood vessels whether to widen or constrict. They tell platelets whether to aggregate. They tell immune cells whether to recruit, attack, engulf, clear, or stand down. They tell endocrine tissues how to coordinate long-range adaptation. They tell cells internally whether to grow, divide, move, survive, shut down, or repair. Their power comes from their position at the intersection of structure and action. They are generated from built material, and once generated they change what the system does. That makes them uniquely important. They are not external regulators dropped into biology from above. They are the instructions that emerge from the body's own architecture.

Why These Roles Must Stay Balanced

The structural, energetic, and signaling roles of lipids cannot be treated as separate categories that can each be optimized independently. They are physically connected inside the same organism, often inside the same molecules, and the body depends on them remaining proportionate to one another. A lipid that stabilizes a membrane today may become signaling substrate tomorrow. A lipid stored for energy may alter signaling tone through its rate of mobilization, its intermediates, or the tissue stress created when its oxidation outpaces mitochondrial control. A signaling lipid released during inflammation may reshape future structure by altering membrane turnover, oxidative load, gene expression, and tissue remodeling. Because of that, lipid balance is not just about having enough of each role present somewhere in the system. It is about keeping the three roles coordinated so that structure supports function, fuel use supports stability, and signaling supports adaptation without dissolving into chronic activation.

The structural role must remain primary because it sets the conditions under which the other two roles can operate safely. If membranes are unstable, overly oxidizable, excessively rigid, or compositionally disordered, then the energetic role becomes harder to execute cleanly and the signaling role becomes harder to control precisely. Receptors misread. Gradients leak. Mitochondria lose efficiency. Barrier tissues become more permissive than they should be. The body can still mobilize fuel and generate signals under those conditions, but the outputs become noisier and more expensive. Energy production creates more strain. Inflammatory activation becomes easier to initiate than to resolve. The organism begins reacting through weakened surfaces. This is one reason a body can appear chemically active yet physiologically unstable. It has signaling and fuel flux, but the structural platform needed to govern both has degraded.

The energetic role must also stay in proportion because lipids used as fuel can support stability or overwhelm it depending on context. A well-regulated lipid fuel system provides continuity across fasting, sustained activity, and the intervals between meals. It reduces the need for constant external intake and supports long-duration energy production in tissues designed for oxidative metabolism. But when lipid mobilization exceeds oxidation capacity, or when fat is stored efficiently but processed poorly, energetic lipids begin to spill into other roles in damaging ways. Incomplete oxidation products accumulate. Lipid intermediates interfere with signaling. The liver becomes overloaded with lipid traffic it cannot direct cleanly. Oxidative stress rises. Membranes may be remodeled under inflammatory pressure rather than under controlled maintenance. The system then stops using fat as a stable reserve and starts experiencing it as metabolic burden. The same lipid pool that should support resilience begins generating distortion because the energetic role has lost coordination with structure and signal timing.

The signaling role is the most volatile of the three, which is exactly why it must remain tied to the other two. Signaling lipids move quickly. They can amplify, recruit, constrict, dilate, sensitize, activate, terminate, or resolve within short windows. That speed is useful during injury, infection, stress, and tissue adaptation, but it also means signaling lipids can dominate the system if the structural reservoir and energetic environment are biased in the wrong direction. A membrane built from unstable or heavily pro-inflammatory substrate can produce signaling outputs that favor escalation more than resolution. A body under chronic energetic strain can convert fuel imbalance into inflammatory language through redox stress, lipotoxicity, and altered mediator synthesis. A system that repeatedly activates without structurally rebuilding will slowly turn signaling into its default mode. At that point, the body is no longer using lipid signals as precise instructions. It is living in a state of continuous lipid-derived interpretive pressure.

Balance matters because each role protects the others when properly aligned. Structural integrity limits signaling noise. It keeps receptors organized, barriers intact, gradients preserved, and activation thresholds meaningful. Clean energetic handling reduces unnecessary stress on membranes and decreases the likelihood that stored lipid will become a source of toxic overflow rather than useful ATP. Well-regulated signaling helps the body respond proportionately and then return to baseline, which protects structure from prolonged inflammatory damage and prevents energy systems from remaining trapped in expensive defensive states. When these roles cooperate, the organism gains something more important than isolated biochemical efficiency. It gains coherence. Inputs are interpreted clearly. Fuels are used without destabilizing the tissues using them. Stress responses begin and end on time. Recovery is possible because the body is not consuming its own architecture while trying to defend itself.

When these roles fall out of balance, chronic disease becomes much easier to understand. A person may have enough stored fuel yet feel underpowered because energetic lipids are not being oxidized cleanly. They may have abundant signaling activity yet poor adaptation because the signals emerging from membranes are biased toward escalation. They may have tissues that are constantly inflamed not because the body lacks defensive ability, but because structural lipids have been remodeled into surfaces that interpret ordinary life as repeated threat. In another case, a person may improve energy transiently through increased fat mobilization but worsen inflammatory tone because the structural and signaling consequences of that flux were not contained. Or they may consume more omega-3 expecting resolution benefits while ignoring the fact that highly unsaturated structure introduced into an unstable oxidative environment can become fragile before it becomes helpful. These contradictions are not contradictions once the three roles are viewed together.

They are what happens when one lipid function is pushed without regard for the others.

This is especially important in the context of omega-3 and omega-6 biology. Omega-3 is often discussed as if increasing it is automatically beneficial because of its signaling potential and its role in resolution pathways. That can be true, but only if structural incorporation is supported and oxidative handling is sufficient. Omega-6 is often discussed as if it exists only as a source of inflammatory excess, but some omega-6-derived signaling is normal and necessary when proportional and properly terminated. The real issue is not moral classification of fats. It is the relationship between structural incorporation, mediator production, and metabolic environment. If a tissue contains excessive pro-inflammatory signaling substrate, unstable membranes, poor antioxidant defense, and high energetic strain, then simply adding more of one lipid class does not guarantee balance. The architecture has to be rebuilt in a way that allows all three roles to re-enter coordination.

The body is healthiest when lipids remain obedient to hierarchy. First they must build stable surfaces. Then they must support controlled fuel handling through those surfaces. Then they must generate signals that reflect real needs and resolve once those needs have been met. If signaling outruns structure, the body becomes reactive. If energetic flux outruns structure, the body becomes unstable. If structure is built without sufficient dynamic capacity, the body may become rigid and unresponsive. Real health is not produced by maximizing any one role. It is produced by maintaining proportion among them. That proportion is what allows a membrane to remain both stable and interpretable, a fuel reserve to remain both available and non-toxic, and a signaling system to remain both responsive and finite.

This is the deeper lesson of lipid biology. Lipids do not just do three different jobs. They create a three-part system that has to remain coordinated if the organism is to function with precision over time. When that coordination is present, energy becomes steadier, signaling becomes cleaner, immunity becomes more discriminating, and tissues recover with less collateral damage. When that coordination breaks, the body begins to fragment into the familiar modern pattern of fatigue, inflammation, metabolic dysfunction, barrier weakness, vascular instability, neural irritability, and poor recovery. The failure is rarely in one isolated pathway. The failure is in lipid role balance itself.

PART II

THE OMEGA SYSTEM

Chapter 4

What Omega-3 and Omega-6 Really Are

Omega-3 and omega-6 are usually presented as if they are supplements, categories on a nutrition label, or opposing health teams competing for moral approval. That framing is too crude to explain what they actually are. Omega-3 and omega-6 are families of polyunsaturated fatty acids defined by the position of the first double bond relative to the methyl end of the fatty acid chain. That chemical distinction sounds small, but it changes how the molecule behaves inside the body, how enzymes process it, what kinds of membranes it helps build, and which signaling mediators can later be derived from it. These are not just fats in the dietary sense. They are structural and signaling substrates that enter phospholipids, alter membrane behavior, and later serve as raw material for inflammatory and pro-resolving chemistry. To understand them correctly, they have to be pulled out of the supplement aisle and put back into physiology.

The reason these fatty acids matter is not simply that they are polyunsaturated. It is that the body uses them as part of its surface architecture and signaling reservoir. Once incorporated into phospholipids, omega-3 and omega-6 fatty acids become part of membranes, where they influence packing, flexibility, oxidative susceptibility, enzyme access, receptor environment, and the kinds of lipid mediators that can be generated when the cell is activated. This means they are not passive inputs. They shape the interpretive surface of the cell and the chemical options available once signaling begins. A membrane containing different proportions of omega-3 and omega-6 is not just chemically different on paper. It behaves differently under stress, produces different mediator profiles when phospholipases release fatty acids from the membrane, and changes how easily inflammation escalates and how effectively it can later resolve.

Omega-6 fatty acids are often discussed in a distorted way because they are associated with inflammatory signaling, but that association gets oversimplified into the idea that omega-6 is inherently harmful. That is not biologically accurate. Omega-6 fatty acids are normal structural and signaling components of human tissues. Linoleic acid is the main dietary omega-6 fatty acid, and from it the body can produce longer-chain derivatives such as arachidonic acid, which becomes one of the major membrane substrates for eicosanoid signaling. Arachidonic acid is not a mistake. It is part of how the body mounts acute responses to injury, infection, vascular disruption, and local stress. Prostaglandins, leukotrienes, and thromboxanes derived from arachidonic acid help control blood flow, pain signaling, immune recruitment, platelet behavior, and multiple forms of defensive activation. The problem is not that omega-6 exists. The problem begins when its structural and signaling dominance becomes disproportionate, when initiation chemistry outruns resolution, and when the body builds membranes that are more prepared to escalate than to finish.

Omega-3 fatty acids are distorted in the opposite direction. They are usually marketed as anti-inflammatory nutrients, as though their main role is to suppress symptoms. That is too shallow. Alpha-linolenic acid is the plant-derived short-chain omega-3, while EPA and DHA are the longer-chain omega-3 fatty acids most directly involved in membrane function and specialized signaling in human tissues. EPA and DHA matter not because they are universally calming molecules, but because they alter membrane composition and provide substrate for mediator families that help shift inflammation toward completion. EPA can contribute to eicosanoid competition and to the generation of E-series resolvins. DHA contributes to membrane properties, especially in neural tissue, and serves as a precursor for D-series resolvins, protectins, and maresins. These are not simple anti-inflammatory agents in the blunt sense of shutting the immune system down. They are part of the machinery that helps the body stop recruiting unnecessary damage once defense has served its purpose. Omega-3 therefore matters less as a suppressor than as a participant in better inflammatory sequencing.

This is why omega-3 and omega-6 should not be understood as opposites in a simplistic nutritional battle. They are parallel substrate families entering overlapping structural and enzymatic systems. Both are polyunsaturated. Both can be built into membranes. Both can be mobilized from phospholipids during signaling. Both influence the physical state of the membrane. Both compete, directly or indirectly, for elongation, desaturation, incorporation, and downstream enzymatic conversion. The real issue is proportion, placement, turnover, and context. When omega-6-derived substrate dominates tissue composition and inflammatory tone is chronically high, the body tends to generate a signaling environment more heavily biased toward initiation and amplification. When omega-3 incorporation improves, especially in the presence of better overall lipid stability and oxidative control, the membrane environment and downstream mediator pool can begin shifting toward a more balanced inflammatory pattern. But even that statement needs care. Omega-3 does not erase the need for omega-6, and omega-6 does not automatically create disease. The deeper question is what kind of membrane and what kind of signaling reservoir the organism has built from the total lipid environment it has been given.

The chemistry also matters because these fatty acids are more fragile than more saturated lipid structures. Multiple double bonds create flexibility, but they also create susceptibility to oxidation. This makes omega-3 and omega-6 biologically powerful and biologically vulnerable at the same time. A membrane enriched in polyunsaturated fatty acids can support dynamic signaling behavior and provide a broad mediator substrate pool, but if oxidative protection is weak, if inflammatory load is high, or if membrane repair cannot keep pace, those same lipids can become sites of peroxidative damage. This is one reason the conversation around these fats becomes misleading when it is reduced to simple intake targets. The value of a polyunsaturated fatty acid depends on the membrane it enters, the tissue using it, the oxidative environment surrounding it, and the broader lipid architecture that stabilizes or destabilizes its presence. Flexibility without protection becomes fragility.

Tissue specificity adds another layer that is usually ignored in mainstream discussions. DHA is especially important in neural tissue, retinal tissue, and other highly specialized membranes where curvature behavior, receptor function, excitability, and long-horizon structural maintenance depend on very particular lipid environments. EPA is often discussed more heavily in relation to circulating inflammatory balance and mediator generation. Arachidonic acid remains central in immune and vascular signaling because rapid local inflammatory response still requires substrate for initiation. Different tissues therefore use omega-3 and omega-6 differently, and the body is not trying to make every membrane composition identical. It is solving tissue-specific structural problems. The brain does not need the same membrane behavior as a neutrophil. The retina does not need the same signaling timing as a platelet. The intestine does not need the same lipid surface as skeletal muscle. What matters is not a universal ratio imposed onto every cell. What matters is whether the organism is remodeling tissues toward a coherent and functional lipid distribution rather than toward chronic interpretive instability.

This is also where the distinction between dietary precursor and tissue-active form becomes important. Short-chain plant omega-3 in the form of alpha-linolenic acid is not the same thing as preformed EPA and DHA in terms of tissue effect, because conversion is limited and variable. The body can elongate and desaturate alpha-linolenic acid, but in many people the production of EPA is modest and DHA is even more constrained. Linoleic acid conversion toward arachidonic acid is also regulated rather than automatic, but the modern environment often supplies omega-6 substrate so abundantly that tissue competition shifts over time. This means the question is not merely whether someone consumes omega-3 or omega-6 in any form. The question is which forms are entering tissue, how much competition exists at the enzyme and membrane level, and what kind of long-term remodeling that intake pattern creates. Nutritional labels flatten this into grams. Biology turns it into structure and signal probability.

The phrase essential fatty acid comes from this reality. Certain polyunsaturated fatty acids or their precursor classes are called essential because the body cannot synthesize them de novo and must obtain them from diet. But essential does not mean unlimited, and it does not mean that all downstream outcomes are automatically beneficial. It means the body needs access to these lipid families because they are part of membrane construction and signaling capability. Without them, the organism loses important structural and communicative functions. With them in excess or imbalance, especially in unstable metabolic conditions, the organism can build membranes that are chemically reactive, signaling-heavy, and difficult to regulate under chronic stress. The same feature that makes these fats necessary also makes them capable of distorting physiology when proportion and context are lost. That is why they have to be understood mechanistically, not ideologically.

What omega-3 and omega-6 really are, then, is not a pair of health trends or a ratio to memorize. They are families of membrane-active, signal-generating polyunsaturated fatty acids that shape how the body builds surfaces and how it responds when those surfaces are activated. They are part of the material from which inflammation begins and part of the material from which it can later be resolved. They contribute flexibility, but they also introduce oxidation risk. They expand signaling possibility, but they also require structural balance and protective context. Once this is understood, the usual public conversation begins to look incomplete. The important question is no longer whether omega-3 is good or omega-6 is bad. The important question is what kind of body these fats are helping to build, what kinds of signals that body is prepared to generate, and whether its membranes have been remodeled toward proportionate response or toward chronic biochemical overreaction.

Polyunsaturated Fatty Acids as Signal Substrates

Polyunsaturated fatty acids are not important only because they become part of membranes. They are important because once they are built into membranes, they create a stored substrate pool from which signals can later be generated. This gives them a role that is structurally deeper and temporally longer than most signaling molecules. A cytokine or neurotransmitter is often synthesized, released, degraded, and cleared within a relatively narrow window. A polyunsaturated fatty acid can sit inside a membrane phospholipid for extended periods, shaping membrane behavior quietly, until a stimulus arrives that causes it to be released and converted into active mediators. That means the body stores part of its future signaling language in its membranes. Signal potential is built into tissue architecture before the signal is ever needed. The membrane is therefore not only an interface and not only a structural boundary. It is also a reservoir of conditional instructions waiting for the right trigger.

This matters because signaling does not begin at the moment of conversion. It begins earlier, at the level of substrate selection and tissue incorporation. When a membrane is enriched with certain polyunsaturated fatty acids, it is being preloaded with certain signaling possibilities. Arachidonic acid built into phospholipids creates one kind of inflammatory and vascular response potential. EPA and DHA built into phospholipids create another. These are not abstract biochemical options sitting in a textbook. They are physical realities built into tissue. When phospholipase activity is triggered by injury, infection, receptor activation, oxidative stress, or mechanical disruption, those stored fatty acids are released from the membrane and handed to enzymatic systems such as cyclooxygenases, lipoxygenases, and cytochrome-dependent pathways. What comes out next depends partly on what was sitting in the membrane in the first place. A cell cannot generate a given class of lipid mediator in meaningful amounts if the substrate pool for that class has not been built into its surfaces over time.

This is one reason polyunsaturated fatty acids occupy such a powerful position in inflammatory biology. They do not just influence signaling from the outside by arriving in circulation. They influence signaling from the inside by being stored within the very structures from which signaling is launched. Arachidonic acid released from membranes can be converted into prostaglandins, thromboxanes, leukotrienes, and other eicosanoids that help coordinate acute inflammatory recruitment, vascular changes, pain signaling, platelet activity, and local defense. EPA can enter related pathways and shift some of those outputs while also giving rise to E-series resolvins. DHA can contribute to membrane structure and, once released, serve as substrate for D-series resolvins, protectins, and maresins, which participate in resolution, tissue protection, phagocytic efficiency, and restoration of order after inflammatory work has been done. The point is not that one substrate family is simply inflammatory and another is simply anti-inflammatory. The point is that polyunsaturated fatty acids supply the raw material from which inflammatory sequence is written. They influence how the response begins, how intensely it develops, and whether the system has the substrate available to move toward completion instead of remaining trapped in activation.

Because of this, polyunsaturated fatty acids should be understood as conditional signaling material rather than passive dietary fats. Their double bonds give them flexibility within membranes, but those same double bonds also make them chemically reactive enough to participate in rapid enzymatic transformation when released. This is part of their biological value. The body uses their reactivity to generate fast, local, potent messages. But that same feature also creates vulnerability. A membrane heavily enriched in polyunsaturated material is carrying a larger reservoir of signal substrate, yet it is also carrying a larger reservoir of oxidation-sensitive matter. Under well-regulated conditions, this allows dynamic signaling and adaptive response. Under poorly regulated conditions, especially when oxidative stress is high and structural protection is weak, those same polyunsaturated lipids can become sources of peroxidative injury, reactive aldehyde formation, distorted membrane behavior, and signaling spillover. The same chemistry that makes them useful as signal substrates also makes them dangerous when control is lost.

This is why substrate balance matters so much. The body is not just choosing whether to signal. It is choosing from which stored material signaling will emerge. If membranes are dominated by substrates that favor strong initiation chemistry, then the body will tend to enter inflammatory response with that material. If membranes are remodeled to include more substrates that support mediator classes involved in resolution and restoration, the body gains access to a different downstream language once activation begins. This does not mean structure disappears once signaling starts. Structure remains upstream the entire time, because the membrane is where the substrate was housed, and the membrane's composition determines the probabilities of future mediator production. A tissue that has been rebuilt under chronic inflammatory pressure may therefore become easier to activate not only because receptors are altered, but because its stored substrate reservoir has also shifted. The next signal is shaped by the last remodeling cycle.

Polyunsaturated fatty acids as signal substrates also help explain why chronic disease often has a delayed, cumulative character. A person does not need an immediately obvious inflammatory crisis to be changing their future inflammatory behavior. Repeated dietary exposure, repeated oxidative injury, repeated phospholipid remodeling, and repeated immune activation can gradually alter the substrate landscape sitting in membranes across many tissues. Over time, that changes how the body is primed to respond. One tissue may become more likely to generate pain-amplifying mediators. Another may become more likely to sustain vascular irritation. Another may remain poor at generating the mediator profile required for efficient resolution. The person experiences the output as chronic inflammation, poor recovery, recurrent symptoms, or exaggerated sensitivity, but underneath those patterns is a membrane-level change in what signaling material is available when the next trigger arrives. The body carries its recent history inside its phospholipids.

This also clarifies why the phrase inflammatory fat is often too blunt to be useful. A polyunsaturated fatty acid does not carry a moral identity. It carries structural and signaling potential. Arachidonic acid is necessary because acute defense requires initiation chemistry. EPA and DHA are important because control over inflammatory timing also requires access to substrate that can help shift the sequence toward resolution. The real issue is whether the stored substrate pool is proportionate to the demands being placed on the body and whether the broader structure can handle the reactivity built into those lipids. A membrane overloaded with highly oxidizable polyunsaturated material in a high-stress, poorly protected environment may become volatile. A membrane with too little dynamic signaling substrate may become structurally durable but less capable of proper adaptive signaling. Biology is not trying to maximize one category. It is trying to maintain a signal substrate pool that permits precise activation and clean exit without chronic overshoot.

The importance of polyunsaturated fatty acids as signal substrates reaches beyond classical inflammation. These lipids also influence vascular tone, platelet aggregation, endothelial behavior, nociception, immune cell chemotaxis, barrier repair, microglial activation, and multiple forms of intracellular stress signaling. Even when they are not being directly released into well-known mediator pathways, their presence in the membrane changes the local environment in which receptors and enzymes operate. That means they participate in signaling both by becoming mediators and by shaping the surfaces through which mediator-generating events are interpreted. Their role is therefore double-layered. They are stored instruction sets and they are part of the physical medium through which those instructions are triggered.

Seen clearly, polyunsaturated fatty acids are not merely fats with multiple double bonds. They are reserve signaling substrate built into living structure. The body uses them to preload future inflammatory, vascular, neural, and reparative responses into its own membranes. That is why they matter so much in a book about omega-3, omega-6, and resolution biology. They explain how diet becomes tissue, how tissue becomes signal, and how signal becomes behavior. Long before a symptom appears, the substrate pool is already being written. Long before inflammation begins, the membrane has already decided what kind of language that inflammation will have available.

Essential Fatty Acids and Their Pathways

The term essential fatty acid is often repeated without explaining what makes a fatty acid essential in the first place. A fatty acid is called essential when the body cannot synthesize it de novo and therefore must obtain it from diet. In humans, this applies to two parent polyunsaturated fatty acids: linoleic acid, the primary omega-6 essential fatty acid, and alpha-linolenic acid, the primary omega-3 essential fatty acid. The body can elongate and desaturate these parent molecules into longer-chain derivatives, but it cannot create the omega-6 or omega-3 double bond pattern from scratch because it lacks the enzymatic machinery to insert double bonds beyond certain positions in the carbon chain. That limitation forces dependence on dietary intake. Essential does not mean that every downstream product will be produced in ideal amounts or that intake of the parent fatty acid automatically guarantees optimal tissue composition. It means the pathway has to begin with raw material the body cannot manufacture on its own.

Once these parent fatty acids enter the body, they do not remain metabolically static. They enter elongation and desaturation pathways that can convert them into longer and more functionally specialized molecules. Linoleic acid can move through a sequence involving gamma-linolenic acid, dihomo-gamma-linolenic acid, and eventually arachidonic acid. Alpha-linolenic acid can move through stearidonic acid, eicosatetraenoic acid, EPA, docosapentaenoic acid, and ultimately DHA through a more complex sequence that includes elongation, desaturation, and peroxisomal steps. These pathways matter because the parent essential fatty acids are not the end of the story. The longer-chain derivatives are often the tissue-active forms most directly involved in membrane composition, inflammatory mediator production, neural structure, retinal function, and resolution biology. What the body can do with essential fatty acids therefore depends not only on intake but on pathway efficiency, tissue demand, and metabolic competition.

That competition is one of the most important features of these pathways. Omega-3 and omega-6 families share parts of the same enzymatic machinery, especially desaturase and elongase systems. This means the body is not processing each family on separate rails. They interact. High flux through one family can affect the handling of the other, not because one is inherently illegitimate, but because both are drawing from overlapping conversion capacity. In practical terms, the relative availability of linoleic acid and alpha-linolenic acid influences how much pathway attention each family receives. This is one reason simple dietary presence is not enough to explain tissue outcomes. A person may consume some alpha-linolenic acid, but if conversion pressure, competition, or metabolic conditions limit downstream production, tissue EPA and DHA status may remain modest. The pathway exists, but its throughput is not unlimited.

The omega-6 pathway deserves precision because it is often discussed only through the lens of excess inflammation. Linoleic acid is the dietary starting point, but its biological significance depends on what happens after incorporation and conversion. Through desaturation and elongation, it can contribute to the formation of arachidonic acid, which then becomes a major membrane substrate for eicosanoid production. Arachidonic acid is central to acute inflammatory signaling, vascular control, pain pathways, and multiple forms of local immune activation. It is not a pathological accident. It is part of the body's normal capacity to respond rapidly to tissue disruption and threat. The problem begins when pathway dominance, membrane enrichment, and inflammatory conditions together bias the organism too heavily toward initiation chemistry without equally competent termination and repair. In that case the omega-6 pathway is not wrong, but it becomes overrepresented in a system that has lost proportionality.

The omega-3 pathway is often misunderstood in the opposite direction. Alpha-linolenic acid is the essential dietary precursor, but the longer-chain products EPA and DHA are the forms most directly associated with membrane remodeling, neural tissue composition, retinal structure, and specialized pro-resolving mediator generation. The conversion from alpha-linolenic acid to EPA is limited in many humans, and conversion to DHA is more constrained still. This is why the distinction between precursor omega-3 and tissue-active omega-3 matters. A diet may technically contain essential omega-3 while still supplying relatively little preformed EPA and DHA to tissues. From a pathway perspective, that means the organism has the raw starting material but may not be generating downstream products in the quantity or distribution needed to significantly reshape membrane composition or signaling capacity. Essentiality alone does not guarantee sufficiency at the endpoint.

These pathways also operate within tissue-specific priorities. The body is not trying to convert every essential fatty acid into the same downstream product everywhere. Some tissues require more arachidonic acid for acute signaling readiness. Others require more DHA because membrane curvature, excitability, photoreceptor function, or neural stability depend on it. The liver plays a central role in handling, modifying, packaging, and redistributing fatty acids, but tissue uptake, remodeling, and retention determine where those molecules ultimately matter. A pathway on paper is therefore not the same as a pathway expressed in living tissue. The body does not simply manufacture EPA, DHA, or arachidonic acid and leave them floating in abstraction. It incorporates them into phospholipids, stores them in particular membrane pools, and then draws on those pools later under stress, signaling demand, or structural turnover.

This is one reason essential fatty acid pathways have to be understood as both structural and signaling systems at once. The pathway does not end when a fatty acid reaches its longer-chain form. That product then enters membranes, changes membrane behavior, and becomes part of the substrate reservoir for future mediator synthesis. Arachidonic acid stored in phospholipids later becomes available for prostaglandin, thromboxane, and leukotriene production. EPA and DHA stored in phospholipids later become available for alternative eicosanoid profiles and for specialized pro-resolving mediator families. The pathway therefore determines not just what the tissue is made of today, but what kinds of inflammatory and reparative language it will be able to generate tomorrow. Essential fatty acid metabolism is stored future behavior.

The oxidative vulnerability of these pathways also has to be considered. As the fatty acids become more unsaturated, they become more chemically flexible but also more susceptible to peroxidation. This gives the body a tradeoff. Longer-chain polyunsaturated products expand structural nuance and signaling capacity, but they also require better containment, better antioxidant protection, better membrane repair, and better control over inflammatory timing. A tissue enriched in highly unsaturated products without adequate protection is carrying more signaling potential and more chemical fragility at the same time. That is why pathway support cannot be reduced to the idea of making more long-chain polyunsaturated fatty acids at all costs. The question is whether the organism can incorporate and protect them within a stable architecture.

Seen clearly, essential fatty acids and their pathways are not just nutrient conversion charts. They are the route by which diet becomes membrane composition, and membrane composition becomes inflammatory potential, neural behavior, vascular signaling, and resolution capacity. Linoleic acid and alpha-linolenic acid are essential because the body cannot begin these families without outside input, but what happens after intake depends on conversion, competition, tissue demand, oxidative context, and long-term remodeling. The real significance of these pathways is not that they turn one fatty acid into another. It is that they determine what kind of body gets built from the input. They determine which substrates are stored in membranes, which mediator families are available during stress, and whether the organism is being equipped more heavily for initiation, for adaptation, or for balanced completion.

Why the Body Requires Both

The body requires both omega-3 and omega-6 because they are not interchangeable and they do not build the same signaling and structural possibilities. Each family contributes a different kind of material to membranes and a different set of downstream options once those membranes are activated. The mistake is to imagine that one family is the legitimate one and the other is a biological error. That is not how the system is built. The body needs initiation as well as resolution. It needs dynamic signaling as well as controlled shutdown. It needs membrane flexibility, tissue-specific responsiveness, vascular control, immune recruitment, neural function, growth, repair, and protection against overreaction. No single fatty acid family can carry all of those requirements alone. The body uses both because it is not trying to create one uniform lipid effect. It is trying to build a signaling-capable organism that can enter stress responses when necessary and leave them when appropriate.

Omega-6 is required because acute biology must be able to mobilize quickly. Arachidonic acid-derived signaling is part of how the body generates pain sensitivity when tissue is damaged, changes vascular behavior when injury occurs, recruits immune cells when threat is detected, and coordinates local defense when disruption has to be contained. These are not optional functions. A body that could not initiate inflammation, alter blood flow, activate platelets, or recruit defensive cells would not be healthier. It would be less able to survive ordinary challenges. Omega-6-derived pathways are part of how the body responds with speed and force when a rapid local reaction is needed. That role becomes dangerous only when it becomes disproportionate, prolonged, or insufficiently opposed by pathways that help complete the response once its useful phase is over.

Omega-3 is required because initiation alone is not enough. A body that can start inflammation but cannot guide it toward completion becomes trapped in its own defense chemistry. EPA and DHA matter because they alter membrane composition and because they provide substrate for mediator families involved in de-escalation, debris clearance, tissue protection, and restoration of order after inflammatory work has been done. This does not make omega-3 a passive calming agent. It makes it part of the machinery that prevents acute defense from becoming chronic damage. The body requires omega-3 because tissue protection, neural stability, membrane behavior, and inflammatory resolution all depend on having access to substrate that does more than intensify response. Without omega-3, the organism loses part of its ability to finish what omega-6 helps begin.

The structural role also makes both families necessary. Membranes are not built from one kind of fatty acid because different tissues require different physical behavior. Some membranes need rapid signaling flexibility. Some need specialized curvature. Some need highly tuned excitability. Some need a signaling reservoir rich enough to support local inflammatory language. Others need a stronger contribution from lipids that support resolution-oriented mediator production or neural membrane behavior. DHA, for example, is especially important in tissues such as the brain and retina because those membranes require specific physical properties that shorter or less unsaturated fatty acids do not reproduce in the same way. Arachidonic acid remains important in tissues that need immediate signaling readiness. The body requires both families because it is solving multiple structural problems at once, not building one generic membrane repeated across all tissues.

Both are also required because signaling in real physiology is sequential. Acute initiation without later resolution is destructive, but resolution without the ability to mount a proper early response is also dysfunctional. The body has to move through phases. First it must detect disruption, then contain it, then recruit the appropriate machinery, then clear what needs clearing, then stop the escalation, then rebuild. Omega-6-derived substrate contributes strongly to the early and middle phases of this sequence. Omega-3-derived substrate contributes strongly to the later phases and to the membrane conditions that make proportionate signaling more likely in the first place. The body therefore requires both because biological control depends on sequence, and sequence depends on having access to different classes of substrate at different stages of the same event.

This is why the real problem is not the existence of either family but the loss of proportion between them. If omega-6-derived structure and substrate dominate too heavily, the organism becomes better prepared to escalate than to resolve. If omega-3 availability is too low, the body loses part of its capacity to complete inflammatory events cleanly and to maintain certain specialized membrane properties over time. On the other hand, simply adding omega-3 without regard for oxidative stability, membrane protection, and the broader lipid environment does not automatically restore balance. The goal is not to replace one family with the other. The goal is to restore coordination so that initiation chemistry remains available when needed, resolution chemistry remains available when needed, and membrane structure remains capable of supporting both without falling into chronic volatility.

The body therefore requires both omega-3 and omega-6 for the same reason it requires acceleration and braking, activation and restraint, entry into defense and exit from defense. These are not opposing moral categories. They are complementary parts of a controlled biological sequence. Omega-6 helps the organism respond with force. Omega-3 helps the organism recover with intelligence. Both enter membranes. Both shape signaling. Both become part of tissue behavior over time. Health depends less on choosing sides than on rebuilding the relationship between them so the body can defend itself without becoming trapped in defense.

The Myth of "Good vs Bad"

One of the most damaging habits in nutrition is the tendency to sort molecules into moral categories. A fat becomes good, another becomes bad, and the discussion ends before physiology has even begun. That habit makes marketing easier, but it makes understanding harder. The body does not use lipids according to moral identity. It uses them according to structure, context, timing, tissue demand, enzymatic access, oxidative environment, and the sequence of events the organism is trying to carry out. A fatty acid can be useful in one role and harmful in another. It can support membrane function in one tissue and become excessive signaling substrate in another. It can be necessary in acute defense and destructive in chronic dysregulation. Once that is understood, the good-versus-bad frame starts to collapse because it was never precise enough to describe lipid biology in the first place.

Omega-6 is one of the clearest examples of this distortion. It is often treated as the villain because arachidonic acid-derived mediators participate in inflammation, pain, platelet activity, and acute vascular response. But those pathways exist for reasons. The body has to be able to respond when tissue is damaged, when pathogens are present, when bleeding has to be controlled, or when local defense must be mobilized quickly. Without omega-6-derived signaling, the organism would not become cleaner or calmer. It would become less competent. The real problem is not that omega-6 exists or that it participates in inflammatory signaling. The problem is that in many modern conditions, omega-6-derived structure and signaling become overrepresented in a body already under chronic oxidative, metabolic, and inflammatory strain. The issue is not moral corruption of one fat family. The issue is disproportion inside a system that has lost control of sequence.

Omega-3 is distorted just as badly, but in the opposite direction. It is turned into the heroic fat, the universally beneficial input that can be added to almost any health problem as though it carries its own built-in corrective intelligence. That is too simple. Omega-3 can be extremely important, but its value depends on what kind of membrane it enters, what oxidative conditions surround it, how much of it is actually incorporated into tissue, how much competing substrate is already present, and whether the body has the enzymatic and structural capacity to use it well. EPA and DHA can support membrane behavior and contribute to resolution-oriented signaling, but they are still highly unsaturated molecules. In unstable oxidative environments, that unsaturation can also become a liability. That does not make omega-3 bad. It means even a valuable lipid can create vulnerability if it is introduced into the wrong architecture without the stability required to protect it.

This is why isolated praise and isolated blame both fail. Arachidonic acid is not bad because it helps generate inflammatory mediators. Those mediators are part of normal defense. DHA is not good simply because it is found in neural tissue and resolution pathways. It still has to be handled, incorporated, protected, and balanced. Saturated fats are not bad because they reduce membrane fluidity relative to polyunsaturated fats. In many contexts they contribute structural stability and resistance to peroxidative damage. But that does not mean all membrane behavior improves by maximizing rigidity. Cholesterol is not bad because it appears in cardiovascular discourse as a risk marker. It is also a membrane organizer and steroid precursor without which cellular architecture and endocrine biology would collapse. The body does not experience these molecules as brand identities or online arguments. It experiences them as materials with specific physical consequences.

The good-versus-bad framework also fails because it ignores role switching. The same lipid can serve different purposes depending on state. A polyunsaturated fatty acid stored in a membrane today may later become inflammatory or pro-resolving substrate tomorrow. A triglyceride stored as fuel can later influence signaling through the conditions of its mobilization. A structural lipid can become part of a signaling cascade once released. A signaling event can alter future structure by changing how membranes are remodeled after stress. In biology, lipids are not trapped in one category. They move between architecture, fuel handling, and communication. Once molecules are understood as role-shifting components inside a dynamic system, simplistic labeling becomes less useful. The real question is never whether a lipid belongs on the good list or the bad list. The real question is what it is doing in that tissue, at that time, under those conditions.

This moral framing also hides one of the central truths of chronic disease, which is that harm often emerges from imbalance, misplacement, overrepresentation, or failed sequencing rather than from the mere presence of a molecule. The body does not usually break because it encountered one evil nutrient in isolation. It breaks because structural ratios shift, signaling timing deteriorates, membranes become easier to oxidize, mitochondrial handling becomes less efficient, and inflammatory pathways lose their ability to end cleanly. In that situation, even normal biological components can participate in pathological outcomes because they are being used inside a disordered system. Arachidonic acid can contribute to chronic inflammation when resolution fails. Highly unsaturated omega-3 incorporation can become fragile when antioxidant protection is weak. Saturated structures can become limiting if adaptability is lost in certain membrane contexts. None of this is captured by calling one molecule clean and another toxic. The system has to be read as a system.

The language of good and bad also encourages people to think in terms of elimination instead of architecture. They look for the enemy fat to remove or the hero fat to add, as though the body were waiting for a single dietary verdict. But the organism is trying to maintain surfaces, gradients, receptor function, barrier control, signaling reserve, mitochondrial performance, and immune timing all at once. That means the relevant question is compositional. What kind of membrane is being built. What kind of signaling reservoir is being stored. What kind of oxidative burden is the system carrying. What kind of structural protection surrounds highly reactive lipids. What kind of inflammatory sequence is the body equipped to generate and complete. Those questions are harder than simply asking which fat is good, but they are the questions that actually correspond to physiology.

This is especially important when discussing omega-3 and omega-6 together. The body does not require a hero and a villain. It requires a relationship. Omega-6 helps create rapid local response capacity. Omega-3 helps shape membrane behavior and expand access to mediator families involved in completion and repair. Both are necessary. Both can become problematic in the wrong context. Both derive their meaning from proportion, tissue placement, and system state. The problem begins when one family dominates structural incorporation and downstream signaling to the point that the organism becomes better at escalation than at closure, or when the attempt to correct that imbalance ignores the oxidative and architectural conditions required to make the correction hold. The issue is never simply one good input rescuing the body from one bad input. It is whether the lipid environment has been rebuilt into something coherent enough to support proportionate biological behavior.

A more honest framework is to stop asking whether a lipid is good or bad and start asking what problem it solves, what liability it introduces, and what conditions determine which side of that balance becomes dominant. Every meaningful lipid does both. Polyunsaturated fats provide signaling flexibility and mediator diversity, but they also introduce oxidation risk. More saturated structures provide durability and resistance to peroxidation, but they can reduce flexibility if not balanced appropriately. Cholesterol stabilizes and organizes membranes, but excessive mismanagement of cholesterol traffic within broader metabolic dysfunction can still reflect deeper systemic problems. Biology does not eliminate tradeoffs. It manages them. A useful nutritional framework has to do the same.

The myth of good versus bad survives because it is emotionally satisfying. It offers a simple map in a system that is actually conditional, layered, and physically constrained. But the body is not asking for moral clarity. It is asking for proportion, sequence, and structural coherence. Lipids are not saints or villains. They are materials. Some build faster signals. Some build stronger surfaces. Some provide substrate for escalation. Some provide substrate for resolution. Some do more than one of these at the same time. Health depends on how they are arranged, not how they are judged. Once that becomes the frame, the conversation improves immediately. It stops being about choosing the righteous fat and starts being about rebuilding the body's lipid architecture so that defense, energy, and recovery can occur without turning against the organism itself.

Chapter 5

Arachidonic Acid and the Initiation of Inflammation

Arachidonic acid sits near the center of inflammatory biology because it is one of the body's main stored substrates for rapid defensive signaling. It is not floating around as a random irritant waiting to cause trouble. It is built into membrane phospholipids, especially at positions where it can be released when the cell detects injury, threat, mechanical disruption, immune activation, or other stress signals. That placement is important because it means arachidonic acid is part of the body's prepared response system. The membrane is not only a boundary and not only a signaling surface. It is also a loaded reservoir of potential inflammatory chemistry. When the right trigger arrives, enzymes such as phospholipase A2 liberate arachidonic acid from the membrane, and once released, it becomes available to cyclooxygenase, lipoxygenase, and related enzymatic pathways that rapidly generate a large family of mediators. Those mediators are what give inflammation much of its early direction, force, vascular character, and local urgency. To understand why inflammation starts the way it does, arachidonic acid has to be understood first as stored architecture and then as mobilized instruction.

This point matters because inflammation is often described as if it begins with immune cells deciding to become aggressive. In reality, the sequence is more physical and more immediate. A tissue is disturbed. Receptors sense damage-associated signals, microbial signals, oxidative stress, or mechanical disruption. Membrane-associated enzymes are activated. Arachidonic acid is released from phospholipids. Enzymatic conversion begins. Blood vessels change tone. Endothelial permeability shifts. Platelets may become more active. Pain signaling is amplified. Immune cells are recruited. What looks like one event called inflammation is actually a coordinated cascade launched from stored lipid substrate. That does not make arachidonic acid a pathological molecule. It makes it one of the body's main acute response materials. Without it, the organism would struggle to generate the speed and local intensity required to contain injury, respond to infection, or coordinate early tissue defense. Inflammatory initiation is not an accident. It is a built-in capacity, and arachidonic acid is one of its key fuels.

The reason arachidonic acid is so effective in this role is that it occupies a middle ground the body can use efficiently. It is reactive enough to be rapidly converted into potent local mediators, but stable enough to remain stored within membranes until release is needed. Once liberated, it enters pathways that produce prostaglandins, thromboxanes, leukotrienes, lipoxins, and related eicosanoid molecules. Each of these mediator families influences different parts of the inflammatory sequence. Some increase vascular permeability so plasma proteins and immune cells can reach the site of disruption. Some alter vasodilation or vasoconstriction depending on tissue context and timing. Some recruit leukocytes and intensify chemotaxis. Some increase pain sensitivity so damaged tissue is protected behaviorally. Some affect platelet aggregation and hemostatic coordination. In other words, arachidonic acid does not create one generic inflammatory signal. It creates a language of local control, and that language is how the body translates tissue disruption into organized reaction.

This is why arachidonic acid has to be discussed carefully. In popular nutrition language, it is often treated as if it were synonymous with harmful inflammation, but that interpretation confuses function with excess. The body needs initiation chemistry. If blood vessels could not change permeability, immune cells could not be recruited effectively, and damaged tissue could not generate a local alarm state, defense would fail before resolution was ever relevant. The real problem begins when arachidonic acid-derived initiation becomes chronically dominant, when the substrate reservoir is disproportionately weighted toward escalation, or when later phases of inflammatory sequencing fail to shut down the reaction once the useful work has been done. Arachidonic acid is not the problem because it starts inflammation. The problem is what happens when starting becomes easier than finishing.

The structural origin of arachidonic acid also explains why inflammatory tone is partly predetermined before any acute event occurs. A tissue that has incorporated substantial arachidonic acid into its membrane phospholipids is not simply resting in a neutral state. It is holding a certain kind of future signaling potential. If phospholipase activation occurs, that tissue is prepared to generate a particular range of eicosanoid outputs. This means chronic remodeling of membrane composition changes not only how the membrane behaves mechanically and electrically, but also what kind of inflammatory response becomes likely under stress. The tissue carries its future reaction within its own surface structure. A membrane more enriched in arachidonic acid is more prepared for strong initiation chemistry. That can be useful when acute responsiveness is needed. It becomes a liability when stress is chronic, oxidative damage is ongoing, immune activation is frequent, and the body repeatedly draws from the same initiation-heavy reservoir without adequately rebuilding the larger sequence toward closure.

The vascular effects of arachidonic acid-derived signaling show how quickly this chemistry can alter local reality. Prostaglandins can expand or contract vessels depending on subtype and context. Endothelial surfaces can become more permissive, allowing immune cells and plasma factors to exit circulation and enter tissue. Platelet-derived thromboxanes can influence aggregation and clot formation. These are not minor side effects of inflammation. They are core parts of the body's decision to convert a stable tissue environment into an acute response zone. Once these vascular shifts begin, the tissue is no longer operating under ordinary homeostatic rules. Fluid dynamics change. Cellular traffic changes. Pressure relationships change. Local oxygen delivery and nutrient exchange can change. Pain sensitivity changes. The site becomes metabolically and immunologically different. Arachidonic acid is one of the molecules that makes this transition possible, which is why it has such importance at the very start of inflammatory events.

Pain is another major part of this initiation sequence. Arachidonic acid-derived prostaglandins sensitize nociceptors and make tissue disturbance more behaviorally obvious. This is often viewed negatively because pain is unpleasant, but the biology behind it is protective. The body uses pain to alter movement, reduce load on injured structures, and increase awareness of tissue damage or irritation. Inflammation without pain would often lead to continued use of compromised tissue and greater structural injury. Again, the issue is not that arachidonic acid produces pain-related mediators. The issue is whether those mediators remain proportionate to the problem they are signaling and whether the system can later reverse sensitization once repair is underway. When inflammatory sequencing fails, pain remains after utility has ended. At that point the body is no longer using arachidonic acid-derived signals intelligently. It is repeating initiation chemistry without successfully completing the transition into restoration.

The immune recruitment side of arachidonic acid biology is equally important. Leukotrienes and related mediators help direct immune cells toward disturbed tissue, increase adhesion interactions, and intensify local defensive behavior. This is useful when there is genuine infection, tissue damage, or a need for rapid containment. But because these mediators can strongly amplify local immune traffic, they also contribute to the shift from proportionate acute inflammation into chronic inflammatory persistence when regulatory balance is lost. A tissue repeatedly generating arachidonic acid-derived recruitment signals can remain stuck in a state of cellular arrival without efficient debris clearance, resolution signaling, and return to baseline. The immune system then appears overactive, but in structural terms the tissue is repeatedly drawing from an initiation-centered substrate pool and failing to transition into the later phases that would complete the job.

This is one reason arachidonic acid has to be understood inside a sequence rather than in isolation. It belongs to the beginning of inflammation far more than to the end. It helps establish the early local conditions of defense. It changes vascular access, pain sensitivity, platelet behavior, and immune recruitment. It is part of how the body says something is wrong here and resources need to move now. That role is legitimate and necessary. But if the sequence stops there, initiation becomes self-damaging. Tissues remain permeable too long. Nociceptors remain sensitized too long. Immune cells remain recruited too long. Reactive oxygen species and proteolytic activity remain elevated too long. At that point the body is not suffering because arachidonic acid exists. It is suffering because initiation has been decoupled from resolution.

This chapter therefore establishes a crucial principle for the rest of the book. Inflammation begins with lipid mobilization from membranes, and arachidonic acid is one of the main early substrates that gives inflammation its force. That makes it essential, not optional. But because it is essential, it also has to be matched by equally competent systems that can contain, redirect, and terminate the response once the need for escalation has passed. Arachidonic acid explains how the body launches defense. It does not explain how the body safely exits defense. That distinction is where much of modern chronic illness begins. The organism is still capable of initiating. It is no longer as capable of completing. Once that happens, arachidonic acid stops looking like part of a healthy sequence and starts looking like chronic inflammatory burden, even though the deeper failure is not in the existence of initiation chemistry itself. The deeper failure is in what does or does not come after it.

Omega-6 as an Activation Signal

Omega-6 functions as an activation signal because it helps load tissues with the substrate needed to begin rapid response when disturbance occurs. This does not mean omega-6 itself is always circulating as an alarm molecule. It means omega-6-derived fatty acids, especially arachidonic acid, are built into membrane phospholipids in a way that prepares the cell for future activation. The signal is stored before it is expressed. When receptors detect tissue injury, immune challenge, oxidative stress, mechanical disruption, or other forms of danger, phospholipases release omega-6-derived substrate from the membrane, and that release creates immediate access to a family of mediators that can change vascular tone, increase permeability, recruit immune cells, amplify pain sensitivity, and intensify local defensive activity. Omega-6 is therefore an activation signal in reservoir form. It is part of how the body keeps early inflammatory potential embedded in tissue architecture rather than waiting to build it from scratch after the problem has already begun.

This stored activation capacity is one reason omega-6 is biologically necessary. A body that could not rapidly generate local inflammatory signaling would be slow to contain injury, slow to recruit immune help, slow to alter blood flow at damaged sites, and slow to protect tissue behaviorally through pain and sensitization. Acute defense requires molecules that can move quickly and act locally, and omega-6-derived mediators provide much of that early language. Prostaglandins, leukotrienes, and thromboxanes do not emerge from nowhere. They emerge from omega-6 substrate already positioned inside membranes, ready for mobilization once threshold is crossed. That makes omega-6 less like a generic dietary fat and more like a preloaded ignition system. Under the right conditions, it helps the body say something is wrong here, pay attention here, send resources here, and change behavior here.

What makes omega-6 especially powerful in this role is that it links structure to urgency. A membrane enriched in omega-6-derived substrate is not just a membrane with different physical properties. It is a membrane carrying a certain future inflammatory bias. Once activated, it can rapidly generate signals that expand the reaction outward from the initial point of disturbance. Blood vessels can widen or change permeability. Endothelial surfaces can become more adhesive to immune cells. Platelets can become more reactive. Pain thresholds can drop. Immune cells can be drawn into tissue with greater force. This is how local tissue disruption becomes organized inflammation rather than isolated biochemical noise. Omega-6 gives the body a way to convert damage detection into a coordinated state change. Activation is not just turned on. It is assembled through mediator families built from omega-6 substrate already present in the membrane.

This is also why omega-6 should not be described as inflammatory in a purely negative sense. Inflammation at the initiation stage is not inherently pathological. It is one of the main ways the body protects itself. Without it, tissue damage would spread more easily, microbial intrusion would be less contained, and repair would begin too late or too weakly. Omega-6-derived signaling is part of how the body prioritizes a problem. It makes the site metabolically louder. It changes blood flow, sensation, cellular traffic, and biochemical activity so the tissue is no longer treated as normal background terrain. The body requires this activation logic. The problem begins only when activation continues after it has served its purpose, or when the membrane reservoir has been remodeled so heavily toward initiation that even modest disturbances produce excessive inflammatory output.

That shift from useful activation to chronic overactivation is where context becomes critical. Omega-6 as an activation signal is healthy when it appears in proportion to real need and when the organism retains the ability to move into later stages of inflammatory sequencing. If the tissue can recruit, contain, clear, and then resolve, omega-6 has done its job. But if the body repeatedly mobilizes omega-6-derived substrate in response to ongoing metabolic stress, gut-derived immune irritation, oxidative burden, mechanical strain, or unresolved tissue damage, then activation becomes a chronic state rather than a temporary phase. The membrane remains loaded with initiation material, the system keeps drawing from it, and the person begins living inside repeated low-grade alarm signaling. At that point omega-6 is not acting as a faulty molecule. It is acting as an overused one inside a sequence that is no longer being completed.

This is one of the main reasons the modern conversation around omega-6 becomes confused. People see the effects of chronic inflammatory activation and assume omega-6 itself is the enemy. That interpretation mistakes function for imbalance. The body needs omega-6 because it needs to be able to respond rapidly when something goes wrong. But a body built under chronic stress, oxidative instability, poor resolution capacity, and disproportionate membrane loading with omega-6-derived substrate will naturally behave as though activation is easier than recovery. The real issue is not that the ignition system exists. The issue is that the brakes, steering, and shutdown sequence are no longer proportionate to the power of ignition. Omega-6 becomes dangerous when activation dominates the organism's operating style.

The signaling role of omega-6 also extends beyond obvious inflammation. Activation includes vascular change, platelet behavior, nociceptive sensitization, epithelial response, immune recruitment, and shifts in tissue metabolism. These are all part of the body's decision to move from ordinary maintenance into active defense. In that sense, omega-6 is not simply a trigger for swelling or redness. It helps move tissue into a different operational mode. The body reallocates attention, resources, and biochemical priority. That mode is useful when short-lived and harmful when persistent. It is adaptive when paired with completion and destructive when left open-ended. Omega-6-derived activation is therefore best understood as necessary early-phase biological force. It gives the system the capacity to react decisively. The danger appears when decisiveness becomes default rather than temporary.

Seen clearly, omega-6 as an activation signal is one of the central truths of inflammatory biology. The body builds part of its emergency language directly into its membranes, and omega-6-derived fatty acids are a major part of that language. They prepare tissues to escalate when escalation is justified. They help transform cellular detection into tissue-wide response. They make defense possible. But because they are so effective at beginning the sequence, they also reveal the deeper problem in chronic illness. Many people still have strong activation capacity. What they lack is equally strong completion capacity. The body can still say go. It has become less able to say enough.

Eicosanoid Cascades

Eicosanoid cascades are the biochemical expansion system that turns membrane disturbance into organized inflammatory action. They begin when polyunsaturated fatty acids, especially arachidonic acid and in some contexts EPA, are released from membrane phospholipids by phospholipase activity after a trigger has been detected. That trigger may be tissue injury, immune receptor activation, oxidative stress, mechanical damage, endotoxin exposure, cytokine signaling, ischemia, or another form of biological disruption. Once the fatty acid is liberated from the membrane, it enters enzymatic pathways that convert stored structural substrate into highly active local mediators. This is what makes the term cascade useful. The system does not produce one signal and stop. It branches outward into multiple mediator families, each affecting blood flow, vascular permeability, pain sensitivity, leukocyte trafficking, platelet behavior, smooth muscle tone, oxidative activity, and the timing of the inflammatory sequence itself. The cascade is how the body scales up a local trigger into a tissue-level state change.

The first major feature of an eicosanoid cascade is speed. The body does not need to synthesize an entirely new structural platform before reacting. The substrate is already present in the membrane, and the enzymes required for conversion are either present, inducible, or rapidly mobilized. That allows an injured or activated tissue to move quickly from detection into action. A membrane phospholipid loses arachidonic acid. Cyclooxygenase enzymes may begin converting that arachidonic acid into prostaglandin intermediates. Lipoxygenase pathways may begin producing leukotriene or lipoxin precursors. In some tissues, cytochrome-dependent routes contribute additional oxidized lipid products with their own local effects. The tissue then stops behaving like resting tissue and starts behaving like activated tissue. Vessels change. Immune traffic changes. Sensory thresholds change. Cellular recruitment begins. The key point is that the eicosanoid cascade is not separate from membrane biology. It is membrane biology becoming inflammatory instruction.

The cyclooxygenase branch is one of the main early arms of this cascade. Through COX enzymes, arachidonic acid is converted into unstable intermediates that are then processed into prostaglandins, prostacyclin, and thromboxanes. These are not redundant molecules. They handle different parts of the local response. Some prostaglandins increase pain sensitization, alter vascular tone, raise local temperature, or influence immune activity. Prostacyclin can affect vascular behavior and platelet restraint in certain settings. Thromboxanes push in a different direction by promoting platelet aggregation and influencing vascular constriction. The meaning of the cascade therefore depends on tissue context and mediator mix. The body is not simply making inflammation stronger. It is changing the operating rules at the site. It is determining whether blood should flow more freely, whether clotting should increase, whether nerves should become more sensitive, whether local tissue should swell, and whether immune cells should interpret the area as an active zone requiring attention.

The lipoxygenase branch extends the cascade into immune recruitment and inflammatory amplification. Through lipoxygenase activity, arachidonic acid can be converted into leukotrienes and related compounds that intensify leukocyte chemotaxis, alter bronchial tone, increase vascular permeability, and strengthen the recruitment logic of acute inflammation. This is one reason inflammatory tissue begins attracting more cells into itself once the cascade is underway. The tissue is not merely damaged. It is broadcasting. Leukotrienes help generate that broadcast by increasing the biochemical force pulling immune cells toward the site and by reshaping the local environment so that immune traffic becomes easier and more sustained. This is useful when real containment is needed. It becomes destructive when the recruitment phase stays active longer than the problem justifies or when the tissue never transitions cleanly into later stages of debris clearance and shutdown.

The cascade is also self-amplifying in practice, even when it is tightly regulated in design. Eicosanoid production can increase vascular permeability, and increased permeability can increase exposure of tissue to circulating immune components and inflammatory signals. Recruited immune cells can generate additional cytokines, reactive oxygen species, proteases, and lipid mediator production, which can further stimulate phospholipase activity and additional arachidonic acid release from nearby membranes. Pain sensitization changes behavior, which alters tissue use and sometimes tissue loading. Platelet activation changes microvascular conditions. Endothelial shifts alter trafficking patterns. In this way the cascade does not simply spread chemically. It changes the local physical environment so that more inflammatory events become likely. That is why initiation can become disproportionate so easily in a stressed system. Once the cascade starts, it creates conditions that favor its own continuation unless counter-sequencing mechanisms come online.

This is where balance becomes crucial. Eicosanoid cascades are supposed to be phase-specific. Their purpose is to initiate and organize early response, not to remain dominant indefinitely. Arachidonic acid-derived eicosanoids are especially powerful because they help the body create urgency, but urgency is only useful if it is time-limited. Once microbial containment, hemostasis, or acute damage signaling has been established, the tissue needs to move toward clearance, repair, and reduction of collateral injury. If the eicosanoid cascade keeps running without appropriate containment, the same mediators that originally protected tissue begin contributing to pain persistence, vascular dysfunction, leukocyte overrecruitment, oxidative injury, and barrier breakdown. The problem is then not that the cascade exists. The problem is that it has remained in command after the job requiring command has changed.

EPA can also enter eicosanoid pathways, and this matters because it slightly alters the character of the cascade. EPA-derived eicosanoids often have different biological potency and different downstream consequences than their arachidonic acid-derived counterparts. This does not erase inflammatory initiation, nor should it. It changes substrate competition and can shift the mediator field toward a somewhat different signaling profile. That shift is part of why omega-3 incorporation matters upstream. The membrane reservoir partly determines which version of the cascade becomes available once phospholipase activity begins. A membrane storing more EPA relative to arachidonic acid is not identical in inflammatory potential to one storing mostly arachidonic acid. The difference is not absolute replacement. It is altered probability within the cascade. The tissue has slightly different words available when it begins speaking inflammatory language.

Eicosanoid cascades also explain why chronic disease can feel like repeated false emergency. The body does not need a dramatic acute injury every day to keep these pathways partially active. Chronic endotoxin exposure, adipose-derived inflammation, barrier dysfunction, oxidized lipids, repetitive mechanical strain, unresolved infection, mitochondrial stress, and persistent cytokine signaling can all maintain enough phospholipase activity and enzymatic throughput to keep eicosanoid output elevated or repeatedly re-triggered. The person then lives inside a body that keeps converting membrane substrate into activation chemistry. Pain persists. Vascular tone becomes less stable. Immune cells continue arriving. Recovery remains incomplete. The body acts like it is still in the early-middle phase of response because, biochemically, it often is.

This is why understanding eicosanoid cascades is so important for the rest of the omega-3 and resolution discussion. They show how initiation actually happens in material terms. Membrane structure is disrupted or signaled. A fatty acid is released. Enzymatic branches convert that fatty acid into local instructions. Those instructions alter the tissue environment and recruit a larger defensive state. Nothing about this is abstract. It is physical, stored, triggered, and amplified. Eicosanoid cascades are the mechanism by which lipid architecture becomes inflammatory behavior. They explain why the body can respond so quickly, why imbalance becomes so consequential, and why changing membrane composition over time can alter not only structural behavior but the very language the body uses when something goes wrong.

Necessary vs Chronic Inflammation

Inflammation is not a design flaw. It is a controlled emergency program built into tissue so the body can respond when normal conditions are broken. Without it, injury would spread more easily, pathogens would gain territory more easily, damaged structures would persist without coordinated cleanup, and repair would begin too late or too weakly. Necessary inflammation is the form that serves a clear purpose and remains tied to sequence. It begins when tissue disruption, infection, toxic exposure, or structural injury creates conditions that cannot be handled by ordinary maintenance alone. Local vessels change behavior. Permeability shifts. Immune cells are recruited. Damaged material is identified. Pain sensitivity may rise so the injured area is protected from further use. Oxidative chemistry may increase because microbes or damaged components have to be contained and dismantled. This is not pathological simply because it is uncomfortable. It is the body moving from background maintenance into active defense because the situation requires more than quiet homeostasis can provide.

What makes necessary inflammation healthy is not the absence of force. It is the presence of direction. The response is matched to a real disturbance, and each phase helps prepare the next one. Initiation chemistry opens access. Recruitment brings in the machinery. Clearance removes threats and debris. Then the system shifts. The same tissue that intensified blood flow, immune traffic, and pain signaling has to begin reducing those outputs once their job is done. Macrophages change behavior. Dead cells and spent inflammatory material are cleared. Barrier integrity begins to restore. Pro-inflammatory mediator dominance gives way to pro-resolving signaling. Pain sensitization declines. Vascular permeability tightens back down. Tissue no longer behaves like an emergency zone because the emergency sequence has been completed. Necessary inflammation is therefore not defined by mildness. It is defined by completion. It does work, then it exits.

Chronic inflammation is different because it has lost that sequence. It may still use many of the same molecules and cell types, but it no longer behaves like a temporary program moving toward closure. Instead, the body remains trapped in repeated initiation, incomplete clearance, unresolved tissue signaling, or ongoing low-grade recruitment. The system keeps spending resources without finishing the task those resources were meant to accomplish. Blood vessels may remain too permissive. Nociceptors may remain sensitized. Immune cells may keep arriving while debris clearance stays inefficient. Oxidative stress may continue damaging tissue faster than repair can stabilize it. The membrane reservoir keeps being drawn upon for inflammatory signaling, but the later phases that should terminate the response never fully dominate. At that point inflammation stops being a response to a contained event and becomes part of the tissue's background operating style.

This is why chronic inflammation is not simply more inflammation. It is inflammation that has become structurally mismanaged. The body still knows how to start. In many cases it is very good at starting. The deeper failure is that the body is no longer coordinating the transition from activation to resolution. A tissue may continue generating arachidonic acid-derived signals because the trigger has not truly been removed, because barrier dysfunction keeps supplying new immune stimuli, because mitochondrial stress keeps generating danger chemistry, because damaged membranes keep releasing reactive substrate, or because the signaling environment has been remodeled to favor escalation more than completion. In each case the result feels similar. The response remains open. The body lives in a state of unfinished defense.

That unfinished state changes the meaning of symptoms. In necessary inflammation, pain, swelling, fatigue, heat, and local sensitivity are part of a temporary biological logic. They help alter behavior, allocate resources, and protect tissue during a defined period of work. In chronic inflammation, the same outputs no longer reflect an intelligent time-limited sequence. They become evidence that the system has failed to return to baseline. Pain persists after useful protection has ended. Fatigue continues because the body remains metabolically expensive. Swelling continues because vascular control remains altered. Immune signaling continues because the tissue is still being read as unfinished business. The body is no longer simply defending itself. It is being held inside defense.

This distinction is one of the most important in modern health because many people try to suppress all inflammation as though the goal were silence. Total suppression is not the solution. A body incapable of mounting necessary inflammation would be weak, slow to recover, and poor at containing real threats. The goal is not to abolish inflammatory capacity. The goal is to preserve acute inflammatory competence while restoring the ability to resolve. That requires more than blocking one mediator. It requires membranes that can support proper signaling sequence, immune cells that can shift phenotype after acute work is done, barrier systems that stop feeding repeated triggers into tissue, mitochondria that stop generating excess distress signals, and a lipid substrate environment that does not keep loading the system toward endless initiation. Resolution is not the absence of inflammation. It is the successful completion of inflammation.

This is where omega-3 and resolution biology become so important in the broader argument of the book. Chronic inflammation is often treated as though the body has too much inflammatory force and too little suppression. In many cases the more accurate description is that the body has enough force to begin but insufficient structural and signaling conditions to end well. Necessary inflammation depends heavily on omega-6-derived initiation chemistry because early defense must happen quickly. Chronic inflammation develops when that early chemistry is repeatedly mobilized without sufficient downstream transition into cleanup, restraint, and tissue restoration. The body does not only need to turn inflammation on correctly. It needs to turn it off correctly, and not by bluntly disabling the immune system, but by completing the biological job in the right order.

Seen clearly, necessary and chronic inflammation are not distinguished by whether inflammation exists. They are distinguished by whether the sequence remains intelligent. Necessary inflammation is specific, proportionate, and finite. Chronic inflammation is repetitive, poorly terminated, and structurally self-sustaining. One protects tissue by temporarily changing its state. The other damages tissue by keeping that state active after its useful phase has ended. That is why the real question is never simply how much inflammation the body has. The deeper question is whether the body still knows how to move from alarm to repair without getting trapped in alarm itself.

The Problem of Over-Initiation

The problem of over-initiation begins when the body becomes too ready to start inflammatory defense and not ready enough to control where that defense stops. Initiation is supposed to be sharp, local, and temporary. It exists to mark disruption, change tissue conditions quickly, recruit the right cellular machinery, and create enough force to contain a problem before it spreads. But when the threshold for activation drops, or when tissues are repeatedly loaded with triggers that keep crossing that threshold, initiation stops behaving like an emergency response and starts behaving like a default posture. The body begins reacting to ordinary biological friction as though it were exceptional danger. Membranes release substrate too easily. Receptors amplify too quickly. Vascular changes happen too often. Immune cells are summoned too readily. Pain pathways stay too close to the surface. The result is not simply inflammation. It is a body that has become primed to enter inflammation faster than it can justify or complete.

This can happen for several reasons at once. Membrane composition may become biased toward activation-heavy substrate, especially when arachidonic acid-rich signaling potential is repeatedly mobilized without sufficient counterweight from resolution capacity. Barrier tissues may begin leaking signals that should have remained outside, forcing the immune system to respond to a steady stream of low-grade provocation. Mitochondria under stress may generate danger chemistry that keeps tissues biochemically loud even in the absence of obvious injury. Oxidative damage may alter membranes so they become easier to disturb and more likely to release inflammatory substrate. Adipose tissue may add background inflammatory pressure through chronic excess signaling. Repeated mechanical strain, poor recovery, persistent endotoxin exposure, unresolved infection, or metabolic instability can all keep the initiation machinery partially engaged. None of these conditions require dramatic acute injury. They only require enough repeated disturbance to teach the body that activation is normal.

Once over-initiation takes hold, the entire inflammatory sequence becomes distorted. Early-phase chemistry starts appearing in places and at times where it should have remained minimal. The tissue becomes more vascularly reactive, more permeable, more sensitive, and more crowded with immune traffic. Nociceptors are sensitized more often, so discomfort appears sooner and lasts longer. Cytokines and eicosanoids are generated more readily, which feeds forward into additional phospholipase activity and more substrate release from nearby membranes. The tissue environment becomes easier to ignite with each cycle because initiation itself remodels the local structure. Oxidative stress increases. Membrane damage increases. Barrier precision declines. Cellular debris accumulates faster than it can be cleared. The body is no longer merely responding to a problem. It is becoming easier to trigger into response as part of its new baseline.

This creates one of the most important asymmetries in chronic illness. Starting inflammation is usually easier than finishing it. Initiation chemistry is fast, forceful, and heavily supported by built-in substrate reservoirs. Resolution is more demanding. It requires proper timing, phenotype switching in immune cells, successful clearance of damaged material, intact barrier restoration, enough metabolic energy to rebuild, and access to the signaling environment that tells the body the acute phase is over. When over-initiation dominates, those later steps never gain full control. The body keeps arriving at the early-middle phase of inflammation and re-entering it before closure has taken place. In practical terms, this means the organism is always spending on defense and never fully collecting on repair. The tissue becomes trapped in repetition.

Over-initiation also changes how the body interprets normal life. Inputs that should have been handled quietly begin generating disproportionate reaction. Food components provoke more immune attention than they should. Exercise creates more inflammatory residue than the recovery systems can clear cleanly. Minor stressors trigger outsized systemic consequences. Mechanical pressure produces longer-lasting pain. Small injuries take too long to stop feeling active. The immune system becomes less discriminating because the thresholds governing activation have shifted downward. This does not mean the body has become irrational. It means the surfaces and signaling systems through which it reads the world have been remodeled into a more defensive state. Reality begins to look more threatening to the organism because its membranes, receptors, and mediator reservoirs are configured to escalate quickly.

This is one reason simple anti-inflammatory suppression so often disappoints. If the deeper problem is over-initiation, then silencing one branch of inflammatory output may reduce symptoms temporarily without changing the tissue state that keeps generating new activation. The body remains easy to trigger. The membrane reservoir remains biased toward early-phase signaling. Barrier problems continue feeding immune provocation. Mitochondrial stress continues generating internal alarm chemistry. Oxidative instability continues lowering the threshold for membrane disruption. The visible fire is dampened, but the ignition conditions remain intact. This is why chronic inflammatory states often return as soon as suppression is removed. The sequence was not completed. The tissue was only muted while the architecture of over-initiation remained in place.

The role of omega-6 biology becomes especially important here. Omega-6-derived substrate is necessary for acute defense, but when tissues are repeatedly drawing on that substrate without adequate resolution and reconstruction, the body becomes too fluent in the language of escalation. It knows how to increase permeability, recruit cells, amplify pain, and alter vascular tone. It becomes less capable of stopping those actions once they are no longer useful. Over-initiation is therefore not just a signaling problem. It is a structural memory problem. The tissue keeps carrying the material and the interpretive habits of early-phase defense. Each new trigger enters an environment already prepared to overreact.

This is where the next part of the lipid story becomes essential. A body suffering from over-initiation does not just need less inflammation in the blunt sense. It needs restoration of threshold, proportion, and sequence. It needs membranes that are less easily pushed into reactive instability. It needs less constant release of activation substrate and better access to the lipid mediators that help terminate inflammatory programs once the necessary work has been done. It needs immune behavior that can still mobilize decisively when required but no longer treats every disturbance as grounds for prolonged escalation. Over-initiation is the problem because it turns an intelligent defense system into a chronic mode of operation. The body keeps pressing go, and each time it does, it becomes slightly less able to remember how to stop.

Chapter 6

Omega-3 as Resolution Substrate

Omega-3 becomes most biologically meaningful when it is understood not as a generic anti-inflammatory nutrient, but as substrate for the completion phase of inflammation. That distinction matters because it changes the entire frame. Anti-inflammatory is often used to imply suppression, as though the goal were simply to turn down symptoms, dampen immune activity, or block the body from expressing force. Resolution is different. Resolution is not the absence of inflammation and it is not passive fading. It is an active, energy-dependent, signal-dependent sequence in which the body stops unnecessary recruitment, clears inflammatory debris, removes dead cells, restores barrier integrity, reduces pain sensitization, reorganizes vascular behavior, and returns tissue to a state that can support ordinary function again. Omega-3 matters here because EPA and DHA are part of the substrate pool from which the body can generate mediator families involved in that transition. They do not merely calm tissue in the abstract. They help provide the molecular material through which tissue can move from escalation toward completion.

This makes omega-3 fundamentally different from the way it is usually marketed. Most public discussion treats it as a beneficial input that reduces inflammation, supports the brain, helps the heart, or improves general wellness. Those claims are not entirely wrong, but they stay too close to the symptom layer. The deeper reason omega-3 matters is that it changes what kind of membrane and what kind of signaling reservoir the body is building over time. EPA and DHA enter phospholipids. Once incorporated, they alter membrane behavior, change local lipid organization, and become available for later release when tissues are activated. When the body needs to transition out of acute inflammatory intensity, those stored omega-3 substrates can be enzymatically converted into mediator families that do not simply blunt force, but help redirect the sequence. The body begins reducing neutrophil recruitment, increasing efferocytosis, improving clearance efficiency, and restoring tissue order. Omega-3 is therefore not just helpful because it makes inflammation smaller. It is helpful because it makes inflammatory sequencing more complete.

That idea only becomes clear once inflammation is seen as a timed event rather than as a quantity problem. If inflammation were simply too much immune activity, then suppression would look like the obvious solution. But much of chronic inflammatory illness is not caused by the mere existence of inflammatory force. It is caused by incomplete inflammatory sequencing. The body still initiates. It still recruits. It still produces pain sensitization, vascular change, and immune traffic. What it does poorly is exit. Tissue remains open, noisy, metabolically expensive, and structurally unresolved. In that setting, omega-3 becomes important because it contributes to the substrate environment required for tissues to stop living in early-phase chemistry. It gives the body a way to generate different downstream instructions from the same activated membrane environment. The tissue does not just stop. It begins doing different work.

EPA and DHA are not identical in this regard, and their distinction matters. EPA can enter eicosanoid pathways and alter the mediator profile generated during inflammatory activation. In some cases it produces related mediator families with different biological intensity or different downstream implications than arachidonic acid-derived products. EPA also serves as substrate for E-series resolvins, which participate in the later phases of inflammatory control. DHA contributes strongly to membrane structure in specialized tissues, especially neural and retinal tissues, but it is also a major substrate for D-series resolvins, protectins, and maresins. These mediator families are not simply weaker inflammatory signals. They carry a different kind of instruction. They help limit further neutrophil influx, promote macrophage-driven clearance of dead cells and debris, reduce unnecessary tissue injury, and improve the transition from defense to repair. This is why the term resolution substrate is more accurate than anti-inflammatory fat. Omega-3 is not just turning inflammatory volume down. It is helping write the exit sequence.

This has major consequences for how chronic disease should be understood. A tissue with low omega-3 incorporation and poor access to resolution-mediating substrate may still initiate inflammation very effectively. In fact, many chronically ill tissues do exactly that. They are good at escalation. They are chemically prepared to recruit, amplify, and sensitize. But when acute work should begin handing off to cleanup and restoration, the signaling environment is weaker, the membrane reservoir is biased toward early-phase chemistry, and the body has fewer tools available to terminate the sequence intelligently. The result is persistence. The tissue continues behaving as though the emergency is still unfolding because it has not been given the molecular instruction set required to complete what it started. Omega-3 matters because it helps restore part of that missing instruction set, but only if it is actually incorporated into the tissue and only if the surrounding architecture can protect and use it.

That last condition is essential, because omega-3 is not magic. EPA and DHA are highly unsaturated molecules, and that unsaturation gives them flexibility and signaling value, but it also makes them chemically fragile. A body under high oxidative stress, poor antioxidant protection, chronic membrane damage, or heavy inflammatory load may incorporate omega-3 into an environment that cannot yet protect it well. In that case, the person may not experience the full benefit expected from simple supplementation. Some may feel only modest changes. Some may feel unstable responses. Some may improve only after broader structural conditions begin to change. This is one reason fish oil discussions have become so confused. People expect omega-3 to behave like a pharmacologic override when in reality it behaves more like structural preparation for a different signaling outcome. Resolution substrate only matters if the tissue can hold it, preserve it, release it properly, and move through the downstream sequence it supports.

This also explains why omega-3 belongs inside the membrane story rather than floating above it as a separate nutrient topic. Resolution does not begin with a capsule. It begins with tissue remodeling. EPA and DHA have to enter phospholipids, influence local membrane conditions, compete within the substrate environment, and become part of the body's stored response potential. That takes time. It depends on turnover. It depends on transport. It depends on the larger lipid environment, including what kinds of omega-6-derived substrates dominate the membrane, what oxidative pressure the tissue is under, how well mitochondria can support the energy cost of repair, and whether barrier systems are still feeding repeated activation into the same tissue. Omega-3 works inside architecture. It is not outside architecture. That is why the benefits of omega-3 often appear inconsistent when the architecture surrounding it is ignored.

The phrase resolution substrate also makes clear that omega-3 does not eliminate the need for initiation. The body still requires omega-6-derived activation chemistry. It still needs arachidonic acid to generate early inflammatory force when injury, infection, or real tissue disruption occurs. Omega-3 does not replace that need. It complements it by helping the body avoid permanent residence in that early phase. A healthy organism requires both entry into defense and exit from defense. Omega-6 helps heavily with the first. Omega-3 helps heavily with the second. That is why the relationship matters more than the slogan. The body is not healthiest when it suppresses all initiation. It is healthiest when it can initiate proportionately and then resolve completely. Omega-3 earns its place not because it opposes inflammation as such, but because it helps protect the body from becoming trapped in inflammation after the necessary phase has passed.

Once this is seen clearly, many familiar contradictions start to resolve. A person can have inflammatory symptoms despite taking omega-3 because substrate incorporation alone does not guarantee full resolution if the tissue remains barrier-disrupted, oxidatively unstable, or repeatedly re-triggered. Another person may improve substantially because their tissues were able to remodel, protect, and use the new substrate environment effectively. A third person may notice neurological or mood-related improvement because DHA-dependent membrane behavior in neural tissue shifted before obvious systemic inflammatory markers changed. These are not random outcomes. They reflect the fact that omega-3 is acting as part of tissue architecture and downstream mediator availability, not merely as a universal symptom-lowering chemical.

The central point of this chapter is that omega-3 should be understood as material for inflammatory completion. EPA and DHA are built into membranes, stored in tissues, and later converted into mediator families that help the body shift out of escalation and into cleanup, repair, and restored control. That makes omega-3 biologically decisive, but only within a larger structural logic. Resolution requires substrate, but it also requires energy, timing, immune phenotype change, barrier repair, and a membrane environment that can support the sequence without falling back into repeated initiation. Omega-3 is one of the body's major resources for that work. It does not force resolution from the outside. It equips the body to generate resolution from within.

EPA and DHA as Precursors, Not Endpoints

EPA and DHA are often discussed as though their biological importance ends once they are present in the blood, the capsule, or even the membrane. That framing is incomplete. EPA and DHA matter precisely because they are not endpoints. They are precursors. They are upstream material that the body can incorporate, store, release, and convert into later functions depending on tissue state and inflammatory timing. Their presence alone does not equal resolution. Their intake alone does not equal repair. Even their incorporation into phospholipids is still only part of the story. What makes them decisive is what the body is then able to do with them. They become part of membrane architecture, yes, but they also become part of future signaling possibility. They are reserve material for downstream mediator production, reserve material for altered receptor environments, reserve material for a different inflammatory sequence than the one dominated by repeated omega-6 initiation.

This matters because modern supplement language tends to treat EPA and DHA as finished therapeutic agents. One hears that EPA lowers inflammation, DHA supports the brain, and the implication is that once these molecules are consumed, the work is largely done. But biology does not work that way. A molecule can be present and still remain underused, misused, oxidized, poorly incorporated, or functionally muted by the surrounding architecture. EPA and DHA have to enter the body, survive digestion, be absorbed, be transported, be incorporated into the right phospholipid pools, and then be retained in tissues long enough to alter membrane behavior and future signaling output. Even after that, their deepest effects still remain conditional. A tissue under inflammatory challenge must be able to release them at the right time, route them into the right enzymatic pathways, and convert them into mediator families that help redirect the sequence toward completion. EPA and DHA are therefore potential, not guarantee. They are substrate, not finished result.

EPA shows this especially clearly because much of its importance lies in what it can become under activated conditions. Once incorporated into membranes, EPA can compete within eicosanoid pathways and shift the character of the lipid mediators generated when phospholipases release fatty acids from phospholipids. It can also serve as precursor for E-series resolvins, which help reduce unnecessary neutrophil trafficking, improve clearance behavior, and move tissues away from repeated escalation. That means EPA is valuable not simply because it exists in the membrane, but because it changes the options available once the membrane is mobilized. It alters the future chemistry of inflammation. Its role is therefore prospective. The body stores EPA now so that later, under conditions of activation, different instructions can be generated from the same surface.

DHA is similar, but its role carries an even stronger structural component in certain tissues. DHA is heavily incorporated into neural and retinal membranes, where its effects on curvature behavior, receptor environment, excitability, and membrane dynamics are especially important. But even here, DHA is not the endpoint. It is precursor to additional levels of function. Once released from membranes under the right conditions, DHA can be converted into D-series resolvins, protectins, and maresins, mediator families associated with inflammatory resolution, tissue protection, phagocytic efficiency, and restoration of tissue order. In other words, DHA does not only help build a different membrane. It helps build a membrane capable of supplying a different downstream language during stress and repair. Its importance lies not just in what it is, but in what it enables.

This distinction between precursor and endpoint also explains why omega-3 results are often delayed, inconsistent, or context-dependent. If EPA and DHA were endpoints, their presence alone should generate uniform outcomes. But they are not endpoints. They are integrated into systems that have to process them correctly. A person may consume omega-3 yet remain in a tissue environment dominated by repeated oxidative injury, ongoing barrier dysfunction, excessive arachidonic-acid-driven initiation, poor mitochondrial support, or weak enzymatic conversion into pro-resolving mediators. In that setting, EPA and DHA can still be biologically valuable, but their value may not be fully expressed because the sequence they are meant to support keeps getting interrupted. The substrate is present, but the downstream machinery is not yet coordinating around it. This is why omega-3 cannot be judged only by intake or blood level. The real question is whether the body is using EPA and DHA as precursors to a different kind of tissue behavior.

Thinking of EPA and DHA as precursors also keeps the timing of physiology clear. They do not act like fast-acting suppressive drugs. They act more like strategic construction material that changes future response capacity. First they alter membrane composition. Then that new composition changes receptor environment, substrate balance, and membrane behavior. Later, under activation, it changes what kinds of mediators can be generated and in what proportion. Later still, those mediators influence immune cell trafficking, debris clearance, vascular normalization, pain de-sensitization, and barrier recovery. This is a long chain. It begins with intake, but it does not end there. The endpoint is not EPA or DHA sitting in tissue. The endpoint is improved sequence: better transition from initiation to resolution, better cleanup, better recovery, better return to baseline.

This is one reason the language around omega-3 has to become more exact. When people say omega-3 is anti-inflammatory, they often imagine the molecule itself as the final actor. In reality, EPA and DHA are more like upstream raw material for a body trying to become better at its own later-stage work. They are part of the preconditions for resolution. They help create a membrane environment that can behave differently, and they help supply the fatty acid substrate from which later pro-resolving mediators can be generated. That is a more powerful role than the usual supplement narrative allows, but it is also a more conditional one. A precursor is only as useful as the system that converts it into action.

This brings the structural logic of the book back into focus. The body does not heal by possessing the right molecules in abstraction. It heals by building them into the right places, releasing them under the right conditions, and converting them into the right outputs at the right phase of a biological sequence. EPA and DHA belong to that logic. They are not endpoints because biology rarely ends at the molecule. Biology moves through architecture, activation, conversion, and consequence. EPA and DHA matter because they sit near the beginning of that chain. They are part of what the body must have on hand before it can resolve intelligently later.

Seen clearly, this makes omega-3 more important and less magical at the same time. More important, because EPA and DHA are upstream determinants of what kinds of inflammatory and reparative chemistry become possible. Less magical, because they do not bypass structure, oxidation, transport, membrane remodeling, immune phenotype shifts, or the energy cost of repair. They are not the finished answer. They are the starting material for a better answer. The body requires them not because they are the final form of health, but because without them, one of the major biochemical roads toward completion remains underbuilt from the start.

The Limitation of "Anti-Inflammatory" Thinking

The phrase anti-inflammatory sounds useful because it appears to offer a clear goal. Inflammation is associated with pain, swelling, fatigue, tissue irritation, vascular dysfunction, and many chronic disease states, so anything described as anti-inflammatory is assumed to be beneficial almost by definition. But that language creates a major conceptual error. It treats inflammation as though the main problem were simply excess quantity, as though the body were generating too much force and the solution were therefore to reduce that force as directly as possible. In many real biological situations, that is not the deepest problem. The deeper problem is failed sequencing. The body is often able to initiate inflammation quite effectively. What it does poorly is complete the process and restore tissue order once the useful phase has ended. Anti-inflammatory thinking reduces this entire sequence to a volume knob. Resolution biology shows that the real issue is often not volume, but timing, direction, and exit.

This matters because inflammation is not inherently pathological. Acute inflammation is one of the main ways the body protects itself. It increases vascular access, recruits immune cells, changes pain thresholds, mobilizes local defenses, and creates the conditions needed to contain damage or infection. A body incapable of mounting inflammation would not become healthier. It would become vulnerable, slow, and unable to protect its own structure under stress. The anti-inflammatory frame often forgets this and encourages people to think that less inflammatory activity is always better. That is not true. The body does not need less inflammation in the abstract. It needs the right inflammation at the right time for the right duration, followed by the right transition into clearance, repair, and normalization. Once that is understood, the inadequacy of anti-inflammatory thinking becomes obvious. It aims at suppression when the body often requires orchestration.

The problem becomes especially clear in chronic illness. Many chronic inflammatory states are not driven by a simple surplus of inflammatory ability. They are driven by tissues that remain trapped in early-phase inflammatory logic. The body keeps recruiting, sensitizing, leaking, signaling, and amplifying because the later phases that should terminate the response have not gained control. Debris remains uncleared. Barrier function remains weak. Macrophages do not transition efficiently into restorative behavior. Pro-resolving mediator production remains inadequate relative to the scale of initiation. Oxidative stress continues damaging membranes, which then continue releasing more substrate for early-phase chemistry. In that setting, calling the problem inflammation and looking for an anti-inflammatory solution misses the central failure. The system is not merely too active. It is unfinished.

This is one reason blunt suppression often produces incomplete results. If a person lowers one branch of inflammatory output but does nothing to restore membrane composition, improve barrier integrity, reduce repeated triggers, support mitochondrial stability, or supply substrate for resolution-mediating pathways, then the visible intensity of inflammation may drop while the underlying tissue state remains unresolved. Symptoms quiet temporarily, but the system remains easy to re-ignite because the architecture of over-initiation has not changed. The body is still loaded with activation substrate, still structurally unstable, still poor at clearance, and still unable to complete the sequence that suppression interrupted rather than finished. This is not an argument against symptom relief. It is an argument against mistaking symptom reduction for biological completion.

The language of anti-inflammatory also flattens the role of omega-3 into something smaller than it actually is. EPA and DHA are often described as anti-inflammatory fats, which makes them sound like biological dampers whose main value lies in turning inflammatory chemistry down. That description misses the deeper reason they matter. Omega-3 functions as resolution substrate. It changes membrane composition, alters the pool of releasable fatty acids during activation, and provides precursor material for mediator families that help reduce neutrophil recruitment, improve efferocytosis, limit collateral injury, and restore tissue order. These are not simply weaker inflammatory signals. They are part of a different phase of the sequence. Anti-inflammatory language makes omega-3 sound suppressive when in reality its most important role is often transitional. It helps the body move from defense toward completion.

There is also a practical limitation built into anti-inflammatory thinking because it encourages people to judge success too early and too narrowly. If the goal is only to lower inflammatory markers or reduce discomfort, then any intervention that decreases visible output may appear successful even if the tissue remains metabolically expensive, structurally fragile, and dependent on ongoing suppression. A more serious biological standard asks a different set of questions. Has neutrophil recruitment decreased because the problem resolved, or because signaling was blocked while debris remained? Has pain decreased because tissue normalized, or because sensitization was muted while the underlying trigger persisted? Has cytokine output fallen because inflammatory sequencing completed, or because the immune system was restrained without barrier repair and cleanup? Anti-inflammatory thinking does not force these distinctions. Resolution thinking does.

This is why the body should be understood as needing inflammatory competence plus resolution competence, not simply lower inflammatory tone. It must be able to mount force when force is necessary. It must also be able to withdraw that force without leaving behind damaged tissue, trapped immune cells, oxidized membranes, persistent nociceptive signaling, or open vascular and epithelial barriers. The healthier body is not the body that never inflames. It is the body that inflames proportionately, clears efficiently, and exits cleanly. Once this becomes the frame, many familiar contradictions disappear. It becomes easier to understand why chronic disease can coexist with immune activation and poor healing at the same time, why symptom suppression can fail to restore baseline, and why omega-3 matters more as a precursor to completion than as a generic anti-inflammatory badge.

The limitation of anti-inflammatory thinking, then, is that it mistakes a phase for the whole process and a symptom strategy for a systems strategy. It is built around the assumption that inflammation is the enemy rather than recognizing that unfinished inflammation is the enemy. The real problem in many chronic conditions is not that the body can still generate force. It is that it has become less able to close the loop once force has been used. A more accurate framework is therefore not anti-inflammatory but pro-resolution, structure-aware, and sequence-aware. That framework does not ask only how to make inflammation smaller. It asks how to make the body better at finishing what it starts so tissue can return to order instead of remaining suspended in defense.

The Requirement for Downstream Conversion

EPA and DHA do not resolve inflammation simply by being present. They have to be converted downstream into usable biological action, and that requirement is one of the main reasons omega-3 is so often misunderstood. Intake is upstream. Tissue incorporation is upstream. Even membrane enrichment is still upstream. The body only benefits fully when those stored omega-3 molecules are taken from structural presence into functional sequence. That means release from phospholipids at the right time, enzymatic handling through the right pathways, generation of mediator families capable of changing inflammatory behavior, and successful execution of the processes those mediators are meant to direct. Without downstream conversion, omega-3 remains potential sitting in tissue. It may still influence membrane properties to some extent, but its most important role in resolution biology remains underexpressed. This is why the presence of substrate should never be confused with completion of the pathway that substrate is meant to support.

The body treats EPA and DHA as raw material for later instruction. Once inflammatory activation has already begun, those fatty acids have to be liberated from membrane phospholipids and then routed into the enzymatic systems that can generate resolvins, protectins, maresins, and related mediator classes. That step is not automatic in the simplistic sense. It depends on timing, tissue state, enzyme availability, redox environment, the local presence of competing substrates such as arachidonic acid, and the broader structural condition of the tissue undergoing inflammation. A body can contain EPA and DHA yet still fail to convert enough of them into meaningful pro-resolving output if the inflammatory environment remains dominated by initiation chemistry, if oxidative damage is distorting enzymatic behavior, or if the tissue is repeatedly re-triggered before the later phases of the sequence can establish control. In practical terms, this means omega-3 status alone cannot tell the whole story. The real question is whether the tissue can use omega-3 as precursor rather than merely store it as decoration.

This requirement for conversion is one of the main differences between structural presence and signaling consequence. A phospholipid containing DHA in a neural membrane may already alter curvature behavior, receptor environment, and excitability even before any enzymatic release occurs. That is real and important. But the deeper resolution role of DHA only appears when the body is able to transform that substrate into the downstream mediator language required for inflammatory completion and tissue protection. The same applies to EPA. Its incorporation can alter membrane behavior and substrate competition, but its most decisive role in resolution depends on what happens after activation. The body must turn stored omega-3 into instruction. If it cannot, then inflammation may continue to begin with force while the exit chemistry remains too weak to take command. This is one reason the benefits of omega-3 often appear incomplete in chronically stressed or metabolically unstable tissue. The substrate entered the system, but the sequence that should follow it remained underbuilt.

Downstream conversion also makes clear that resolution is an active process, not a passive decline in inflammatory noise. Pro-resolving mediators do not simply allow inflammation to fade from lack of stimulation. They help direct specific forms of work. They reduce further neutrophil recruitment. They encourage macrophages to engulf apoptotic cells and debris more efficiently. They help limit unnecessary tissue damage. They support restoration of barrier integrity, normalization of vascular behavior, and the withdrawal of alarm signaling once the relevant task has been completed. All of that requires actual biochemical instruction. The body does not drift into order by accident. It has to be told, through the right mediator environment, that the emergency phase is over and that cleanup and rebuilding now have priority. EPA and DHA matter because they help supply that later instruction, but only if the body completes the conversion from precursor to mediator.

This is why simply labeling omega-3 as anti-inflammatory creates confusion. That phrase makes it sound as though EPA and DHA should directly suppress inflammatory output by their mere presence, and when that does not happen uniformly, people assume the concept itself is weak or overstated. In reality, the issue is often that the body has not completed the necessary downstream work. A person may increase omega-3 intake, but if membrane incorporation remains limited, if the inflammatory environment remains saturated with repeated omega-6-driven initiation, if oxidative stress keeps damaging membranes faster than they can be remodeled, or if immune cells do not transition efficiently into pro-resolving phenotypes, then conversion into meaningful resolution output may remain poor. The intervention then appears weaker than expected, not because omega-3 lacks importance, but because precursor alone does not replace pathway competence.

Competition also matters here. EPA and DHA do not enter an empty enzymatic landscape. They enter tissues where arachidonic acid, oxidative stress, cytokine signaling, phospholipase activity, and multiple enzyme systems are already shaping what kinds of mediators are most likely to be produced. If the membrane substrate pool remains heavily weighted toward initiation chemistry, the body may continue defaulting toward early-phase eicosanoid production even while omega-3 is present in meaningful amounts. The issue is not simple exclusion. It is proportion and pathway priority. A tissue repeatedly mobilized into early inflammatory behavior will keep behaving according to the substrate and enzymatic dominance built into that state. For omega-3 to express its full resolution value, the system has to shift far enough that downstream conversion into pro-resolving mediator classes can actually influence the sequence rather than remain biochemically possible but biologically minor.

The requirement for downstream conversion also explains why time matters so much in omega-3 biology. Structural remodeling takes time. But beyond remodeling, tissues also need time to enter inflammatory events with a different substrate environment and to allow that environment to generate different downstream consequences. This is slower than a drug effect because it is not a direct override. It is a change in how the body is prepared to respond the next time activation occurs. First the membrane changes. Then the substrate reservoir changes. Then, under future challenge, the mediator output can begin changing. Then immune behavior, clearance, pain signaling, and tissue restoration can begin shifting. The real endpoint is not higher intake or even higher membrane incorporation. The real endpoint is a different inflammatory trajectory once the body is stressed again.

Seen clearly, downstream conversion is the step that separates nutritional presence from physiological consequence. EPA and DHA are necessary because they provide raw material the body cannot easily replace from nothing, but their necessity is only fully expressed when that material is transformed into action. The body needs more than omega-3 stored in tissue. It needs omega-3 released, enzymatically processed, translated into pro-resolving mediator families, and then followed by the actual cellular work of clearance, restraint, repair, and return to baseline. That is why omega-3 should never be understood as a finished answer. It is upstream material for a sequence the body still has to know how to run. When that sequence is intact, omega-3 becomes one of the most important resources for inflammatory completion. When that sequence is impaired, omega-3 may still help structurally, but its deepest value remains only partially expressed because the body is holding the precursor without fully converting it into resolution.

Setting the Stage for Resolution

Resolution does not begin at the moment the body decides to stop inflammation. It begins earlier, in the way tissue is built, the way activation is sequenced, and the way damage is handled while the inflammatory response is still underway. This is one of the biggest reasons resolution is so often misunderstood. People imagine it as a passive settling phase that follows once the provoking stimulus fades or once enough inflammatory force has been blocked. Real biology is more demanding than that. A tissue can only resolve well if it has preserved enough structural order during activation to support the transition out of activation. It has to retain membrane integrity, enough energetic capacity to carry out cleanup, enough vascular control to stop oversupplying the inflammatory zone, enough immune precision to shift from recruitment into clearance, and enough stored substrate to produce the mediator language that tells the system the early phase is over. Resolution is therefore not an afterthought added to inflammation. It is the later half of the same sequence, and its success depends on what conditions were preserved or lost during the beginning.

This means the stage for resolution is set first in membranes. The membrane determines which substrates are available once phospholipases are activated, which receptors amplify early-phase chemistry, how much oxidative fragility the tissue carries into stress, and whether the cell has access to omega-3-derived precursors that can later be converted into pro-resolving mediators. A membrane overloaded with activation-heavy substrate, structurally unstable under oxidative strain, or chronically remodeled by repeated inflammatory cycles does not enter tissue stress neutrally. It enters already biased toward escalation. That bias matters because the same membrane that releases arachidonic acid during initiation must later provide EPA and DHA if the tissue is going to shift toward completion. The membrane is therefore not only the place where inflammation starts. It is the place where the possibility of ending inflammation is either preserved or weakened before the event has fully unfolded.

The stage is also set by whether the tissue can contain damage without turning every local signal into a system-wide problem. Barrier integrity matters here in a very literal sense. If intestinal barriers remain permeable, microbial fragments and incompletely excluded materials continue feeding immune provocation into the organism. If endothelial barriers remain overly permissive, immune traffic, plasma proteins, and inflammatory signals keep entering tissue spaces that should already be returning to tighter control. If cellular membranes remain oxidatively unstable, danger chemistry continues leaking out of damaged compartments and telling surrounding cells that disruption is still active. Resolution requires that inputs sustaining initiation begin to fall. That only happens when boundaries start holding again. A body cannot exit inflammation cleanly while still receiving repeated evidence, real or perceived, that the problem is ongoing.

Immune cell behavior is another major part of this preparation. Early in inflammation, neutrophils and related acute responders are necessary because speed matters. But resolution cannot occur if the tissue stays dominated by recruitment logic. Macrophages have to shift from aggressive inflammatory participation toward efferocytosis, debris handling, and orchestration of repair. That transition is not cosmetic. It changes the tissue from a site of attack into a site of controlled dismantling and reconstruction. Dead cells must be recognized and removed without spilling their contents further into the environment. Extracellular debris has to be cleared before it becomes a new inflammatory trigger. Local cytokine tone has to change. Lipid mediator output has to change. This is one reason the body needs omega-3-derived downstream conversion. Without the mediator environment that supports this handoff, immune activity often remains stuck in the earlier logic of arrival and force rather than moving into containment and cleanup.

Energy availability also determines whether resolution can happen at all. Cleanup is expensive. Membrane repair is expensive. Rebuilding junctions, reorganizing tissue architecture, restoring ion gradients, recycling damaged components, and supporting phenotype shifts in immune cells all require functioning mitochondrial output. A body already living near its energetic limit may still initiate inflammation because initiation can be driven by stress chemistry and stored substrate release, but it may fail when the time comes to pay for completion. This creates one of the hidden asymmetries of chronic inflammation. The organism still has enough force to begin but not enough organized energy to finish. Resolution therefore depends not only on having the right signals, but on having enough mitochondrial integrity and metabolic stability to carry out the labor those signals demand.

Timing is part of the stage as well. Resolution is not supposed to begin before initiation has done its necessary work, but it is also not supposed to wait indefinitely. The system has to know when enough recruitment has occurred, when the threat is controlled enough, when collateral damage is beginning to outweigh benefit, and when the tissue must change priorities from force to restoration. That timing is created through mediator shifts, receptor signaling shifts, immune cell phenotype shifts, substrate availability, and local tissue feedback. A body trapped in over-initiation loses this timing. It keeps treating the tissue as though more recruitment is still the answer. Setting the stage for resolution therefore means preserving the ability to change phases. The tissue must remain capable of hearing a new instruction rather than repeating the old one more loudly.

This is where anti-inflammatory thinking fails most clearly. It assumes the solution is to turn inflammatory intensity down, when in reality the body needs conditions that allow phase transition. Lowering output without improving membrane substrate balance, barrier repair, immune cleanup behavior, mitochondrial capacity, and downstream omega-3 conversion may reduce visible inflammation while leaving the tissue unable to truly resolve. The stage has not been set. The actors have only been quieted. Real resolution requires a tissue environment that can stop recruiting, start clearing, and then rebuild in a way that reduces the likelihood of immediate reactivation. That is a much deeper biological achievement than symptom suppression, and it depends on structure as much as it depends on signaling.

Seen clearly, setting the stage for resolution means preparing the body to finish what inflammation begins. It means membranes that carry not only activation substrate but completion substrate. It means barriers that can close again after they open. It means immune cells that can shift from combat to cleanup. It means mitochondria that can fund repair after stress. It means tissue architecture stable enough to survive the inflammatory phase without collapsing into ongoing danger signaling. Resolution is not an accidental fade-out at the end of inflammation. It is a built capacity, and like every other meaningful capacity in physiology, it has to be prepared in advance.

PART III

SPMs: THE BIOLOGY OF RESOLUTION

Chapter 7

What Are Specialized Pro-Resolving Mediators (SPMs)?

Specialized pro-resolving mediators are the lipid-derived signals the body uses to actively complete inflammation without simply shutting immunity off. That definition has to be stated carefully because SPMs are often misunderstood from the start. They are not the same thing as general anti-inflammatory compounds. They are not blunt suppressors. They do not function by making the immune system weak, silent, or indifferent. They function by changing the phase of the inflammatory response. They help move tissue out of recruitment, escalation, permeability, and collateral damage, and into clearance, containment, repair, and restored control. In practical terms, SPMs are part of the body's exit intelligence. They are how the organism stops behaving like it is still in the middle of an emergency when the useful work of that emergency has already been done.

The phrase specialized matters because these mediators are not generic background lipids. They are produced through defined enzymatic pathways from specific polyunsaturated fatty acid precursors, especially EPA, DHA, and in some cases n-3 DPA. They belong to distinct mediator families such as resolvins, protectins, maresins, and lipoxins, each of which contributes to different parts of the transition from inflammatory force to inflammatory completion. The phrase pro-resolving matters because they do not merely reduce signal intensity. They direct work. They reduce further neutrophil recruitment when further neutrophil recruitment is no longer useful. They enhance efferocytosis, the macrophage-driven clearance of apoptotic cells and inflammatory debris. They help restore barrier integrity, limit unnecessary tissue damage, reduce persistent pain sensitization, and support the return of tissue from emergency metabolism toward normal function. The phrase mediator matters because these are real signaling molecules, not vague wellness concepts. They carry instruction through receptor-mediated biological effects, and those instructions change what cells do next.

This is what separates SPMs from the older and much more limited view of inflammation as a process that simply rises and then fades. For a long time, inflammation was described as though it naturally burned out once the provoking stimulus weakened or once enough anti-inflammatory pressure was applied. That picture left out one of the most important discoveries in modern inflammatory biology, which is that resolution is not passive. It is an organized biochemical phase with its own signals, its own timing, its own receptor systems, and its own cellular tasks. Tissue does not automatically return to baseline just because the early inflammatory burst slows down. Dead cells still have to be removed. Extracellular debris still has to be cleared. Vascular permeability still has to normalize. Nociceptive amplification still has to be withdrawn. Immune traffic still has to stop arriving in excess. Barriers still have to be rebuilt. SPMs are part of what makes that happen.

Their importance becomes obvious once chronic inflammation is viewed correctly. Many chronically inflamed tissues are not failing because they lack activation chemistry. They are often rich in activation chemistry. They can recruit, amplify, leak, sensitize, and escalate with impressive consistency. The deeper problem is that they do not transition well. They remain suspended in inflammatory mid-process. Neutrophils continue arriving or continue leaving behind unresolved debris. Macrophages fail to clear efficiently or fail to shift fully into restorative phenotypes. Cytokine tone remains elevated. Oxidative chemistry remains active. Membranes remain unstable and continue releasing more substrate for early-phase signaling. The tissue behaves as though the emergency is still open because, in biochemical terms, the signals required to close that emergency have not gained enough control. SPMs matter because they are part of the signal system that closes the loop.

This also explains why SPMs should never be framed as simple immune suppressors. Suppression reduces force. Resolution redirects force. That distinction is central to this entire book. A suppressed immune system may produce less overt inflammatory output, but that does not mean tissue has been cleared, danger has been removed, or repair has begun correctly. In some situations suppression can even delay completion by muting signals without restoring the cleanup phase that must follow them. SPMs do something more precise. They reduce the continuation of unnecessary recruitment while increasing the efficiency of clearance. They restrain collateral damage without preventing the body from defending itself. They help terminate pain-promoting chemistry while encouraging removal of the dead cells and debris that would otherwise keep generating that chemistry. They do not erase inflammation as a concept. They help finish it as a sequence.

Because they are lipid-derived mediators, SPMs also reinforce one of the major themes of the book: the body stores part of its future inflammatory and reparative language inside membranes. EPA and DHA are not valuable only because they improve membrane composition in a static sense. They are valuable because, once incorporated into phospholipids, they provide precursor material from which pro-resolving mediators can later be generated. This means the capacity to resolve is partly built ahead of time. A tissue carrying more useful omega-3-derived substrate is carrying more of the raw material required for later exit signals. That does not guarantee successful resolution on its own, because downstream conversion, oxidative stability, immune phenotype shifts, and sufficient metabolic support are all still required. But it does mean the ability to produce SPMs is rooted in prior structural conditions, not just in the heat of the moment.

SPMs also clarify why the common phrase anti-inflammatory is too blunt to describe what many tissues actually need. A tissue trapped in chronic inflammatory activation does not only need less inflammatory signaling. It needs better inflammatory sequencing. It needs the later instructions that tell neutrophils to stop arriving in excess, tell macrophages to increase efferocytosis, tell the vascular bed to stop behaving like an emergency corridor, and tell nociceptive systems that the phase of heightened protection can now be withdrawn. That is the territory of SPMs. They belong to the completion phase, not merely the silencing phase. They represent one of the clearest examples in biology of how the body solves problems not just by turning processes on and off, but by moving them through phases in the correct order.

The different SPM families also matter because resolution is not one task. It is many tasks coordinated together. Resolvins help reduce ongoing inflammatory cell recruitment and influence multiple parts of tissue de-escalation. Protectins are associated with tissue protection, especially in neural and other specialized contexts, and with limiting inflammatory injury. Maresins are strongly linked to macrophage-mediated repair, efferocytosis, and restorative tissue behavior. Lipoxins, though often derived through different precursor relationships than the omega-3-derived families, are also part of the pro-resolving landscape and demonstrate that the body has multiple routes for signaling that the acute inflammatory phase must not remain dominant. The point is not that each family should be memorized as a separate trivia category. The point is that the body has built an entire class of mediators whose function is to end inflammatory work intelligently rather than merely to oppose inflammation in the abstract.

This chapter matters because it marks the transition from talking about omega-3 as substrate to talking about what that substrate can become. EPA and DHA are not the finished answer. They are upstream materials. SPMs are part of the downstream answer, because they are among the mediators generated from those materials that actively help the body regain order after disruption. They reduce unnecessary continuation. They improve cleanup. They protect tissue from prolonged inflammatory injury. They help restore the structural and signaling conditions that ordinary function depends on. In a body that can still initiate strongly but resolve poorly, SPMs help explain what is missing. The organism does not only need less force. It needs the biochemical intelligence required to know when force has done enough.

Resolvins

Resolvins are one of the clearest examples of why inflammation cannot be understood only through the language of suppression. Their role is not simply to make inflammatory signals smaller. Their role is to help the body change phases. They are lipid mediators generated from omega-3 fatty acid precursors, mainly EPA and DHA, and they belong to a class of signals produced after those fatty acids have already been incorporated into membranes, released under the right conditions, and converted through downstream enzymatic pathways. This makes resolvins part of the body's active exit strategy. They do not erase the need for early inflammation. They begin to matter when early inflammation has already done enough and the tissue now needs to stop recruiting damage faster than it can clear it. In that sense, resolvins are not peacekeeping molecules in the sentimental sense. They are operational molecules that reduce unnecessary continuation and improve the conditions required for completion.

The name itself is instructive. Resolvins are called resolvins because they participate in resolution, not because they merely lower inflammatory intensity in a vague way. They help reduce further neutrophil infiltration once the useful phase of neutrophil-heavy recruitment is ending. They influence macrophage behavior in ways that improve debris clearance and support the removal of apoptotic cells before those cells break down and become new inflammatory fuel. They help limit collateral tissue injury caused by prolonged inflammatory traffic. They can reduce pain-promoting signaling and help shift vascular and tissue behavior away from open emergency mode. This is what makes them biologically important. A tissue trapped in chronic inflammatory repetition often does not need weaker immunity. It needs better instructions for when to stop escalating and start clearing. Resolvins belong to that instruction set.

There are two major families typically emphasized in this context: E-series resolvins, which are derived from EPA, and D-series resolvins, which are derived from DHA. That distinction matters because EPA and DHA do not simply duplicate one another. Each supplies a different precursor pathway and therefore contributes to a somewhat different mediator landscape once conversion begins. E-series resolvins represent one route by which EPA-based incorporation can later become pro-resolving signaling. D-series resolvins represent one route by which DHA-based incorporation can later become pro-resolving signaling. The practical point is not that one family must be treated as superior in the abstract. The practical point is that omega-3 in tissue becomes more biologically meaningful when it is understood as stored precursor for families like these, rather than as a static nutrient badge. The membrane holds the possibility. The resolvin is one form that possibility can take once the body is ready to move from force toward restoration.

Resolvins also show why timing is everything in inflammatory biology. A molecule that reduces neutrophil recruitment too early could impair useful defense. A molecule that reduces neutrophil recruitment after adequate early-phase work has been done can prevent unnecessary tissue damage and help the system move into cleanup. Resolution is therefore not the opposite of immunity. It is immunity shifting tasks. Resolvins do not tell the body to ignore disruption. They tell the body that further escalation is no longer the smartest use of energy and tissue. That distinction is central. In chronic inflammatory states, the problem is often not that the body cannot defend itself. It is that the body cannot stop defending as though the emergency were still expanding. Resolvins begin correcting that error by changing what kind of work inflammatory cells are being asked to do.

This is why resolvins matter so much in the broader logic of omega-3 biology. EPA and DHA are not endpoints. They are upstream structural and signaling precursors. Resolvins are one of the downstream mediator families that show what omega-3 is for. It is for building a body that can still initiate when necessary, but does not remain trapped in initiation when the relevant phase has passed. A membrane reservoir containing omega-3-derived substrate carries more than a nutritional fact. It carries future access to mediators like resolvins that can help the body reduce further inflammatory recruitment, improve clearance, protect local tissue, and regain order. Without that downstream possibility, omega-3 remains only partly expressed. With it, the tissue gains one of the main biochemical tools required to finish what inflammation began.

Protectins

Protectins are DHA-derived specialized pro-resolving mediators that help defend tissue during and after inflammatory stress without relying on blunt suppression. Their name reflects that role. They are called protectins because they participate in tissue protection, especially when inflammatory activity, oxidative stress, or cellular injury threatens to convert a necessary response into unnecessary damage. This makes them especially important in a book like this, because they show clearly that resolution is not just about making inflammation smaller. It is about preserving tissue while the inflammatory sequence is being brought under control. A response can begin appropriately and still become destructive if the tissue undergoing that response is not protected from prolonged exposure to its own defense chemistry. Protectins belong to the part of the body's mediator system that helps prevent that slide.

Like other SPMs, protectins do not appear from nowhere. They depend on prior membrane incorporation of DHA, later release of DHA from phospholipids under the right conditions, and downstream enzymatic conversion into a mediator form the tissue can actually use. That makes protectins a good example of why DHA should never be treated as a finished endpoint. DHA is valuable structurally, especially in neural and retinal tissue, but its value also lies in what it can become. When tissue is under stress, protectin generation gives the body access to a class of signals that can reduce unnecessary inflammatory injury, influence leukocyte behavior, and support the shift away from open-ended inflammatory escalation. In that sense, protectins are not just downstream products. They are part of the reason storing DHA in membranes matters in the first place.

Their protective role is especially important in tissues where inflammatory collateral damage is costly. Neural tissue is the clearest example. The nervous system can tolerate remarkably little disorder before function begins to degrade. Excess immune recruitment, persistent oxidative chemistry, excitotoxic stress, prolonged membrane disruption, and unresolved debris can all damage signaling precision and structural continuity in ways that do not stay local for long. Protectins are important here because they help create conditions under which tissue can survive inflammation without remaining trapped in inflammatory injury. They belong to the logic of controlled defense rather than runaway defense. The body still responds, still detects danger, still performs cleanup, but it does so with more regard for preserving the integrity of the tissue that has to remain functional afterward.

This is also why protectins should not be understood as simply weaker inflammatory mediators. They are not watered-down versions of initiation signals. They represent a different phase and a different set of priorities. Early inflammatory mediators help recruit, amplify, and alter tissue conditions quickly. Protectins help reduce the continuation of that damage when continuation is no longer useful. They support the turn from disruption toward containment and preservation. In practical terms, they help the body limit how much of the tissue has to be sacrificed in order to solve the problem that triggered inflammation in the first place. That is a very different job from merely lowering inflammatory volume. It is a job of strategic restraint in service of repair.

Protectins also reinforce one of the most important themes running through this manuscript, which is that membrane composition determines future behavior. A tissue enriched in DHA is not only building a certain kind of membrane. It is building a certain kind of future response potential. If inflammatory stress occurs, the tissue has more access to DHA-derived downstream mediator families such as protectins. If that substrate is sparse, or if oxidative damage keeps destabilizing the membrane environment in which it is stored, the tissue may remain relatively poorer in the signals that help protect it during the later phases of inflammation. This is one reason chronic inflammatory environments are so destructive. They do not only activate too much initiation chemistry. They often fail to generate enough preservation chemistry to prevent the inflammatory process from injuring the tissue it is supposed to protect.

Seen clearly, protectins help explain why DHA matters beyond the familiar language of brain support or membrane fluidity. DHA is not valuable only because it sits inside neural tissue. It is valuable because under the right conditions it can be converted into mediator classes that help defend that tissue from the consequences of unresolved inflammatory stress. Protectins are part of the body's way of saying the response must now become more selective, less damaging, and more compatible with long-term tissue survival. They do not eliminate immune activity. They help refine it so that defense does not continue shredding the environment it was meant to preserve.

Maresins

Maresins are DHA-derived specialized pro-resolving mediators produced primarily through macrophage-centered pathways, and they are especially important because they connect resolution directly to cleanup and repair. Their name comes from macrophage mediator in resolving inflammation, which is exactly what makes them so useful conceptually. They show that resolution is not merely the decline of inflammatory intensity. It is organized work carried out by cells that have shifted roles. Early in inflammation, immune activity is dominated by recruitment, containment, and force. Later, if the sequence is functioning properly, macrophages begin taking on a different kind of responsibility. They clear apoptotic cells, remove debris, help limit ongoing tissue damage, and support the transition into reconstruction. Maresins belong to that later phase. They are part of the signal language through which the tissue begins moving from combat into restoration.

This macrophage connection matters because macrophages sit at the hinge point between unresolved inflammation and genuine repair. A tissue can recruit neutrophils rapidly, generate eicosanoids efficiently, and still fail to heal if the macrophage phase never becomes effective enough to clear what the early phase left behind. Dead cells that are not removed become new inflammatory stimulus. Damaged membrane fragments, oxidized lipids, extracellular debris, and unresolved microdamage all keep telling the tissue that the emergency is still active. Maresins help interrupt that cycle by supporting the kind of macrophage behavior that closes inflammatory work rather than perpetuating it. They improve efferocytosis, support debris handling, and help reorient the tissue away from continued escalation. This makes them central to the argument of the book, because chronic inflammation often persists not only from too much initiation, but from too little successful cleanup.

Like resolvins and protectins, maresins depend on prior DHA availability. They are downstream products, not spontaneous events. DHA must first be incorporated into membranes, stored within phospholipid architecture, and then released and converted under the right conditions. That means maresin biology begins long before a macrophage starts clearing anything. It begins with tissue composition. A membrane environment that contains usable DHA is carrying part of the precursor pool needed for later restorative signaling. This is why omega-3 should never be understood as a finished answer at the moment of intake. Its value lies partly in what it can later become once the body enters the stage of inflammation where cleanup and repair must take priority. Maresins are one expression of that later value. They are what DHA can become when the tissue is ready not merely to stop inflammatory recruitment, but to start resolving the structural consequences of what recruitment has already done.

What makes maresins distinct is their strong association with tissue restoration rather than with de-escalation alone. Resolvins are often discussed in relation to limiting further inflammatory recruitment. Protectins are often emphasized for their role in preserving tissue from inflammatory injury. Maresins, while overlapping with both, point even more clearly toward rebuilding conditions. They belong to the biology of repair-compatible resolution. A tissue cannot truly resolve if it only stops bringing in new inflammatory cells. It also has to remove what has accumulated, restore local order, and reduce the debris burden that would otherwise keep provoking the next round of inflammatory activity. Maresins help create that transition. They make inflammation more finishable.

This is especially important in chronic disease states where tissue seems to remain stuck in a loop of irritation, partial damage, incomplete recovery, and rapid reactivation. In many of those settings, the body is still capable of signaling danger, but it is less capable of clearing the aftermath of danger. Macrophages remain present, but their behavior may stay skewed toward inflammatory participation rather than restorative clearance. The tissue remains chemically noisy because the remnants of previous inflammatory cycles have not been removed well enough to let the next phase begin cleanly. Maresins matter here because they are part of the downstream signal environment that helps turn macrophages into better finishers. They improve the quality of the handoff between defense and reconstruction.

Seen clearly, maresins reinforce one of the deepest ideas in this book: resolution is labor, not silence. The body does not return to health by merely reducing inflammatory output. It returns by clearing the remains of what inflammation did, restoring structural order, and reducing the likelihood that leftover damage will become the trigger for another round of activation. Maresins are part of the biochemical language that supports that work. They are DHA-derived instructions for a tissue trying to regain coherence after stress. They help explain why omega-3 matters not simply for calming the body, but for helping the body clean up after itself well enough that it no longer has to keep acting inflamed.

Derived from EPA and DHA

Specialized pro-resolving mediators are derived from EPA and DHA because these long-chain omega-3 fatty acids serve as the stored precursor pool from which the body builds part of its resolution chemistry. That point is more important than it first appears. It means the body does not improvise resolution from nothing after inflammation has already caused enough disruption. It has to enter the inflammatory sequence already carrying the structural material required for a controlled exit. EPA and DHA must first be absorbed, transported, incorporated into membrane phospholipids, and retained in tissue long enough to become part of the cell's future signaling reserve. Only then can they be released under the right conditions and converted into mediator families that help reduce continued neutrophil recruitment, improve macrophage-driven clearance, protect tissue from excess collateral damage, and restore local order. Resolution therefore depends on prior membrane composition. The tissue can only derive these signals if it was built with the right precursor material before the need for those signals became urgent.

EPA and DHA do not generate the same downstream products, and that difference matters because it shows that omega-3 biology is not one undifferentiated category. EPA is the precursor for E-series resolvins, which participate in reducing ongoing inflammatory recruitment and shifting the character of inflammatory signaling away from simple continuation. DHA is the precursor for D-series resolvins, protectins, and maresins, which extend the resolution program into tissue protection, efferocytosis, and repair-compatible macrophage activity. This means EPA and DHA are related, but they are not functionally identical. Each supplies a different branch of the downstream mediator landscape, and those branches help solve different parts of the same biological problem. The body is not just trying to make inflammation weaker. It is trying to change what the tissue does next. That requires more than one kind of precursor input.

This precursor relationship also explains why omega-3 should never be mistaken for an endpoint. EPA and DHA are upstream molecules. Their presence in tissue matters because of what they make possible later. First they change membrane behavior. Then they change substrate availability. Then, under activation, they can be released and enzymatically converted into SPMs. Then those SPMs can change immune cell behavior, vascular behavior, nociceptive signaling, clearance efficiency, and tissue recovery. The real biological effect is therefore layered across time. A person does not benefit from EPA and DHA simply because the molecules are present in circulation or because they appear on a lab panel. The body benefits when those molecules have been incorporated deeply enough, preserved well enough, and converted effectively enough to alter the trajectory of an inflammatory event once that event begins.

This is one reason omega-3 results are often less immediate and less uniform than supplement language implies. If SPMs are derived from EPA and DHA, then several things must already be true for that derivation to matter. The tissue must contain the substrate. The membrane must be able to release it appropriately. The enzymatic environment must be able to convert it into useful mediator classes. The inflammatory sequence must reach a point where those mediators can actually shift the tissue away from continued escalation. A chronically stressed tissue can fail at any of these stages. It may incorporate too little DHA or EPA. It may remain dominated by arachidonic-acid-heavy initiation signaling. It may suffer enough oxidative damage that highly unsaturated membrane lipids become fragile before they become useful. It may remain too repeatedly re-triggered for the later resolution phase to gain command. In those cases, the limitation is not the concept of omega-3 itself. The limitation is that precursor availability has not been successfully translated into downstream resolution behavior.

Seen clearly, the phrase derived from EPA and DHA carries a much larger meaning than a simple biochemical source note. It means resolution is built from stored membrane material. It means the body's capacity to exit inflammation depends partly on what kinds of fatty acids have already been loaded into tissue. It means omega-3 matters because it provides the raw material for mediator families that help inflammation finish rather than simply intensify. And it means the quality of the body's recovery is partly determined long before recovery begins, because the membrane already contains, or fails to contain, the precursor pool from which the exit chemistry must later be made.

Not Suppressive — Actively Resolving

One of the most important distinctions in this entire subject is that specialized pro-resolving mediators are not suppressive in the blunt pharmacologic sense. They do not solve inflammation by simply shutting the immune system down, muting all defensive signaling, or forcing tissue into artificial silence. Suppression reduces output. Resolution changes the phase of the response. That difference is not semantic. It is biological. A suppressed inflammatory system may produce fewer visible signals, but that does not mean damaged material has been cleared, dead cells have been removed, vascular permeability has normalized, pain sensitization has been withdrawn intelligently, or tissue architecture has begun rebuilding in an orderly way. A response can be quieter and still remain unfinished. Specialized pro-resolving mediators matter because they do something more precise. They help the body complete the inflammatory sequence rather than merely dull its expression.

This is why the word actively matters. Resolution is work. Neutrophil recruitment has to stop when further recruitment is no longer useful. Macrophages have to increase efferocytosis so apoptotic cells are cleared before they break apart and become fresh inflammatory stimulus. Debris has to be removed from the extracellular environment. Barrier integrity has to be restored. Vascular behavior has to shift from emergency access back toward controlled selectivity. Pain-amplifying chemistry has to be withdrawn once its protective role is no longer justified. These are not passive events that happen automatically once inflammatory force declines. They require instruction. SPMs are part of that instruction. They do not merely make inflammation weaker. They help direct the biological labor that turns an inflamed tissue back into a functional one.

This distinction is what separates resolution from anti-inflammatory suppression. Suppression is often useful for symptom control, but it does not necessarily tell the body how to finish what it started. It may reduce cytokine output, reduce pain, or reduce swelling, while leaving unresolved debris, barrier failure, immune mis-sequencing, and tissue instability still in place underneath the quieter surface. An actively resolving tissue is different. It is not just less inflamed. It is moving toward completion. Cellular traffic changes. Cleanup improves. Collateral damage falls. The tissue is no longer organized around escalation. It is organized around exit. That is why SPM biology is so important. It restores the idea that the goal is not simply to make inflammation smaller. The goal is to make it finish properly.

Seen in this light, omega-3-derived resolution pathways are not valuable because they sedate the immune system. They are valuable because they help the immune system stop behaving as though the emergency is still expanding when the relevant phase has already passed. They preserve host defense while reducing unnecessary continuation. They support immune competence while improving inflammatory termination. They do not cancel the defensive sequence. They complete it. That is the deeper meaning of not suppressive, actively resolving. The body does not heal by being silenced. It heals by being guided out of emergency with enough precision to clear the damage, preserve the tissue, and return to order without remaining trapped in defense.

The Missing Half of Inflammation Biology

For decades, inflammation biology was taught and discussed as though the main story ended with activation. A trigger appeared, inflammatory pathways turned on, immune cells were recruited, vascular tone changed, permeability increased, pain sensitization rose, and the task of medicine became identifying how to reduce or block those outputs. That framework captured the beginning of the sequence, but it left out the second half, which is why so much modern thinking about chronic disease remains incomplete. Inflammation does not become pathological simply because it exists. It becomes pathological when it cannot finish. The missing half of inflammation biology is the biology of resolution: the active, signal-dependent, substrate-dependent process by which the body stops further unnecessary recruitment, clears cellular debris, removes dead cells, restores barrier integrity, reduces collateral damage, and returns tissue to a state that can support normal function again. Without that half, the picture of inflammation is structurally broken from the start.

This omission matters because it changes what chronic inflammation appears to be. If the only biology that matters is initiation, then persistent inflammatory disease looks like a problem of excess force. The body seems to be overreacting, overproducing inflammatory mediators, and overactivating immunity, so the obvious solution becomes suppression. But once the missing half is restored to the model, a different interpretation becomes possible and often more accurate. Many tissues in chronic disease are not failing because they cannot generate activation. They are often very capable of activation. They fail because activation is not being handed off to completion. Neutrophils continue arriving or continue leaving behind material that has not been cleared. Macrophages do not fully transition into effective efferocytosis and restoration. Membranes remain damaged and keep supplying new initiation substrate. Barriers remain open and continue feeding fresh triggers into the system. The body is not simply too inflamed. It is caught in unfinished inflammation.

This is why so many symptom-centered strategies fall short. If the missing half of inflammation biology is ignored, treatment naturally gravitates toward turning early-phase chemistry down. That can relieve pain, swelling, heat, or biochemical markers of inflammatory output, and sometimes that is necessary. But it still does not answer the deeper question of whether the tissue has completed the inflammatory job. Has the debris been cleared. Has the vascular bed normalized. Has the nociceptive amplification been withdrawn because danger has truly decreased, or because signaling was muted while the underlying problem remained. Has the barrier been repaired. Has the membrane reservoir shifted away from automatic re-initiation. Has the tissue regained the structural conditions needed to remain quiet without constant intervention. Without the resolution half of the model, these questions disappear, and with them disappears the difference between silence and completion.

The discovery and elaboration of specialized pro-resolving mediators changed this landscape because it showed that resolution is not passive decay. It is an active program. The body generates specific mediator families from stored lipid precursors, especially EPA and DHA, that help shift immune behavior, reduce ongoing recruitment, improve efferocytosis, protect tissue, and restore local order. This means inflammatory completion is not a fortunate accident. It is built into the same biological intelligence that built inflammatory initiation. The body has start signals and finish signals. It has escalation chemistry and closure chemistry. It has molecules that open emergency access and molecules that tell the emergency machinery when to stand down and clear the site. The missing half of inflammation biology is therefore not a side note. It is the exit architecture without which the entry architecture becomes dangerous by default.

This missing half also explains why omega-3 has been so persistently misunderstood. When inflammation is viewed only through the initiation lens, omega-3 is interpreted as anti-inflammatory, which makes it sound like a nutrient that somehow turns inflammatory volume down from the outside. But within the fuller model, omega-3 becomes something more important and more coherent. It is resolution substrate. It provides precursor material for mediator families that help the body complete what arachidonic-acid-heavy early-phase signaling helped begin. That does not make omega-3 the opposite of inflammation. It makes omega-3 part of the later sequence of inflammation. The absence of that conceptual shift is one reason the public conversation has stayed shallow for so long. The real value of omega-3 cannot be understood until inflammation itself is understood as a two-phase problem: initiation and completion.

Seen clearly, the missing half of inflammation biology is the reason chronic disease so often feels stuck. The body still knows how to enter defense. It no longer exits efficiently. It continues recruiting, leaking, sensitizing, oxidizing, and signaling as though the event were still active because the later biology required to terminate that state has not taken command. Once resolution is restored to the model, many modern pathologies start to make more sense. Chronic pain is not just excessive nociception. It can be persistent failure to withdraw protective amplification after useful danger has passed. Chronic vascular irritation is not just excessive inflammatory tone. It can be repeated failure to normalize permeability and endothelial behavior. Chronic immune activation is not just an overzealous system. It can be a system repeatedly beginning without successfully finishing. The missing half is what explains why the body can be both highly reactive and poorly healed at the same time.

That is why this half of the story changes everything. It moves the question from how to silence inflammation to how to make inflammation finish properly. It reframes omega-3 from supplement mythology into substrate physiology. It shifts attention from simple blockade toward structural remodeling, mediator balance, barrier repair, membrane composition, mitochondrial support, and immune phenotype transitions. Most importantly, it restores the idea that the body is not designed only to defend. It is designed to defend and then return to order. When that second design is ignored, medicine sees only half the event. When it is restored, inflammation stops looking like a one-way march toward damage and begins to reveal its real architecture: a sequence that is only healthy when it has an exit.

Chapter 8

The Resolution Phase of Inflammation

The resolution phase of inflammation is the part of the sequence in which the body stops treating the tissue as an active battlefield and begins converting that same tissue into a site of clearance, containment, and restoration. That description sounds simple, but the biology underneath it is exacting. Resolution is not the passive fading of inflammatory noise once the initial trigger becomes weaker. It is a coordinated phase change. The system has to stop further unnecessary recruitment, limit ongoing collateral damage, remove dead cells before they rupture into new inflammatory fuel, clear extracellular debris, normalize vascular permeability, restore barrier behavior, withdraw pain amplification that is no longer protective, and rebuild enough structural order that the tissue no longer presents itself as unfinished danger. Every one of those tasks requires signals, energy, timing, and substrate. That is why the resolution phase deserves to be treated as its own chapter rather than as the endnote of inflammation. It is not the quiet part after the important work. It is the important work that determines whether the earlier phase leaves behind healing or persistence.

This shift in phase changes the meaning of the inflammatory environment. During initiation, tissues become more permeable, more vascularly reactive, more chemically loud, and more permissive to immune traffic because the body is prioritizing access and force. During resolution, those same priorities must begin reversing without losing control of the site. The body cannot simply slam inflammatory activity off. It has to manage the handoff. Neutrophil-heavy recruitment must taper at the right time. Macrophages must become better finishers, not just continued participants in damage chemistry. Cytokine tone has to change from amplifying the event to containing it. Lipid mediator output has to shift from arachidonic-acid-dominant initiation language toward pro-resolving instruction. Endothelial surfaces have to stop behaving like open emergency corridors. Epithelial and tissue barriers have to regain selectivity. The tissue is still active during this phase, but its activity is now aimed at ending the event intelligently rather than extending it by habit.

One reason the resolution phase is so often missed is that it does not always look dramatic from the outside. Early inflammation announces itself through pain, swelling, heat, redness, restricted movement, fatigue, or measurable spikes in familiar inflammatory markers. Resolution is less theatrical. It appears as improved cleanup, reduced inappropriate recruitment, normalized permeability, fading pain sensitization, more efficient debris removal, and a gradual return of tissue control. But those quieter changes are not biologically secondary. They are what determine whether tissue can regain coherence. A wound can stop bleeding and still fail to resolve well. An infection can be controlled and still leave behind immune disorder if the cleanup phase remains poor. A joint can become less acutely swollen and still remain metabolically inflamed if dead cells, oxidized lipids, and extracellular debris are not cleared effectively. Resolution is therefore not defined by the disappearance of symptoms alone. It is defined by the successful completion of tissue-level tasks that make the disappearance of symptoms biologically trustworthy.

At the center of this phase is a change in what cells are being asked to do. Early inflammation is built around access, detection, amplification, and immediate containment. Resolution is built around removal, restraint, and repair-compatible order. Neutrophils, while often necessary early, are not supposed to dominate indefinitely. Their continued arrival and continued presence become damaging if the site no longer requires acute force. Macrophages have to assume a more decisive role, especially through efferocytosis, the engulfment of apoptotic cells before those cells spill their contents and create fresh inflammatory provocation. This single task has enormous importance. If dead cells remain uncleared, the inflammatory site never receives the message that useful work has been completed. Debris remains visible. Damage remains legible to the immune system. The body keeps interpreting the area as active unfinished business. The resolution phase succeeds only when cleanup becomes efficient enough that the tissue stops broadcasting emergency.

This is where specialized pro-resolving mediators become indispensable. Without them, the body still knows how to start inflammation, but it loses much of the biochemical intelligence required to finish it well. Resolvins, protectins, maresins, and related mediator families help reduce ongoing neutrophil influx, improve macrophage-driven clearance, limit unnecessary tissue injury, and support the normalization of the local environment. These are not suppressive effects in the blunt sense. They are transition effects. They tell the tissue that further escalation is no longer the smartest move. They redirect effort away from force and toward completion. Because these mediators are derived from stored omega-3 substrate, the resolution phase also makes plain why membrane composition matters so much. A body cannot generate a strong resolution program from a membrane environment that never carried enough appropriate precursor material to begin with.

The vascular side of this phase is just as important as the immune side. Early inflammation opens access. Resolution has to close it again without trapping unresolved damage inside the tissue. That means endothelial behavior must normalize. Permeability must decrease from emergency levels. Plasma leakage has to fall. Traffic signals that were encouraging cellular entry have to quiet down. Fluid balance has to begin restoring. If vascular behavior remains in the early-phase state, tissue continues to swell, signaling continues to spread, and the local environment remains more permissive to repeated activation. In other words, the body keeps the door open after the relevant surge has passed. Resolution requires that the door begin closing at the same time cleanup becomes more effective. Without that synchronization, the tissue lives in a half-open state where incoming inflammatory pressure and outgoing debris clearance never fully match.

Pain biology also changes during resolution, and this is often overlooked because pain is usually treated only as a symptom to manage rather than a signal to interpret. Early in inflammation, pain sensitization serves a protective purpose. It discourages loading of damaged tissue and marks the area as unsafe for normal behavior. But once useful protection has been achieved, continued pain amplification becomes a sign that the tissue has not completed its return to order. The nervous system remains informed that the site is still dangerous, and that continued message alters movement, stress response, sleep, mood, and systemic energy allocation. Resolution therefore has to include de-sensitization in the proper sequence. Pain does not simply vanish because time passed. It becomes less necessary because the tissue stops generating the inflammatory and structural evidence that justified elevated nociception in the first place. A body that cannot resolve well often becomes a body that cannot stop protecting tissues long after the relevant threat has diminished.

Resolution is also metabolically expensive, which is why mitochondrial capacity and general energetic integrity matter so much here. Cleaning up after inflammation is not passive rest. Phagocytosis costs energy. Rebuilding membranes costs energy. Restoring junctions, re-establishing gradients, processing damaged components, and shifting cell phenotypes all cost energy. A tissue living under mitochondrial strain may still be able to launch inflammatory activation because activation can be driven by stored substrate release, stress signaling, and acute immune mobilization. But that same tissue may fail when it comes time to pay for the labor of closure. The result is one of the defining asymmetries of chronic inflammatory disease: the body still has enough force to begin but not enough organized energy to finish. This is why the resolution phase cannot be treated as merely a signaling question. It is also a question of whether the tissue has the metabolic means to execute the work that the signals are trying to direct.

Barrier restoration belongs to this phase for the same reason. Inflammation often begins by temporarily loosening normal control. That can be useful when access is necessary, but if barriers do not recover, the tissue remains vulnerable to new triggers while still trying to recover from old ones. Intestinal barriers that remain too permeable continue feeding immune-provoking material into the system. Epithelial barriers that remain open continue exposing tissues to unnecessary insult. Cellular membranes that remain oxidatively fragile continue generating danger chemistry and releasing signals that make neighboring cells interpret the area as unstable. The resolution phase has to reduce this constant re-triggering. It has to make the tissue harder to alarm once the acute need for alarm is gone. Otherwise the body gets trapped in a loop where every attempt at completion is interrupted by the arrival of fresh evidence that the emergency is not over.

This is why chronic inflammation is so often better described as failed resolution than as excessive initiation alone. Many chronically ill tissues are highly competent at starting. They release arachidonic acid. They generate eicosanoid cascades. They recruit. They amplify. They sensitize. What they do poorly is carry the event through efferocytosis, barrier restoration, vascular normalization, membrane repair, and immune de-escalation strongly enough that the site stops behaving as a site of threat. The resolution phase is the half of inflammation that has been missing from much of public and even clinical thinking, and without it the entire picture stays distorted. One keeps asking how to reduce inflammation, when the deeper question is how to make inflammation finish. The answer is not simple silence. It is successful sequence.

That is the defining logic of this chapter. The resolution phase of inflammation is the body's method for ending inflammatory work without leaving behind a residue of danger. It depends on specialized mediators, cleanup-capable immune cells, restored vascular control, repaired barriers, sufficient energy, and membranes built from substrate that can support completion rather than only escalation. If that phase succeeds, tissue returns to order with minimal collateral damage. If it fails, the body remains suspended in a state of unfinished defense, where activation continues to recur because the environment never stopped looking like a problem. Resolution is therefore not the fade-out of inflammation. It is the disciplined biological achievement that determines whether inflammation becomes healing or becomes chronicity.

Inflammation Is a Program with an End State

Inflammation is often described as if it were a force that simply rises when the body is threatened and falls when the threat disappears. That description is incomplete because it treats inflammation like a volume change rather than a programmed sequence. In reality, inflammation is a timed biological operation with defined phases, defined goals, and an intended end state. It begins by detecting disruption, shifts tissue into a defensive mode, recruits the necessary cellular machinery, contains damage or threat, clears what must be removed, and then transitions toward restoration. The end state is not merely less inflammation. The end state is recovered order. Vascular permeability returns toward baseline. Neutrophil-heavy recruitment stops. Macrophages clear apoptotic cells and debris. Pain amplification withdraws once protection is no longer needed. Barriers re-form. Membranes stop broadcasting damage. Tissue stops presenting itself as an emergency zone. That is what completion looks like.

This matters because a program is judged by whether it finishes, not merely by whether it starts correctly. A body that can initiate inflammation but cannot reach its end state is not exhibiting too much inflammation in the most meaningful sense. It is exhibiting incomplete inflammation. The difference is critical. If inflammation is seen only as force, the obvious response is suppression. If inflammation is seen as a program, then the more serious question becomes whether the program is moving through its full sequence. Has recruitment given way to clearance. Has activation given way to containment. Has tissue transitioned from damage control into repair-compatible stability. The pathological problem in many chronic conditions is not that the body still has inflammatory capacity. It is that the program keeps restarting or remains stalled before it reaches termination.

The idea of an end state also explains why resolution is not passive. Programs do not complete themselves by drifting. They complete because later instructions become dominant. In inflammation, those later instructions include reduced neutrophil influx, improved efferocytosis, normalization of vascular behavior, restoration of epithelial and endothelial boundaries, and the generation of specialized pro-resolving mediators from omega-3-derived substrate. Without those signals and those tasks, inflammation does not truly end. It only fluctuates in intensity. Tissue may look quieter for a time while remaining structurally unfinished underneath. The real end state is not symptom reduction alone. It is the point at which the tissue no longer requires emergency logic to maintain control.

Once inflammation is understood this way, chronic disease starts to look different. Chronic inflammation is what happens when the program loses its end state. The body still detects. It still recruits. It still amplifies. But it no longer exits efficiently. Debris remains. Barriers remain open. Membranes remain unstable. Immune cells remain in the wrong mode. Signaling remains biased toward continuation rather than completion. The system is not just inflamed. It is stuck inside an unfinished biological script. That is why the goal should not be framed only as reducing inflammation. The deeper goal is restoring the body's ability to let inflammation arrive, do its work, and then terminate in a way that leaves tissue more ordered rather than chronically defended.

Initiation → Amplification → Resolution

Inflammation is best understood as a sequence rather than a state. It begins with initiation, moves through amplification, and is supposed to end in resolution. Each phase has a different job, a different signal logic, and a different cost to the tissue. Problems arise when these phases are collapsed into one vague category called inflammation, because the body does not treat them as interchangeable. Initiation exists to detect disruption and convert it into local action. Amplification exists to expand and coordinate that action so the problem can be contained effectively. Resolution exists to stop the continued use of force once force has done enough, clear what the inflammatory process has produced, and restore tissue conditions that make ordinary function possible again. If the first phase is missing, defense is weak. If the second is missing, defense is too small to contain the threat. If the third is missing, defense becomes chronic damage. The health of the system depends on movement through the whole sequence, not on the isolated strength of any one phase.

Initiation is the moment the tissue decides that ordinary maintenance is no longer enough. Damage signals, microbial patterns, oxidative stress, mechanical disruption, or barrier breach activate receptors and membrane-associated enzymes. Arachidonic acid is released from phospholipids. Early eicosanoid production begins. Vascular tone changes. Permeability shifts. Platelets may become more active. Pain sensitivity rises. The tissue becomes chemically louder because attention and resources need to be redirected there. This phase is rapid by design. The body is not trying to deliberate endlessly. It is trying to mark a site as no longer ordinary and make sure the system notices. Initiation is therefore the phase of recognition and first response. It is where the inflammatory event is launched and where the local environment is altered enough to prepare for the next stage.

Amplification follows because detection alone is not enough. Once the body has identified a meaningful problem, it has to scale the response to a level capable of containment. More immune cells are recruited. Cytokine signals intensify. Additional eicosanoids and related mediators are produced. Endothelial surfaces become more permissive to cellular traffic. Neutrophils and other early responders move into the tissue in larger numbers. Oxidative chemistry increases where microbial control or damage handling requires it. Pain signaling often becomes stronger, not because the body is malfunctioning, but because tissue must be protected behaviorally while the response is underway. Amplification is the phase of force multiplication. It expands the local inflammatory event into something large enough to matter. This is useful when proportional. It becomes dangerous when it continues after the tissue has already crossed the threshold of adequate response.

Resolution is the phase that changes the meaning of everything that came before it. Without resolution, initiation and amplification remain open-ended. With resolution, they become part of a successful sequence. This phase reduces further neutrophil influx, improves macrophage-driven efferocytosis, clears apoptotic cells and extracellular debris, restores endothelial and epithelial control, reduces unnecessary pain sensitization, limits further collateral injury, and moves the tissue out of emergency logic. Specialized pro-resolving mediators derived from EPA and DHA become especially important here because they help provide the biochemical instructions for this handoff. Resolution is not the collapse of the inflammatory response from exhaustion. It is the active conversion of an inflammatory site into a recovering site. The tissue stops asking for more force and starts asking for cleanup, containment, and repair.

The arrow between these phases matters because it shows direction. Initiation is supposed to lead to amplification when the problem requires escalation. Amplification is supposed to lead to resolution when continued escalation would cost more than it would protect. Chronic inflammatory disease often reflects failure of that directional movement. The body initiates correctly enough and amplifies powerfully enough, but the handoff into resolution is weak, delayed, incomplete, or repeatedly interrupted. The result is a tissue that keeps living in the first two phases. It remains recruited, sensitized, permeable, and chemically expensive because the third phase has not taken command strongly enough to finish the event. That is why the full sequence matters more than any single marker of inflammatory output. Healthy inflammation is not low inflammation. Healthy inflammation is inflammation that can move all the way through its own program and arrive at its end state instead of looping inside the middle.

SPMs as the "Stop Signal"

Specialized pro-resolving mediators can be understood as the body's stop signal, but only if that phrase is understood precisely. They are not stop signals in the sense of shutting biology down, freezing immunity, or forcing silence onto tissue that still needs active defense. They are stop signals in the sense of telling the inflammatory program that further escalation is no longer the correct task. That distinction matters because the body does not need inflammation to disappear at random. It needs inflammation to stop expanding once the useful work of initiation and amplification has been done. SPMs provide part of that instruction. They help the tissue shift out of recruitment, permeability, collateral damage, and repeated alarm signaling, and into clearance, containment, and restoration. They do not just make inflammation quieter. They tell the system to stop doing the kind of work that belongs to the earlier phase.

This is why the word signal is more accurate than the word suppressor. A suppressor reduces output whether or not the sequence has been completed. A stop signal changes what the system does next. In the presence of SPM activity, neutrophils are no longer called in excess to a site that has already received enough acute-phase force. Macrophages are pushed toward efferocytosis and cleanup rather than continued inflammatory participation. Endothelial behavior begins moving away from emergency openness. Pain-promoting chemistry begins losing priority as tissue danger decreases. The inflammatory site stops behaving like a place that still needs more reinforcement and begins behaving like a place that needs to be cleared and rebuilt. That is a much more intelligent form of stopping than blunt inhibition. It preserves the logic of the sequence while ending its wasteful continuation.

The stop signal role of SPMs is especially important because inflammation has a natural bias toward continuation once it is underway. Early mediators recruit cells, recruited cells generate more signals, oxidative chemistry damages more structure, and damaged structure creates fresh inflammatory evidence. Without an active signal telling the system that enough force has been applied, the body can remain trapped in recruitment and amplification. SPMs interrupt that loop. They do not deny that the loop was necessary at first. They terminate its dominance once the balance of cost and benefit has changed. That is why they belong to resolution biology rather than to generic anti-inflammatory thinking. They do not oppose inflammation as a category. They oppose the continued use of early-phase inflammatory logic after that logic has already done its job.

Seen clearly, SPMs as the stop signal means they are part of the body's way of closing the inflammatory loop without leaving the site unfinished. They tell the tissue to stop calling for more force and start processing what force has already produced. They are the biochemical instruction that says enough recruitment, enough permeability, enough escalation, now clear, restore, and return to order. Without that signal, inflammation can remain chemically active long after its useful phase has passed. With it, the body gains a way to end defense intelligently rather than merely silence it.

Why Resolution Is an Active Process

Resolution is an active process because the body does not return from inflammation to normal function by waiting. It returns by doing work. That work includes stopping further unnecessary immune recruitment, clearing apoptotic cells before they rupture into fresh inflammatory stimulus, removing extracellular debris, withdrawing pain sensitization that is no longer protective, restoring endothelial and epithelial control, rebuilding damaged membrane structure, and re-establishing the metabolic and signaling conditions that allow the tissue to stop presenting itself as a site of danger. None of that happens automatically just because the initial trigger has weakened or because inflammatory output has been partially reduced. The tissue has to be reorganized. The inflammatory site has to be dismantled. What was opened has to be closed again. What was recruited has to be cleared. What was damaged has to be rebuilt. Resolution is active because order has to be reconstructed, not merely uncovered.

This is one of the most important corrections to the old view of inflammation. For a long time, resolution was treated as a passive fade-out, as if the body simply ran out of inflammatory force and drifted back toward baseline once enough time had passed. That interpretation misses the biological labor involved. Neutrophils do not remove themselves efficiently without consequences if they are not recognized and cleared. Debris does not disappear harmlessly if it is left in tissue. Vascular permeability does not always tighten back to normal if the signaling environment remains stuck in emergency mode. Membranes damaged by oxidative and inflammatory stress do not quietly reset themselves. A tissue can become less dramatically inflamed on the surface while remaining biochemically unfinished underneath. Active resolution is what prevents that unfinished state from becoming chronic. It is the phase in which the body deliberately cleans up after its own defense.

The immune system illustrates this clearly. Early inflammation depends heavily on recruitment and amplification, but those same mechanisms become harmful if they continue after acute needs have been met. Resolution requires an active shift in immune cell behavior. Macrophages, in particular, have to become effective finishers. They must increase efferocytosis, clear apoptotic cells and inflammatory remnants, and help change the local mediator environment away from continued escalation. This is not passive decline. It is a functional reprogramming of the inflammatory site. The body is changing the assignment from attack to cleanup. Without that reassignment, dead cells remain visible, oxidized material remains pro-inflammatory, and the tissue keeps interpreting itself as unfinished danger. Resolution is active because someone has to close the site, and biologically that means cells have to do different work than they were doing at the height of the response.

The lipid side of this process proves the same point. Specialized pro-resolving mediators are not passive indicators that inflammation is fading. They are active instructions derived from omega-3 substrate that help reduce further neutrophil influx, increase debris clearance, protect tissue from excess collateral injury, and restore a more stable local environment. These mediators do not emerge as a sign of exhaustion. They emerge as part of a later-phase program. The body uses them to change what the tissue is being told to do. That is why omega-3 should be understood as resolution substrate rather than as a simple anti-inflammatory tool. The role of SPMs is not to let inflammation expire from neglect. Their role is to drive the transition from inflammatory action into inflammatory completion.

Energy demand is another reason resolution must be active. Cleanup costs ATP. Membrane repair costs ATP. Restoring ion gradients, repairing junctions, phagocytosing debris, processing damaged cellular material, and rebuilding tissue architecture all cost ATP. A tissue under mitochondrial strain may still be able to launch inflammation because early inflammatory force can be driven by acute signaling, stress chemistry, and stored substrate mobilization. But completing the event requires sustained organized work. If energy production is compromised, resolution weakens even if the tissue still has enough force to begin the response. This is one reason chronic inflammatory states often persist in metabolically unstable organisms. The body can afford to ignite. It cannot afford to finish. Active resolution therefore depends not only on the right signals, but on enough energetic capacity to carry out the repair those signals are calling for.

Seen clearly, resolution is active because the body is not merely turning something off. It is changing tissue state. It is moving from permeability to barrier control, from recruitment to clearance, from sensitization to normalized signaling, from damage handling to structural restoration. That requires instructions, cells capable of responding to those instructions, structural substrate that supports the later phase, and energy to carry the labor through. Passive language fails here because it makes healing sound easier than it is. Healing after inflammation is organized reconstruction. The body must actively finish what inflammation began, or the site remains stuck between defense and recovery, never fully dangerous enough to justify acute crisis and never fully restored enough to return to normal.

Chapter 9

Mechanisms of SPM Action

Specialized pro-resolving mediators matter because they do not merely exist as interesting downstream lipid products. They do things. They act through defined biological mechanisms that shift tissue out of inflammatory continuation and into controlled completion. That shift is the central subject of this chapter. If the previous chapters established that SPMs are derived from EPA and DHA and belong to the resolution phase rather than to blunt suppression, this chapter has to explain how they actually achieve that effect inside living tissue. The answer is not that they simply make inflammation weaker. The answer is that they alter cellular behavior at several key control points at once. They reduce further inflammatory cell recruitment when additional recruitment would only increase collateral damage. They change macrophage behavior so cleanup becomes more efficient. They improve the clearance of apoptotic cells and tissue debris before those materials can become new inflammatory triggers. They help normalize vascular and epithelial function. They reduce the persistence of pain-promoting chemistry. They protect tissue while the body is transitioning out of the acute phase. In other words, SPMs are operational signals. They change the work the tissue is doing.

The first major mechanism is receptor-mediated signaling. SPMs are not vague membrane effects acting only through bulk lipid incorporation. They bind to specific receptors or receptor systems and trigger downstream changes in immune behavior, inflammatory mediator production, and cellular movement. That matters because it means resolution is not just a passive drift created by substrate balance. It is directed instruction. Cells receive a new signal environment and begin carrying out different priorities. Neutrophils become less likely to continue moving into a site that has already received enough acute-phase force. Macrophages become more likely to engulf dead cells and inflammatory debris. Endothelial behavior begins shifting away from facilitating high inflammatory traffic. Local cytokine tone changes. The tissue is not simply cooling off. It is being told to reassign effort away from continued escalation.

A central mechanism of SPM action is the reduction of further neutrophil recruitment. Neutrophils are useful early because they provide rapid antimicrobial and damage-response capacity, but they are expensive cells in tissue. They bring oxidative chemistry, proteolytic potential, and the capacity for collateral injury if they remain too long or keep arriving after the acute need for force has passed. SPMs help stop that continuation. They reduce signals that maintain excessive neutrophil trafficking and help interrupt the logic of perpetual reinforcement. This is critical because chronic inflammation often persists not only because old neutrophils remain, but because new neutrophils keep being invited into a site that no longer benefits from their presence. By lowering further influx without abolishing the initial ability to recruit when truly needed, SPMs help preserve host defense while ending wasteful extension of the inflammatory phase.

The second major mechanism is the enhancement of efferocytosis and macrophage-driven clearance. This is one of the most important actions in the entire resolution program. Inflammation cannot end cleanly if apoptotic cells remain scattered through tissue or if inflammatory debris accumulates faster than it is removed. Dead cells left uncleared are not neutral. They become new sources of inflammatory provocation as membranes break down and intracellular contents spill into the extracellular environment. SPMs improve the ability of macrophages to recognize, engulf, and process these materials before they become additional danger signals. This is not a side effect of resolution. It is the center of it. A tissue stops behaving like an emergency zone when the visible evidence of the emergency is actually removed. SPMs help make that removal more efficient.

A third mechanism is the reprogramming of macrophage behavior itself. Macrophages are not simple cells with one fixed inflammatory identity. They can participate in early inflammatory amplification, but they can also become the key finishers of the entire event. SPMs help drive that transition. They encourage macrophages to behave less like amplifiers of recruitment and more like coordinators of clearance, containment, and repair-compatible signaling. This is why the resolution phase depends so heavily on them. Chronic inflammation often reflects a site where macrophages remain present but fail to assume full finishing authority. The tissue is left in a chemically ambiguous state where danger has not been adequately cleared and further amplification remains too easy. SPMs help change that balance by making macrophages more effective at the later tasks that turn inflammation into healing rather than persistence.

SPMs also act by limiting collateral tissue injury during the inflammatory transition. Acute inflammation is useful, but it is inherently dangerous because the same molecules and cells that defend tissue can also damage it if their activity remains excessive or poorly timed. Proteases, reactive oxygen species, inflammatory lipid mediators, and prolonged cellular congestion all threaten the tissue the body is supposedly trying to protect. SPMs do not eliminate defense. They narrow its waste. They help reduce the unnecessary continuation of damaging chemistry once the useful early-phase work has been done. This is especially important in tissues where collateral injury is costly, such as the nervous system, vascular surfaces, epithelial barriers, and delicate organ microenvironments. In these settings, resolution has to be more than the disappearance of inflammatory markers. It has to include preservation of the tissue itself while the response is being wound down.

Another major mechanism is the restoration of barrier and vascular control. Early inflammation often requires increased vascular permeability and greater access for plasma proteins and immune cells. That is useful during initiation and amplification, but if permeability remains elevated, tissue stays metabolically and immunologically open. Fluid continues to shift abnormally. Inflammatory signals continue to spread. Cellular traffic remains too permissive. SPMs help reverse that state. They support the transition back toward controlled endothelial behavior and more selective tissue boundaries. This is crucial because inflammation cannot be considered resolved while the tissue remains physically open to repeated provocation. Resolution requires the body to reduce access at the same time it increases cleanup. SPMs are part of the signaling environment that makes this coordinated closing possible.

Pain modulation is another important mechanism. Pain during early inflammation often has clear biological purpose. It reduces movement, changes tissue loading, and keeps attention focused on the damaged area. But once the useful protective phase has passed, continued nociceptive amplification becomes part of the pathology. SPMs help reduce that persistence. They do not simply numb tissue in a crude way. They help remove the inflammatory conditions that keep pain signaling justified and can directly influence mediator systems that support ongoing hypersensitivity. This matters because chronic inflammatory pain is often not just a sensory problem. It is evidence that the tissue continues to behave as though danger remains active. By helping end the inflammatory conditions that sustain that interpretation, SPMs help withdraw protective pain once it is no longer biologically necessary.

SPMs also act by influencing the broader mediator environment. One of the major problems in chronic inflammation is that the tissue remains dominated by early-phase signaling chemistry. Eicosanoid cascades continue to shape the site as though more recruitment and more amplification are still appropriate. SPMs change that mediator balance. They do not merely subtract inflammatory mediators. They add a different instructional class that tells the system to stop repeating the same early logic. This is why they should not be described as passive offsets. They actively compete at the level of tissue meaning. The site receives a new message about what phase it is in, and that changes what cells interpret as necessary.

An important feature running through all of these mechanisms is that SPMs preserve defense while ending excess continuation. That is what makes them so different from blunt suppression. They do not create a biologically naive tissue. They create a tissue capable of finishing. The body still responds to genuine disruption. It still contains threats. It still uses inflammatory force where force is needed. But once sufficient force has been applied, SPMs help shut the gate on further escalation and turn the system toward removal, preservation, and rebuilding. That makes them mechanistically elegant. They solve the real problem in many chronic inflammatory states, which is not the existence of immune competence, but the lack of immune closure.

This chapter therefore makes one core point. The mechanisms of SPM action all converge on phase transition. They reduce further neutrophil influx, enhance efferocytosis, shift macrophages into cleanup modes, limit collateral damage, restore barrier behavior, reduce persistent pain signaling, and alter the mediator environment so tissue stops acting as though escalation is still required. Every one of those actions helps answer the same problem: how does the body stop an inflammatory event without leaving the tissue unfinished. SPMs are the answer because they do not simply oppose inflammation. They organize its ending. If you want, I'll continue with the first subsection under

Stopping Neutrophil Infiltration

Stopping neutrophil infiltration is one of the most important ways specialized pro-resolving mediators change the direction of inflammation. Neutrophils are essential early responders. They arrive quickly, move aggressively into damaged or infected tissue, release oxidants, proteases, antimicrobial factors, and signaling molecules, and help establish the first wave of acute containment.

That role is useful at the beginning because speed matters. But the same features that make neutrophils valuable early also make them dangerous if their entry continues after the acute need for force has passed. Every additional wave of neutrophil infiltration increases oxidative burden, proteolytic pressure, membrane injury, endothelial disruption, and the amount of cellular debris that must later be cleared. A tissue cannot resolve while it is still being continuously restocked with cells built for early-phase damage control. Resolution therefore requires not only that existing inflammatory material be cleaned up, but that new neutrophils stop being invited in excess.

This is why stopping infiltration is not the same thing as erasing immunity. The body is not trying to prevent neutrophils from ever arriving. It is trying to stop recruiting more of them once enough have already arrived to do the necessary early work. That is a phase decision. Early inflammatory signals encourage neutrophil rolling, adhesion, extravasation, and migration into the tissue through changes in endothelial behavior, chemokine gradients, lipid mediator output, and local vascular dynamics. SPMs help reverse that logic. They reduce the signaling conditions that keep drawing neutrophils inward. They make the tissue less chemically attractive to continued recruitment and less structurally permissive to endless inflammatory traffic. This is not suppression in the blunt sense. It is a controlled withdrawal of the invitation.

The importance of this becomes obvious when chronic inflammation is viewed from the tissue level. A chronically inflamed site often remains metabolically expensive because neutrophil-heavy logic never fully shuts off. Even if individual cells die and are cleared, new cells keep entering. That means fresh oxidants, fresh proteases, fresh membrane damage, and fresh inflammatory residue continue appearing faster than the tissue can finish cleaning up the last round. The site never stops looking active because it never stops receiving new acute-phase machinery. In that setting, stopping neutrophil infiltration is not a minor adjustment. It is one of the core conditions required for resolution to even begin. Cleanup can only dominate if new damage-producing cellular input begins to fall.

This is also where the elegance of SPM biology becomes clear. Specialized pro-resolving mediators do not stop neutrophils by paralyzing the immune system. They stop the continuation of neutrophil entry by changing the local meaning of the tissue environment. The site is no longer treated as one that needs more escalation. Endothelial signals become less recruitment-oriented. Chemotactic pull declines. The inflammatory field starts shifting from a zone of entry toward a zone of processing. This allows existing neutrophils to undergo apoptosis and be cleared by macrophages without being constantly replaced. It is a handoff mechanism. The tissue stops prioritizing arrival and starts prioritizing removal.

That handoff matters because neutrophils are biologically short-lived. In a well-sequenced inflammatory response, they arrive, do acute work, and then are removed before they become a major source of secondary tissue injury. If infiltration continues too long, however, the sheer turnover of dying neutrophils becomes part of the pathology. Apoptotic cells accumulate. Clearance systems become overloaded. If efferocytosis cannot keep pace, those cells break down and spill intracellular contents into the extracellular environment, generating more inflammatory stimulus and reinforcing the impression that the site remains dangerous. Stopping neutrophil infiltration therefore protects the tissue in two ways at once. It reduces immediate collateral damage from new arrivals, and it lowers the future cleanup burden that would otherwise keep the site trapped in inflammatory continuation.

Seen clearly, stopping neutrophil infiltration is one of the first true signs that inflammation is entering resolution rather than merely fluctuating in intensity. The tissue is no longer calling for reinforcement. It is beginning to act as though the acute emergency has been contained well enough that more force would now cost more than it would protect. That is exactly the kind of decision specialized pro-resolving mediators help enforce. They do not deny the need for early neutrophil action. They mark the point at which further neutrophil entry stops serving recovery and starts interfering with it. Without that shift, inflammation remains an open door. With it, the body gains the chance to move from repeated recruitment into actual completion.

Enhancing Macrophage Cleanup (Efferocytosis)

Enhancing macrophage cleanup, especially through efferocytosis, is one of the central mechanisms by which resolution becomes real rather than theoretical. Efferocytosis refers to the recognition, engulfment, and processing of apoptotic cells before they lose membrane integrity and spill their contents into the surrounding tissue. That function sounds technical, but it sits close to the heart of whether inflammation ends cleanly or persists. A tissue cannot resolve simply because recruitment slows down. It has to remove the physical remains of the inflammatory event. Neutrophils that have done their work must be cleared. Damaged cellular fragments must be cleared. Oxidized membrane material, extracellular debris, and the remnants of local tissue injury must be cleared. If that does not happen, the inflammatory site remains full of biochemical evidence that the emergency is still active. Macrophages are the major finishers of this phase, and efferocytosis is one of the main ways they turn inflammatory terrain into recoverable terrain.

This is why macrophages should not be understood only as inflammatory cells. Early in the sequence they can participate in cytokine production, immune coordination, and local amplification, but their deeper importance in resolution comes from their ability to change roles. Once acute force has done enough, macrophages have to become cleaners, sorters, and stabilizers. They identify apoptotic cells through altered surface signals, engulf them without allowing those cells to rupture outwardly, and then process what they have taken up in a way that reduces rather than amplifies further inflammatory provocation. This is a remarkably intelligent biological maneuver. The body is not merely removing waste. It is removing it quietly. The contents of dying cells are contained rather than scattered. Their presence stops serving as open evidence of tissue danger. The tissue begins to look less inflamed because the material that justified ongoing inflammatory interpretation is physically disappearing.

Specialized pro-resolving mediators help enhance this process by improving the efficiency and priority of macrophage cleanup. They do not just reduce inflammatory noise in the abstract. They make macrophages better at the actual labor of ending an inflammatory event. This matters because unresolved inflammation often reflects not only too much initiation, but too little successful removal of what initiation produced. A site may contain large numbers of apoptotic neutrophils, oxidized membrane remnants, damaged extracellular material, and fragments of injured cells. If macrophages clear these efficiently, the tissue can move toward stability. If they do not, those materials remain in place long enough to become new sources of inflammatory stimulus. Efferocytosis is therefore not a cleanup detail added after the main event. It is one of the main events in the transition from active inflammation to restored control.

The word quietly matters here. When apoptotic cells are not cleared in time, they can progress into secondary necrosis, losing membrane integrity and releasing intracellular contents into the extracellular environment. At that point, what could have been removed silently becomes a new inflammatory trigger. Damage-associated molecular patterns spread. Oxidized lipids and proteins remain exposed. Proteases and other degradative contents escape. Nearby cells interpret this as ongoing disturbance, and the inflammatory program is fed another round of evidence that the site is still dangerous. Efficient efferocytosis prevents that conversion. It reduces the chance that yesterday's inflammatory cells become today's inflammatory fuel. In this sense, macrophage cleanup is not only restorative. It is protective against re-initiation.

This mechanism is one reason chronic inflammation so often looks like a failure of finishing rather than a failure of starting. Many chronically inflamed tissues still recruit well. They still produce cytokines, eicosanoids, and vascular changes. What they do poorly is clear the aftermath with enough speed and intelligence to break the loop. Macrophages remain present, but they are either overwhelmed, poorly instructed, metabolically strained, or held in phenotypes that favor participation in inflammatory signaling more than completion of inflammatory work. The site remains crowded with cellular remnants and oxidized structural debris. Even if new triggers stopped arriving, the internal residue would still keep the tissue looking unfinished. Enhancing macrophage cleanup through SPM biology changes that situation by making the tissue better at physically removing the reasons it continues to appear inflamed.

Macrophage cleanup also changes the mediator environment in a self-reinforcing way. Successful efferocytosis does not merely subtract debris. It influences what macrophages do next. As they engulf apoptotic cells and process inflammatory remnants, they shift further away from aggressive inflammatory amplification and further toward repair-compatible signaling, restraint, and tissue support. This means cleanup is not just a terminal act. It reshapes the character of the inflammatory site. A macrophage that is cleaning effectively is participating in resolution at multiple levels at once. It reduces visible inflammatory material, lowers the chance of secondary inflammatory triggering, and helps move the local signal environment toward completion rather than continuation. Efferocytosis therefore acts both as sanitation and as instruction.

This is especially important in tissues where inflammatory debris is costly. In the vascular system, retained inflammatory material can prolong endothelial dysfunction and keep permeability or reactivity elevated. In joints, retained debris can maintain pain and immune activation even after the original acute insult has passed. In neural tissue, poor clearance can be especially damaging because even modest structural disorder can alter signaling precision and microglial behavior. In barrier tissues such as the intestine, unresolved cellular debris can combine with ongoing exposure to luminal triggers and make the site exceptionally difficult to calm. In all of these contexts, improving macrophage cleanup is not optional if the body is to move beyond chronic inflammatory repetition. The tissue has to become physically cleaner before it can become biologically quieter.

Seen clearly, enhancing macrophage cleanup through efferocytosis is one of the most concrete expressions of what resolution actually means. It means the inflammatory site is no longer defined by ongoing arrival of force, but by competent removal of what that force left behind. It means the body is not simply asking inflammatory cells to disappear. It is actively collecting them, processing them, and using that process to transition the tissue toward repair. This is why SPMs matter so much. They help make macrophages better closers. They help transform an inflamed environment from one that remains crowded with the residue of damage into one that can finally stop looking like a problem. Without efferocytosis, inflammation lingers because the evidence of inflammation remains. With it, the body gains one of the main mechanisms by which defense can end without leaving disorder in its wake.

Clearing Cellular Debris

Clearing cellular debris is one of the most decisive tasks in the resolution phase because inflammation cannot end in any meaningful way while the tissue remains physically full of evidence that damage is still present. Cellular debris is not inert clutter. It includes apoptotic cells that have not yet been removed, fragments of damaged membranes, oxidized lipids, denatured proteins, extracellular matrix remnants, microbial remains where applicable, and the biochemical residue left behind by neutrophils, macrophages, and stressed tissue cells. As long as this material remains in place, the inflammatory site continues to look dangerous to the immune system. Receptors keep encountering signals associated with disruption. Oxidative chemistry remains easier to sustain. Additional immune recruitment remains easier to justify. The body therefore cannot move fully into repair while the local environment still resembles a partially dismantled battlefield. Resolution requires the tissue to become physically cleaner, not just chemically quieter.

This is why debris clearance is not a cosmetic finishing step after the real inflammatory work is over. It is part of the real work. The inflammatory response itself creates waste. Neutrophils arrive, carry out acute functions, and then die. Damaged host cells must be removed. Oxidized phospholipids and fragmented membrane components accumulate. Proteases, nucleic acid fragments, and disrupted structural proteins remain in the extracellular space. If these materials are left where they fell, they become a new layer of inflammatory stimulus. Even when they are no longer part of the original threat, they continue to signal that the tissue is unsettled, injured, and biochemically unsafe. The body then keeps behaving as though the inflammatory phase is still needed, because the tissue keeps presenting unresolved evidence that something remains unfinished. Debris clearance is what breaks that illusion and allows the site to transition out of emergency mode.

Macrophages are central to this process, but the mechanism extends beyond simple phagocytosis of whole apoptotic cells. The tissue has to collect and process a wide range of damaged material. Membrane remnants have to be internalized and degraded. Oxidized lipid fragments have to be removed before they continue interfering with nearby membranes or serving as danger signals. Protein debris has to be cleared so it does not remain as extracellular irritant. In some cases, microbial fragments or remnants of damaged barrier contents also have to be managed. The site must be stripped of inflammatory leftovers with enough efficiency that the surrounding cells stop reading the local environment as open damage. This is one reason specialized pro-resolving mediators are so important. They do not only reduce future recruitment. They help improve the tissue's capacity to process what the previous phase already produced.

The importance of this becomes even clearer when debris is not cleared well. If apoptotic cells remain too long, they lose membrane integrity and spill intracellular contents outward. If oxidized membrane fragments remain in tissue, they continue exposing surrounding cells to reactive breakdown products and distorted lipid signals. If extracellular protein debris remains lodged in the tissue matrix, local immune cells continue encountering structural evidence of injury. Each of these failures turns residue into reactivation. The tissue does not move forward because the remains of the last inflammatory cycle become fuel for the next one. This is one of the central reasons chronic inflammation can persist even after the original trigger has weakened. The site is still full of material that tells the body the job is not done.

Debris clearance also reduces collateral damage indirectly by lowering the need for continued inflammatory force. A site that remains crowded with damaged cellular material continues requiring surveillance, continued phagocytic attention, and continued chemical defense. A site that has been cleaned effectively no longer justifies the same level of inflammatory mobilization. This is one of the most practical meanings of resolution. The body can stand down because the environment has changed. The visible and molecular signs of emergency are being removed. Once that happens, vascular permeability can normalize more safely, pain sensitization can start withdrawing, immune recruitment can decline, and tissue repair can proceed without being constantly interrupted by the residue of previous inflammatory activity.

This is especially important in tissues where debris is costly. In joints, retained debris can sustain synovial irritation and pain long after the initial insult. In vascular tissues, retained cellular remnants can keep endothelial surfaces reactive and dysfunctional. In the nervous system, even modest accumulation of inflammatory residue can distort signaling and keep local immune cells in an activated state. In the gut, poor debris clearance can interact with ongoing barrier stress and continuous luminal exposure to make local resolution extremely difficult. In each case, the principle is the same. The tissue cannot fully recover while it is still carrying the remains of unresolved inflammation inside itself.

Seen clearly, clearing cellular debris is one of the ways the body converts an inflammatory site from a place of active danger into a place where repair becomes possible. It is not enough to stop new inflammatory cells from arriving. The tissue must also remove what those cells, and the original injury, have left behind. Until that happens, the local environment continues to advertise unfinished damage. Effective resolution therefore depends on cleanup that is both efficient and quiet. The body has to remove the physical residue of inflammation before it can truly stop behaving inflamed.

Promoting Tissue Repair and Regeneration

Promoting tissue repair and regeneration is one of the clearest signs that inflammation has truly entered its later phase, because repair only becomes possible when the body stops spending most of its resources on recruitment and containment. Early inflammation is designed to control disruption. It opens access, mobilizes force, and marks the tissue as a priority zone. But tissue cannot remain in that state and heal at the same time. Repair requires a different operating environment. Cellular traffic has to become more selective. Debris has to be cleared well enough that new structure is not being laid down into biochemical disorder. Oxidative and proteolytic pressure has to fall. Macrophages and surrounding cells have to shift away from destructive urgency and toward constructive work. Blood flow has to remain sufficient for rebuilding without remaining in a state of inflammatory excess. In that sense, repair is not what happens after inflammation disappears. Repair is what begins when inflammatory logic is successfully reprogrammed into restoration logic.

This is why specialized pro-resolving mediators matter so much in tissue recovery. They do not simply make inflammation smaller. They help create the conditions under which rebuilding can occur without being constantly interrupted by fresh inflammatory damage. By reducing continued neutrophil recruitment, enhancing macrophage cleanup, limiting collateral injury, and changing the local mediator environment, SPMs make the tissue less dominated by emergency chemistry and more capable of restoration. That shift is essential because regeneration and repair require structural coherence. Cells cannot rebuild junctions, restore extracellular matrix organization, normalize membrane behavior, and re-establish communication across the tissue if the site remains chemically loud and physically cluttered with unresolved damage. SPMs help clear the ground so regeneration is not forced to compete with an unfinished inflammatory battlefield.

Macrophages are central to this transition. Once they move into effective cleanup modes, they do more than remove waste. They begin shaping the tissue environment in a way that supports reconstruction. A site that has undergone successful efferocytosis and debris clearance stops broadcasting the same level of threat. That alone changes what neighboring cells do. Epithelial cells can begin restoring barrier structure. Endothelial surfaces can begin tightening control. Fibroblasts and other local structural cells can participate in rebuilding without being continuously driven by inflammatory distortion. The tissue becomes more orderly, and once order begins returning, regenerative work becomes more efficient because it is not constantly being overruled by persistent alarm signaling. This is one of the key principles of resolution biology: cleanup and repair are not separate events. Cleanup is part of what makes repair biologically possible.

Tissue repair also depends on the reduction of unnecessary collateral damage. A site under prolonged inflammatory escalation is continuously exposed to oxidants, proteases, membrane injury, vascular leak, and signaling excess. Even if the original insult has been contained, that ongoing chemistry keeps injuring the same tissue the body is trying to save. Regeneration cannot outrun repeated self-damage forever. The system has to stop destroying structure faster than it rebuilds it. This is another way SPMs promote repair. They help reduce the continuation of inflammatory force once that force is no longer proportionate to need. The tissue then has a chance to stabilize. Stabilization is the beginning of regeneration because cells can only rebuild effectively when the environment stops behaving as though it is still under attack.

Barrier restoration is one of the most practical expressions of this process. In epithelial tissues, endothelial tissues, gut lining, skin, and other surfaces that define biological compartments, repair means more than replacing damaged cells. It means restoring selective control. A barrier that heals poorly continues allowing inappropriate exposure, continued immune activation, and repeated disruption of local structure. A barrier that heals well stops feeding the inflammatory loop. SPM-supported resolution helps this happen by lowering ongoing inflammatory pressure and supporting the phase transition required for cells to re-establish junctions, restore surface integrity, and reduce unnecessary permeability. Repair therefore includes reasserting boundaries. The tissue becomes a better barrier again, and by becoming a better barrier it also becomes harder to re-injure through the same unresolved pathways.

Energy remains a major constraint throughout this phase. Tissue repair is expensive. Membranes have to be rebuilt. Proteins have to be synthesized or reorganized. Junctions have to be restored. Extracellular matrix may need remodeling. Ion gradients must be maintained while damaged structures are replaced. A tissue that lacks energetic capacity may still enter inflammatory activation, but it will struggle to complete the slower and more organized labor of regeneration. This is one reason chronic inflammatory illness so often includes poor healing even when inflammatory activity is obvious. The body still has enough chemistry to defend. It does not have enough organized energy to rebuild well. Repair is therefore not just a signaling event. It is a metabolic commitment. The resolution phase promotes regeneration partly by reducing the wasteful energy drain of chronic inflammatory continuation so that tissue resources can be redirected toward reconstruction.

The word regeneration has to be used carefully because not all tissues regenerate to the same degree and not all repair restores original structure perfectly. Some tissues rebuild with remarkable fidelity. Others repair more by stabilization, compensation, or scar formation. But in all cases, the principle remains the same. The body can only move toward its best available form of restoration when inflammation has been sufficiently completed that rebuilding is no longer being sabotaged by continued recruitment, continued debris accumulation, and continued structural instability. Resolution does not guarantee perfect regeneration. It creates the conditions in which the highest level of recovery available to that tissue becomes possible.

Seen clearly, promoting tissue repair and regeneration is one of the reasons the resolution phase should never be confused with simple anti-inflammatory suppression. Suppression can reduce visible inflammatory output without creating real rebuilding conditions. Resolution, by contrast, changes the tissue state in a way that allows restoration to begin. It reduces unnecessary continuation, improves cleanup, protects structure from further collateral injury, and reorients cellular behavior toward repair-compatible work. That is why SPMs and the broader resolution program matter so much. They do not merely help inflammation stop. They help the tissue become healable again.

Chapter 10

When Resolution Fails

Resolution failure is what turns inflammation from a useful biological program into a chronic operating condition. The body still detects disruption, still initiates defense, still recruits inflammatory cells, still changes vascular tone, still amplifies pain sensitivity, and still mobilizes lipid-derived signaling. In that sense, much of the machinery remains functional. What breaks is the transition. The tissue does not move cleanly from force into cleanup, from cleanup into repair, and from repair into restored control. Instead it remains suspended in an unfinished middle. Recruitment slows but does not truly stop. Debris accumulates faster than it is cleared. Macrophages are present but do not finish effectively enough to empty the site of inflammatory residue. Vascular permeability remains too open. Barrier surfaces remain too compromised. Membranes remain structurally unstable and continue releasing the biochemical evidence of damage. The result is not simply inflammation that lasts too long. It is inflammation that has lost its end state.

This is one of the most important distinctions in modern chronic disease. The body is often not failing because it cannot produce inflammation. In many cases it produces inflammation very well. It can still generate eicosanoids, cytokines, adhesion signals, oxidative chemistry, and acute immune traffic. The deeper failure is that this early and middle phase chemistry is no longer being brought under the command of a competent resolution program. Specialized pro-resolving mediator production may be insufficient relative to the burden of initiation. Omega-3-derived substrate may be too limited, too poorly incorporated, too oxidatively vulnerable, or too weakly converted downstream into useful pro-resolving signals. Macrophage cleanup may be incomplete. Barrier damage may continue feeding fresh triggers into the system.

Mitochondrial stress may limit the energy required for actual tissue repair. In that setting the body keeps re-opening a process it never truly finished the last time.

When resolution fails, one of the first things that happens is that inflammatory evidence stops disappearing. Apoptotic neutrophils are not removed efficiently enough and begin to break down into secondary inflammatory material. Oxidized lipids remain in tissue. Damaged membrane fragments remain visible to immune surveillance. Protein debris and extracellular matrix damage continue distorting the local environment. What should have become quiet removal becomes persistent provocation. The tissue stays chemically legible as a site of active disruption even if the original trigger has diminished. This is why chronic inflammation often feels disproportionate to the current insult. The body is not always responding only to what is happening now. It is often responding to what was never successfully cleared from what happened before.

This unfinished state also changes the behavior of immune cells themselves. Neutrophils may continue to arrive because the site continues broadcasting signals of unresolved damage. Macrophages may remain trapped in inflammatory or mixed phenotypes rather than fully transitioning into high-efficiency cleanup and repair-support roles. Cytokine signaling remains elevated not because the body has chosen meaningless excess, but because the tissue continues to present conditions that justify continued surveillance. A site that has not been cleared cannot persuade the immune system to stand down. The immune system is responding to the fact that the site still looks unfinished. Resolution failure therefore becomes self-reinforcing. The longer the tissue remains unresolved, the more inflammatory logic it continues to justify.

Barrier dysfunction is often central to this process. A tissue cannot resolve while fresh triggers keep entering the site faster than the system can process the previous ones. In the intestine, this may mean microbial products, incompletely contained luminal contents, or recurring epithelial injury continue feeding immune activation. In vascular and tissue barriers, excessive permeability may keep immune traffic and signaling molecules moving into places that are supposed to be closing back down. At the cellular level, oxidatively damaged membranes may continue releasing danger-associated chemistry that makes surrounding cells interpret the environment as unstable. Resolution requires decreasing provocation. If provocation stays constant, the body never receives convincing evidence that the emergency phase can safely end.

Energetic failure compounds this problem. Repair is expensive. Cleanup is expensive. Membrane reconstruction, junctional restoration, re-establishing gradients, recycling damaged components, and shifting immune cell behavior all require organized ATP production. A metabolically strained tissue may still initiate inflammation because initiation can run on stress signaling, stored substrate release, and acute defensive logic. But it may fail during the labor-intensive phase of closure. This creates one of the defining patterns of chronic illness. The body has enough force to begin but not enough integrated energy to finish. Symptoms persist not only because the wrong signals remain active, but because the tissue lacks the energetic margin to execute the work those signals are supposed to direct.

This is also why chronic pain, chronic swelling, chronic fatigue, chronic vascular irritation, and chronic immune activation so often travel together. They are different expressions of the same unresolved tissue state. Pain persists because nociceptive amplification has not been withdrawn from a site still broadcasting damage. Swelling persists because vascular and barrier control have not normalized. Fatigue persists because the body remains metabolically committed to defense and cleanup it has not completed. Immune activation persists because the tissue keeps presenting evidence that the job is unfinished. The person experiences separate symptoms. The underlying failure is often one thing: the body has not successfully converted an inflammatory event into a resolved tissue environment.

Resolution failure also reframes the meaning of treatment failure. If one only thinks in anti-inflammatory terms, then partial symptom reduction may look like adequate progress. But a quieter tissue is not necessarily a resolved tissue. A suppressed site can still be full of uncleared debris, unstable membranes, dysfunctional macrophage behavior, unresolved barrier damage, and ongoing re-triggering. This is why symptoms so often return. The sequence was muted, not completed. The body was not helped into resolution strongly enough to stay there. A true resolution-centered view asks different questions. Has recruitment stopped because the site no longer needs it, or only because a signal was blocked. Has debris actually been removed. Have barrier and vascular controls recovered. Has tissue stopped generating evidence of active danger. Has immune behavior shifted from persistence into completion. Without those transitions, the inflammatory program remains unfinished even when it is less loud.

This chapter matters because it changes the entire emotional and biological meaning of chronic inflammation. The body is not necessarily broken in the sense of losing all defensive intelligence. Often it is defensively overcommitted because it cannot obtain the evidence required to exit. It keeps acting inflamed because unresolved tissue keeps telling it to do so. That means the path forward is not merely reducing inflammatory intensity. It is rebuilding the conditions under which inflammation can end. That includes restoring membrane composition, improving omega-3-derived resolution substrate availability, improving downstream conversion into specialized pro-resolving mediators, strengthening macrophage cleanup, restoring barrier function, lowering repeated triggers, and supporting mitochondrial capacity for repair. Resolution failure is what makes chronic disease chronic. It is the point where the body stops suffering from an event and starts suffering from its inability to complete that event well.

SPM Deficiency

SPM deficiency does not mean the body is incapable of producing inflammation. It means the body lacks enough of the specialized pro-resolving mediator signal environment required to bring inflammation to a proper end. That distinction matters because many chronically inflamed tissues are not weak in initiation. They are often highly competent at initiation. They can release arachidonic acid, generate eicosanoids, recruit neutrophils, alter vascular permeability, amplify pain, and sustain immune traffic. What they lack is sufficient downstream pressure toward closure. In that setting, the tissue remains rich in go signals and poor in stop signals. It is built to escalate more easily than it is built to complete. SPM deficiency therefore describes a state in which the later-phase biochemical intelligence of inflammation is underpowered relative to the force of the earlier phases.

This deficiency can emerge from several levels at once. The first is inadequate precursor availability. If EPA and DHA are not sufficiently incorporated into membrane phospholipids, the tissue simply does not carry enough raw material from which resolvins, protectins, and maresins can later be generated. The second is poor downstream conversion. A person may have some omega-3 in circulation or tissue, yet still fail to derive meaningful pro-resolving output if enzymatic routing, tissue state, or inflammatory timing remain biased toward initiation-heavy pathways. The third is excessive oxidative instability. EPA and DHA are highly unsaturated, which makes them biologically useful but also chemically fragile. If membranes are heavily oxidized, if antioxidant protection is poor, or if inflammatory damage is repeatedly injuring the same tissue, omega-3-derived substrate may be degraded or functionally underexpressed before it can support a strong resolution program. The fourth is chronic re-triggering. Even where some SPM generation exists, repeated barrier leakage, persistent endotoxin exposure, ongoing tissue injury, or mitochondrial distress may keep the inflammatory site under such constant activation pressure that the pro-resolving signal never gains dominance.

The consequences of SPM deficiency are predictable once the sequence is understood. Neutrophil recruitment may begin normally but fail to shut down cleanly. Macrophages may arrive but remain less effective at efferocytosis and debris clearance. Apoptotic cells may accumulate and progress into secondary necrosis, turning what should have been quiet removal into fresh inflammatory provocation. Vascular permeability may stay elevated longer than needed. Nociceptive amplification may remain active after its protective usefulness has ended. Tissue barriers may stay compromised because the local environment never fully exits emergency mode. In this sense, SPM deficiency does not create a lack of inflammatory activity. It creates an excess of unfinished inflammatory activity. The body continues behaving as though more force is still needed because it has not been given enough later-phase instruction to shift decisively toward cleanup and restoration.

This is one reason chronic disease can look paradoxical. A person may have high inflammatory markers, persistent pain, slow recovery, and exaggerated immune reactivity, yet the deeper defect is not simply too much inflammation. It is too little resolution pressure relative to the amount of inflammation being initiated. That imbalance leaves the tissue stuck in a loop. Every inflammatory event creates debris and structural disturbance. Inadequate SPM action means that debris is not cleared efficiently enough. The uncleared debris then becomes part of the reason the next inflammatory event is triggered. The site never becomes convincingly safe enough for the immune system to stand down. SPM deficiency therefore turns inflammation into recurrence. The body keeps re-entering a process it never fully completed the last time.

Seen clearly, SPM deficiency is one of the most useful ways to describe chronic inflammatory biology without collapsing back into vague anti-inflammatory thinking. It points to a missing phase, not merely an excessive volume. It says the tissue is poor at biochemical closure. It says the body still has the machinery of defense, but insufficient mediator strength to redirect that machinery into efficient efferocytosis, tissue protection, barrier restoration, and return to baseline. That is why the solution cannot be reduced to blunting early-phase inflammation alone. The deeper task is to restore the conditions under which SPM biology can become strong enough to matter: adequate EPA and DHA incorporation, enough structural protection for those substrates, competent downstream conversion, reduced re-triggering, effective macrophage cleanup, and enough metabolic capacity for repair. Only then does the body regain more than symptom relief. It regains its missing half of inflammatory intelligence.

Enzymatic Bottlenecks (COX/LOX Pathways)

Enzymatic bottlenecks in the COX and LOX pathways help explain why the presence of omega-3 substrate does not automatically guarantee strong pro-resolving output. EPA and DHA may be present in membranes, but they still have to move through enzyme systems that are shared, competitive, context-dependent, and often already heavily occupied by arachidonic-acid-rich initiation chemistry. Cyclooxygenase and lipoxygenase pathways do not operate in an empty space waiting patiently for omega-3 to arrive. They are already embedded inside inflammatory tissue states shaped by receptor activation, cytokine tone, oxidative stress, membrane composition, and the relative abundance of competing substrates. This means the body can carry the raw material for resolution and still fail to express that material efficiently if the conversion machinery remains bottlenecked at the level of enzyme access, enzyme preference, or phase timing.

The first problem is simple competition. COX and LOX enzymes can act on multiple polyunsaturated fatty acid substrates, but they do not do so under neutral conditions. In a tissue heavily enriched with arachidonic acid, especially one that is repeatedly mobilizing omega-6-derived substrate during chronic inflammatory activation, the enzymatic traffic is already biased toward early-phase eicosanoid production. Arachidonic acid is being liberated, converted, and fed into pathways that sustain vascular change, leukocyte recruitment, pain sensitization, and inflammatory amplification. EPA entering that same environment is not automatically granted equal downstream influence. It is competing for shared enzymatic handling inside a site whose biochemistry may still be organized around initiation. DHA faces a related problem, especially when the tissue has not shifted far enough into the later phase for protectin-, maresin-, and D-series resolvin-generating pathways to become meaningfully dominant. The precursor may be present, but the pathway remains crowded.

The second problem is that enzyme activity changes with inflammatory phase. COX and LOX pathways are not simply on or off. Their behavior is shaped by the kind of tissue event underway. Early in inflammation, the system is built to generate force quickly. That means enzyme activity tends to favor mediator output associated with initiation and amplification. Later, if the sequence is functioning properly, the tissue undergoes what is often described as mediator class switching. The same broad enzymatic landscape begins favoring the production of lipoxins and omega-3-derived pro-resolving mediators rather than remaining locked in early-phase eicosanoid dominance. But if that switch does not occur efficiently, then the bottleneck is not only substrate competition. It is a failure of phase transition. The tissue keeps using its enzymes as if it were still trying to build the front half of inflammation, even when what it actually needs is the back half.

Oxidative stress can worsen this bottleneck by distorting the enzymatic environment itself. A chronically inflamed tissue is not just crowded with competing fatty acids. It is often redox-disturbed, structurally unstable, and repeatedly injured. That environment can alter membrane integrity, enzyme localization, receptor signaling, and the broader organization of the mediator system. Even if omega-3-derived substrate is present, the tissue may remain too chemically disordered to route that substrate efficiently into coherent pro-resolving output. Instead of a clean conversion sequence, the organism experiences partial incorporation, partial conversion, and persistent dominance of early-phase chemistry. This is one reason some people can increase omega-3 intake without immediately obtaining the resolution-oriented benefits expected from a simple nutrient model. The bottleneck is not only at the level of what enters the body. It is at the level of what the inflamed tissue can actually do with what entered.

There is also a spatial dimension to this problem. COX and LOX pathway activity is not occurring in abstraction. It is occurring in membranes, in specific cell types, under specific receptor conditions, and within tissues that have different demands and different substrate pools. A macrophage entering a proper resolution phenotype will not use the same enzymatic landscape in the same way as a neutrophil-heavy inflammatory site still dominated by acute recruitment logic. An endothelial surface under ongoing irritation will not necessarily convert substrate in the same pattern as a tissue beginning true repair. This means bottlenecks are not just global biochemical shortages. They are local failures of access, timing, and phenotype. The right substrate has to be in the right cell, in the right membrane pool, at the right phase, with the right enzyme activity surrounding it. Otherwise resolution remains theoretically possible but biologically weak.

This helps explain why chronic inflammation often reflects not just too much arachidonic-acid-derived signaling, but too little successful enzymatic re-routing toward pro-resolving mediator generation. The tissue keeps producing what it already knows how to produce. It keeps entering familiar eicosanoid cascades because those pathways are well-supported by both substrate abundance and inflammatory context. Meanwhile the omega-3-derived side of the system remains underexpressed, not necessarily because EPA and DHA are absent in absolute terms, but because the conversion bottleneck prevents them from exerting proportionate downstream influence. In this sense, COX and LOX bottlenecks are one of the places where chronic inflammation reveals itself as failed sequencing. The body still has enzymes. It still has substrates. What it lacks is efficient pathway transition.

Seen clearly, enzymatic bottlenecks in the COX and LOX pathways are one of the reasons resolution cannot be reduced to supplementation alone. More precursor helps only if the tissue can route that precursor into the right mediator classes at the right time. If competition remains too strong, if early-phase chemistry remains too dominant, if oxidative instability remains too high, or if immune and tissue phenotypes never shift into the later logic of cleanup and repair, then the bottleneck remains in place. The body continues speaking the language of initiation because its enzymes are still being used as tools of initiation. Resolution begins to recover only when substrate availability, tissue state, and phase transition align strongly enough that those same pathways can begin producing the chemistry of completion instead of repeating the chemistry of escalation.

Chronic Inflammatory States

Chronic inflammatory states are what the body looks like when initiation remains easier than completion for long enough that the tissue begins to organize itself around unresolved defense. This does not mean the body is inflamed every moment at maximal intensity. More often it means the tissue never fully returns to baseline. It remains slightly recruited, slightly permeable, slightly oxidatively stressed, slightly painful, slightly immunologically alert, and slightly structurally unfinished, and those partial deviations accumulate into a persistent biological climate. The key feature is not simply duration. It is failure of closure. A chronic inflammatory state is a tissue condition in which the early and middle phases of inflammation keep reappearing or remain partially active because the resolution phase never gains enough control to complete cleanup, restore barriers, normalize signaling, and remove the evidence of danger that continues to justify further inflammatory behavior.

This is why chronic inflammatory states are better understood as resolution-deficient environments than as mere excesses of inflammatory force. The body in these states still has access to arachidonic-acid-derived eicosanoids, cytokine networks, vascular recruitment signals, neutrophil infiltration, nociceptive amplification, and stress-responsive immune activation. In that sense, the machinery of escalation is often intact. What is missing is the coordinated handoff into efferocytosis, debris clearance, tissue protection, barrier restoration, and stable return to order. Apoptotic cells accumulate or are cleared too slowly. Oxidized membrane fragments remain in the extracellular environment. Endothelial and epithelial surfaces remain too open.

Macrophages remain insufficiently effective as finishers. The inflammatory field therefore never becomes convincingly safe enough for the system to stand down. The body continues acting as though something is still wrong because, at the tissue level, unresolved material and unresolved signals are still present.

These states can be sustained by many sources at once. Barrier dysfunction in the gut can keep feeding immune-provoking material into circulation and local tissue. Mitochondrial stress can keep generating redox signals that mimic ongoing danger. Adipose dysfunction can provide constant low-grade cytokine and lipid signaling pressure. Mechanical overload can keep re-injuring tissue before repair completes. Oxidative instability can keep damaging membranes and producing secondary inflammatory byproducts. Infection, biofilm burden, environmental irritants, poor perfusion, sleep disruption, and metabolic dysregulation can all reinforce the same pattern. What unites them is not their origin but their effect. They keep the tissue from receiving a clean enough environment to finish the inflammatory sequence. The result is repetition. The body restarts defense because the old defense never fully ended.

This is why chronic inflammatory states are so often multisystemic in experience even when they begin locally. A gut barrier problem does not remain only a gut problem if immune activation, oxidative stress, and nutrient handling are altered systemically. Persistent vascular irritation does not remain only a vessel problem if endothelial dysfunction changes tissue perfusion, immune traffic, and signaling access across organs. Chronic joint inflammation does not remain only a local pain issue if nociceptive amplification affects sleep, movement, stress response, and systemic energy allocation. Neural inflammatory tone does not remain only a brain problem if autonomic signaling, immune surveillance, and barrier control begin shifting with it. The body is an integrated membrane-and-signal system, so unresolved inflammation in one domain often propagates cost into others. Chronic inflammatory states therefore feel diffuse because they are diffuse. The same unresolved logic is being expressed through multiple tissues at once.

They also create a false appearance of adaptation. A person may look functional while carrying a body that is metabolically expensive, immunologically noisy, and structurally defensive. Symptoms become normalized. Mild pain becomes background. Digestive instability becomes routine. Brain fog becomes expected. Recovery slows and is interpreted as aging, stress, or overwork. But underneath that apparent adaptation, the tissue remains caught in partial emergency logic. The body is spending energy on surveillance and defense that should have been retired. It is rebuilding too slowly because cleanup is incomplete. It is responding too strongly to minor inputs because thresholds have shifted downward in a persistently unresolved environment. Chronic inflammatory states therefore do not always look dramatic. Often they look like a person slowly living inside the cost of not quite recovering.

This is where SPM biology becomes especially relevant. Chronic inflammatory states often reflect inadequate pro-resolving pressure relative to the amount of inflammatory initiation the tissue is experiencing. Omega-3-derived substrate may be too sparse, too poorly incorporated, too weakly converted, or simply outcompeted inside a site still dominated by arachidonic-acid-heavy signaling. The result is a tissue that remains fluent in escalation and relatively weak in closure. It knows how to call for help. It does not know how to convincingly declare the event complete. That is why these states persist. The stop signals are too weak, too late, or too easily overridden by repeated re-triggering. Without stronger resolution biology, the tissue keeps cycling through incomplete repair.

Seen clearly, chronic inflammatory states are not just prolonged versions of acute inflammation. They are a different tissue reality. Acute inflammation is directional. It starts, amplifies, and is meant to end. Chronic inflammation is circular. It reopens itself because too much inflammatory residue, barrier failure, membrane instability, and unresolved signaling remain in place between episodes. The tissue never becomes clean enough, sealed enough, stable enough, or biochemically quiet enough to stop looking like a problem. That is why the solution cannot be framed only as reduction of inflammatory output. The deeper task is to restore the body's ability to complete inflammation as a program. Until that happens, the chronic state remains what it truly is: not simply too much inflammation, but inflammation that never got all the way home.

Why the Body Gets "Stuck"

The body gets stuck when it can still initiate inflammation but can no longer carry that inflammation all the way through to completion with enough consistency to restore tissue order. That is the central pattern. It is not usually a failure of detection. It is not usually a failure of force. In many chronic conditions, detection is strong and force is abundant. The body sees disruption, releases substrate from membranes, generates eicosanoids and cytokines, recruits immune cells, alters vascular tone, increases permeability, and amplifies pain. The early program still works. What fails is the transition. The site does not become convincingly safe enough, clean enough, sealed enough, or structurally stable enough for the inflammatory program to stand down.

The result is a tissue environment that keeps re-signaling danger even after the original insult should have moved into closure. The body is not choosing chronic inflammation in the abstract. It is remaining inside a loop because the biological evidence required for exit never becomes strong enough.

One major reason for this is persistent debris. Inflammation creates waste. Neutrophils die. Damaged cells fragment. Oxidized lipids accumulate. Membrane remnants, extracellular matrix fragments, and degraded proteins remain in tissue. If macrophage cleanup and efferocytosis do not remove these efficiently, the site continues to display the remains of active damage. That matters because the immune system responds not only to the original trigger, but to what remains afterward. Uncleared apoptotic cells can become secondary necrotic material. Oxidized lipid fragments can continue acting as danger-associated signals. Structural debris keeps the local environment chemically unfinished. The body gets stuck because the site keeps looking like the work is not done, and in a real sense it is not done. Cleanup failure becomes re-initiation fuel.

Barrier failure is another major reason tissues get stuck. A barrier that does not recover keeps letting in the kinds of signals that sustain inflammatory interpretation. In the gut, this may mean microbial products, endotoxin, incompletely excluded food-derived material, or other luminal stimuli continue reaching immune surfaces. In vascular tissues, persistent endothelial dysfunction can keep permeability elevated and tissue exposure abnormal. At the cellular level, damaged membranes can continue releasing distress chemistry that tells neighboring cells the local environment is unstable. The inflammatory sequence can only end if the tissue stops receiving fresh evidence that something is still wrong. When boundaries remain open, the body keeps treating the site as active because new provocation keeps entering faster than the old provocation is being resolved.

The body also gets stuck when the substrate balance remains too heavily weighted toward initiation and too weakly weighted toward completion. If membranes are rich in arachidonic-acid-derived inflammatory potential but relatively poor in EPA- and DHA-derived resolution substrate, then the tissue has more material for escalation than for closure. That does not mean omega-6 is illegitimate. It means the later-phase chemistry is underpowered relative to the force of the earlier phases. Even when omega-3 is present, downstream conversion into specialized pro-resolving mediators may remain weak because of enzymatic bottlenecks, oxidative instability, repeated re-triggering, or poor phase transition. The body gets stuck because its biochemical language is skewed toward go signals and underdeveloped in stop signals.

Energy is another hidden reason. The body can often afford to start inflammation before it can afford to finish it. Initiation is fast and can ride on stress signaling, acute substrate release, and immediate immune mobilization. Resolution is labor. Efferocytosis costs energy. Membrane repair costs energy. Restoring barriers costs energy. Re-establishing gradients, rebuilding structure, and shifting immune cell phenotypes all cost energy. A tissue under mitochondrial strain can therefore remain capable of inflammatory activation while becoming poor at inflammatory completion. The body gets stuck because it has enough power to enter defense and not enough organized metabolic capacity to pay for cleanup and reconstruction afterward.

There is also a signaling memory problem. Once a tissue has been through repeated inflammatory cycles, its membranes, receptors, thresholds, and local immune behavior begin to adapt to that environment. The site becomes easier to trigger. Receptors become more likely to amplify. Nociceptive systems remain sensitized. Endothelial and epithelial behavior normalize more slowly. Macrophages may become less efficient finishers. In other words, the tissue learns chronicity at the structural level. It begins to interpret ordinary inputs through a defensive architecture. The body gets stuck because the tissue no longer requires a dramatic threat to behave as though threat is present. The threshold for returning to emergency mode has fallen, while the threshold for returning to true baseline has risen.

This is why the body often appears trapped in a half-healed condition. Symptoms fluctuate, but the underlying state remains unresolved. A person may feel a little better for a time, then flare again from a minor trigger. That pattern is not random. It reflects a tissue that never fully exited its previous inflammatory event. Enough improvement occurred to reduce intensity, but not enough cleanup, barrier restoration, membrane stabilization, and pro-resolving signaling occurred to create durable closure. The site remained vulnerable to reopening because it never stopped being biologically unfinished.

Seen clearly, the body gets stuck because inflammation is a program that requires a real end state, and that end state depends on multiple things going right at once. Debris has to be removed. Neutrophil recruitment has to stop. Macrophages have to finish well. Barriers have to re-close. Membranes have to stabilize. Omega-3-derived resolution signals have to become strong enough to matter. Energy has to be available for repair. If too many of those conditions fail at once, the body does not return to baseline. It stays in a repeating loop of partial activation, partial cleanup, and rapid re-initiation. That is what stuck really means. The system has not lost its ability to respond. It has lost its ability to convincingly declare the response complete.

PART IV

MEMBRANE COMPOSITION AND IMBALANCE

Chapter 11

How Modern Diet Disrupts SPM Production

Modern diet disrupts specialized pro-resolving mediator production not because it contains one single catastrophic ingredient, but because it gradually rebuilds tissues into a state that is better equipped for initiation than for completion. That shift happens through several overlapping mechanisms at once. Membranes become overloaded with omega-6-rich polyunsaturated substrate relative to omega-3-derived precursor pools. Oxidative burden rises, making highly unsaturated membrane lipids more fragile and less stable as signaling reservoirs. Mitochondrial strain increases, reducing the energetic capacity required for cleanup and tissue restoration. Barrier integrity weakens, feeding repeated inflammatory triggers into tissues that should already be transitioning out of defense. Enzymatic pathways remain crowded by initiation-heavy substrate traffic. The result is not merely more inflammation. The result is poorer inflammatory sequencing. The body still knows how to mobilize arachidonic-acid-driven early-phase chemistry, but it becomes less able to derive strong, sustained, downstream pro-resolving output from EPA and DHA when the moment for resolution arrives.

One of the central distortions comes from the repeated dominance of linoleic-acid-rich industrial seed oils and ultra-processed food systems that supply omega-6 substrate in quantities and contexts far removed from the slower, more structurally balanced patterns under which membranes maintain better signaling proportion. The issue is not that omega-6 itself is illegitimate. The issue is chronic overrepresentation. When tissue phospholipids are built in an environment saturated with omega-6 input while omega-3 incorporation remains comparatively weak, the membrane reservoir shifts toward early-phase inflammatory potential. More of the stored substrate pool is prepared to become arachidonic-acid-heavy eicosanoid signaling once phospholipases are activated. Less of that pool is available for meaningful downstream conversion into resolvins, protectins, and maresins. This is how diet changes future inflammatory behavior long before symptoms become obvious. It alters the stored material from which later phases of the inflammatory sequence must be built.

At the same time, the modern diet does not only distort substrate balance. It also destabilizes the environment in which omega-3-derived resolution signals would need to be generated. Highly processed foods often combine unstable polyunsaturated fats, refined carbohydrates, repeated glycemic load, low micronutrient density, poor antioxidant support, and flavor architectures that encourage chronic overconsumption. That creates oxidative and metabolic conditions hostile to clean resolution biology. A membrane containing EPA and DHA is valuable only if it can preserve those molecules long enough to use them intelligently. In a diet that repeatedly raises oxidative stress and postprandial inflammatory burden, highly unsaturated membrane lipids are exposed to a harsher chemical environment. They become easier to peroxidize, easier to damage, and less reliable as protected precursor stores for specialized pro-resolving mediator production. The diet does not just reduce omega-3 status quantitatively. It degrades the qualitative environment required for omega-3 to function as resolution substrate.

Another major problem is the collapse of food structure into chronic inflammatory signaling. Refined carbohydrates, liquid sugars, emulsified fat-sugar combinations, and hyper-palatable ultra-processed formulations alter insulin dynamics, adipose signaling, hepatic lipid handling, and postprandial immune behavior in ways that keep tissues biochemically louder than they should be. This matters for SPM production because the resolution phase depends on a body that can change phases. A body repeatedly pushed into glycemic volatility, lipotoxic overflow, hepatic stress, endothelial irritation, and adipose-derived inflammatory signaling remains too occupied with ongoing initiation pressure to hand off cleanly into the later logic of repair. Even if EPA and DHA are present, downstream conversion into pro-resolving mediator families may remain functionally weak because the organism is constantly being retriggered into the front half of the inflammatory program. The problem is not just lack of substrate. It is chronic interruption of the phase transition required for that substrate to matter.

Modern diet also damages SPM production through micronutrient dilution and structural insufficiency. Resolution is not driven by fatty acids alone. Enzymatic conversion, membrane protection, mitochondrial function, antioxidant defense, and immune cell phenotype shifts all depend on a broader nutritional context. A diet built from refined calories and chemically simplified food products can provide plenty of energy while providing poor support for the systems that protect membranes, manage oxidative stress, maintain metabolic flexibility, and execute cleanup efficiently. The body may therefore be overfed in caloric terms and underbuilt in functional terms. This is one reason people can consume omega-3 supplements inside an otherwise inflammatory dietary structure and see only partial benefit. Resolution requires more than adding precursor. It requires a tissue environment able to preserve, convert, and act on that precursor.

Barrier injury is another major pathway through which diet disrupts SPM production. Modern processed food patterns often destabilize the intestinal environment through emulsifiers, irritant food structures, repeated glycemic excess, low-fiber patterns, poor bile coordination, and altered microbial ecology. Once intestinal barrier integrity weakens, immune-provoking material continues reaching tissues that should have been allowed to quiet down. Endotoxin burden rises. Immune activation becomes easier to sustain. The liver and vascular system are exposed to repeated inflammatory traffic. Under those conditions, the body remains locked in repeated initiation. The enzymatic and cellular context required for mediator class switching toward pro-resolving output becomes harder to establish because the tissue never receives a convincing enough reduction in upstream provocation. SPM production is therefore disrupted not only by what the diet contains, but by the way the diet prevents the body from ever entering a stable enough state to prioritize completion.

There is also a temporal problem built into modern eating patterns. Resolution biology depends on tissues having the opportunity to complete processes. Constant grazing, repeated exposure to hyper-palatable engineered foods, chronic caloric surplus, and the absence of meaningful metabolic quiet reduce the intervals in which the body can re-establish lower-noise signaling conditions. The organism stays in a near-continuous state of digestive, endocrine, and inflammatory engagement. That does not mean eating itself is harmful. It means a food environment built around perpetual stimulation makes it harder for the body to finish one wave of physiological work before the next one begins. SPM production is impaired in that kind of system because resolution depends on clean transitions, and modern eating patterns often erase transitions altogether.

The modern diet also alters tissue composition over long time horizons in a way that reinforces enzymatic bottlenecks. COX and LOX pathways are shared, competitive, and context-dependent. In a tissue repeatedly loaded with omega-6-dominant membrane substrate and repeatedly activated by dietary inflammatory stress, those enzyme systems remain heavily occupied by initiation-heavy traffic. EPA and DHA are not absent in principle, but they enter a biochemical landscape already biased toward arachidonic-acid-driven mediator production. That means the bottleneck is not just low intake of omega-3. It is low pathway influence of omega-3 inside a tissue whose enzymes are being asked, over and over again, to support early-phase inflammatory chemistry. Modern diet keeps the system practicing escalation, so when the moment for resolution arrives, the enzymatic landscape is still crowded with the habits of initiation.

This is why the phrase anti-inflammatory diet is often too small to describe what is actually needed. The body does not simply need fewer inflammatory foods. It needs a dietary environment that reduces repeated re-triggering, protects membrane integrity, restores a more coherent omega-6 to omega-3 substrate relationship, supports mitochondrial capacity, strengthens barrier function, and allows phase transition into true inflammatory completion. In other words, the real dietary problem is not only that modern food creates more inflammatory signals. It is that it systematically dismantles the structural, energetic, and enzymatic conditions required for SPM biology to become effective enough to close inflammatory events once they have started.

Seen clearly, modern diet disrupts SPM production by attacking the resolution program from every angle at once. It overbuilds initiation substrate, underbuilds omega-3-derived completion substrate, increases oxidative damage to the very membranes that must store that completion substrate, crowds enzymatic pathways with early-phase chemistry, keeps barriers leaky, keeps tissues metabolically noisy, and reduces the organism's opportunity to move from defense into repair. The result is a body that still knows how to inflame but is progressively less capable of deriving the lipid mediators required to stop inflaming well. That is the deeper dietary problem. Modern food does not merely make inflammation more likely. It makes completion less available.

Omega-6 Dominance Blocking Pathways

Omega-6 dominance blocks pathways not because omega-6 is inherently illegitimate, but because enzymatic systems, membrane space, and inflammatory signaling capacity are finite. When tissues are repeatedly built from an environment saturated with omega-6-rich substrate, especially linoleic acid feeding the broader arachidonic-acid-heavy signaling reservoir, the body does not simply store more fat. It changes which inflammatory language is easiest to generate. Membranes become more heavily stocked with substrate for early-phase eicosanoid production, and the shared enzymatic machinery that processes polyunsaturated fatty acids becomes increasingly occupied by the chemistry of initiation. In that setting, omega-3-derived substrate is not always absent, but it is functionally outcompeted. It has less room in the membrane, less relative access to the same conversion systems, and less downstream influence when inflammatory activation begins. The result is a body that is biochemically prepared to escalate faster than it is prepared to resolve.

The first level of blockage happens at the level of membrane incorporation. EPA and DHA do not enter an empty membrane waiting to welcome them. They enter phospholipid pools already shaped by long-term dietary input, endogenous remodeling, oxidative turnover, and tissue-specific demand. If omega-6 input remains chronically dominant, more of the membrane reservoir is allocated to linoleic-acid-derived and arachidonic-acid-related structural potential, which means less relative space is available for EPA and DHA to become a meaningful fraction of the releasable substrate pool. This matters because inflammation later draws from what the membrane already contains. A tissue with omega-6-dominant phospholipid composition is preloaded for one kind of response. Even if omega-3 is later added, it may take time and significant remodeling to shift that stored ratio enough to change future mediator output in a biologically strong way.

The second level of blockage happens at the level of shared enzymatic traffic. Omega-3 and omega-6 families are processed through overlapping elongase, desaturase, cyclooxygenase, and lipoxygenase systems. These pathways are not infinitely available. If a tissue is continually mobilizing arachidonic-acid-heavy substrate and continually using COX and LOX pathways for early-phase inflammatory chemistry, EPA and DHA are forced to compete in an environment already organized around initiation. The issue is not that the enzymes refuse omega-3. The issue is that the biochemical road is crowded. Arachidonic acid is being released, converted, and used at scale, while omega-3-derived substrate remains relatively weaker in both abundance and pathway priority. Under those conditions, the body keeps generating the products it is best prepared to generate. Resolution pathways remain possible, but they are biochemically underpowered.

The third level of blockage is phase dominance. A tissue rich in omega-6-derived inflammatory potential tends to remain more fluent in the front half of the inflammatory program. It enters initiation quickly, amplifies efficiently, and keeps those pathways active because the substrate environment supports them so well. That matters because specialized pro-resolving mediator generation is not just a question of substrate presence. It also depends on mediator class switching, the transition in which the tissue stops prioritizing escalation and begins prioritizing closure. Omega-6 dominance makes that switch harder because the inflammatory environment keeps reinforcing the earlier phase. The body remains chemically convinced that more recruitment, more permeability, and more eicosanoid-driven force are still useful. In that context, omega-3-derived resolution chemistry never gains enough influence to take command.

This is why omega-6 dominance does more than increase inflammatory potential. It narrows inflammatory imagination. The tissue keeps solving problems with the same front-loaded chemistry because that is what the structural reservoir and enzymatic landscape are most prepared to produce. More prostaglandin and leukotriene logic becomes easier than more resolvin, protectin, and maresin logic. More neutrophil recruitment becomes easier than more macrophage-led cleanup efficiency. More pain sensitization becomes easier than more withdrawal of pain once tissue protection is no longer needed. In practical terms, omega-6 dominance blocks pathways by making the body repeatedly choose the inflammatory entrance and struggle to find the biochemical exit.

This does not mean the solution is to eliminate omega-6 completely. The body still needs initiation chemistry. It still needs arachidonic-acid-derived signaling for acute vascular response, immune recruitment, and tissue defense. The real problem is disproportion. When omega-6-derived substrate so heavily outweighs omega-3-derived substrate that membrane composition, enzymatic throughput, and tissue timing all become biased toward escalation, the resolution phase becomes chronically under-supported. The body still inflames efficiently, but it no longer resolves with comparable strength. That is what pathway blocking really means here. Not absolute inhibition, but structural and enzymatic crowding that makes the chemistry of completion too weak relative to the chemistry of initiation.

Seen clearly, omega-6 dominance blocks pathways by controlling all the upstream conditions that decide what inflammation can become. It occupies membrane real estate, competes for shared enzymes, reinforces mediator patterns that favor early-phase activity, and makes the shift into resolution less likely to gain dominance once inflammation is underway. The tissue does not become doomed, but it does become biased. It starts more easily than it finishes. That is the real consequence of omega-6 excess in a modern inflammatory environment. It does not just add more fuel to inflammation. It makes the body less able to access the roads required to bring inflammation to an intelligent end.

Substrate Competition

Substrate competition is one of the central reasons omega-3 and omega-6 cannot be understood as isolated nutrients acting independently inside the body. They share space, they share enzymes, and they compete for influence at the exact points where structure becomes signaling. This competition begins long before a mediator is formed. It begins at incorporation into membranes, continues through storage in phospholipids, persists at the moment of phospholipase release during inflammatory activation, and then intensifies again when cyclooxygenase and lipoxygenase enzymes begin converting available fatty acids into downstream lipid mediators. The body is not choosing between abstract categories. It is working with whichever substrates are most available, best positioned, and most dominant within the membrane environment at the moment the inflammatory sequence is triggered. That means tissue behavior is not determined by the existence of omega-3 or omega-6 in principle. It is determined by their competition in practice.

The first arena of substrate competition is the membrane itself. Phospholipids can only hold so many fatty acids, and those positions matter because they become the reservoir from which later inflammatory and pro-resolving mediators are derived. If tissue is built in a context of chronic omega-6 dominance, then more of those phospholipid pools become enriched with linoleic-acid-derived and arachidonic-acid-related substrate, while EPA and DHA remain relatively underrepresented. When inflammatory activation later occurs, the body can only release what it previously stored. A tissue rich in omega-6 substrate will therefore tend to release more of the material needed for early-phase eicosanoid production. A tissue richer in EPA and DHA will carry more of the substrate needed to support later pro-resolving mediator generation. This is not theory layered on top of the membrane. It is the direct consequence of what the membrane is made from.

The second arena is enzymatic competition. Once phospholipases liberate fatty acids from membrane phospholipids, those fatty acids enter shared processing systems. Cyclooxygenases and lipoxygenases do not belong to one fatty acid family alone. They handle whichever substrate reaches them under the conditions present in that tissue. If arachidonic acid is abundant and repeatedly mobilized, those pathways will tend to generate arachidonic-acid-derived eicosanoids that support initiation, amplification, vascular change, pain sensitization, and immune recruitment. If EPA and DHA are more meaningfully present and the tissue has shifted far enough into the later phase of inflammatory sequencing, then the same broad mediator landscape can begin moving toward resolvins, protectins, maresins, and other products more associated with completion. The point is not that one pathway exists and the other does not. The point is that they are competing for throughput. The body generates more of what its substrate environment most strongly favors.

This competition also changes how inflammation feels and behaves at the tissue level. A membrane dominated by omega-6-derived releasable substrate does not only produce more early-phase mediator potential. It changes the probabilities of what an activated cell will do next. More substrate for arachidonic-acid-heavy eicosanoid cascades means stronger bias toward recruitment, permeability, and inflammatory escalation. More EPA and DHA in the membrane does not automatically erase that, but it does create the possibility for different downstream mediator output and a stronger foundation for later class switching into resolution biology. In this sense, substrate competition is not only about quantity. It is about direction. The body can begin an inflammatory event from several possible biochemical landscapes, and whichever substrate pool dominates will influence whether the tissue moves more easily toward sustained activation or toward timely completion.

Timing makes this even more important. Early in inflammation, the body often draws heavily on whatever substrate is most readily available for fast local signaling, and chronic dietary patterns determine what that available pool looks like before the acute event even begins. This means the inflammatory sequence is partly written in advance. If a tissue has been built over months or years under conditions of omega-6 excess and weak omega-3 incorporation, the competition has already been tilted before the first neutrophil arrives. When the trigger occurs, the body reaches into the reservoir it has. That is why substrate competition is such a powerful explanation for chronic inflammatory bias. The organism is not making inflammatory decisions from scratch in every moment. It is making them from a structural memory stored in the membrane.

Substrate competition also helps explain why simply adding omega-3 sometimes produces gradual or incomplete change. EPA and DHA must do more than appear in circulation. They must displace or meaningfully counterbalance existing membrane composition, survive oxidative conditions long enough to remain useful, and exert enough influence within shared enzymatic systems that the body's downstream mediator profile begins to shift. In a tissue long dominated by omega-6-derived substrate, that is not instantaneous. The membrane has to remodel. The releasable pool has to change. Enzymatic traffic has to become less crowded by early-phase chemistry.

The inflammatory environment has to move far enough toward resolution that omega-3-derived substrate can express more than a minor downstream effect. Until then, the competition remains structurally biased, and the body continues speaking mostly in the older inflammatory language.

Seen clearly, substrate competition is one of the most important hidden rules of lipid biology. It explains why the body can require both omega-3 and omega-6 while still being harmed by disproportion between them. It explains why membrane composition matters so much before symptoms appear. It explains why chronic inflammatory states often feel chemically locked into escalation. And it explains why the path to stronger SPM biology is not merely about supplement intake, but about changing the actual substrate environment from which inflammation and resolution are both built. The body resolves from the materials it has on hand. If those materials are too heavily weighted toward initiation, then competition itself becomes part of the reason the body keeps starting more easily than it finishes.

Oxidative Damage to PUFAs

Polyunsaturated fatty acids are biologically powerful because their multiple double bonds make them flexible, dynamic, and useful as both membrane components and signaling substrates. But those same double bonds also make them chemically vulnerable. This is the core problem of oxidative damage to PUFAs. The very structural feature that allows omega-3 and omega-6 fatty acids to participate in membrane fluidity, receptor environment, and downstream mediator generation also makes them easier targets for free radical attack and lipid peroxidation. A polyunsaturated membrane is not just a signaling-capable membrane. It is also a membrane carrying built-in fragility if the surrounding environment cannot protect it. That fragility matters because once peroxidation begins, the tissue does not simply lose a few fatty acids. It begins to lose structural coherence, signal precision, and the integrity of the very substrate pool from which both inflammatory and pro-resolving mediators are supposed to be generated.

This is especially important in a modern inflammatory environment, where oxidative stress is not a rare event but a repeated condition. Mitochondrial inefficiency, chronic immune activation, glycemic volatility, endotoxin exposure, endothelial irritation, environmental toxins, poor antioxidant capacity, and repeated tissue injury all increase the likelihood that membrane PUFAs will be exposed to reactive oxygen species and related chemical stress. When that happens, polyunsaturated fatty acids are prone to peroxidative chain reactions. One attacked lipid can destabilize neighboring lipids, creating a spreading zone of membrane injury rather than an isolated molecular event. The result is not just chemical damage in the abstract. Membrane permeability can change. Receptor behavior can distort. Ion gradients become harder to maintain. Signaling becomes noisier. The tissue begins making decisions through damaged surfaces.

This problem has a special relevance for omega-3 biology because EPA and DHA are among the most unsaturated fatty acids in human membranes. They are therefore highly valuable as resolution substrate and highly vulnerable as oxidative targets. That combination creates one of the central tensions of this book. The body needs these fatty acids because they provide the precursor pool for resolvins, protectins, and maresins. But if the tissue environment is heavily oxidized, those same fatty acids may be damaged before they can be preserved, released, and converted into useful pro-resolving mediators. In that setting, the issue is not that omega-3 is bad. The issue is that highly unsaturated substrate placed into an unstable oxidative environment becomes fragile. The membrane is carrying the material for resolution, but the chemistry of the surrounding tissue keeps injuring that material faster than it can be used intelligently.

This has consequences at both the structural and signaling levels. Structurally, peroxidized PUFAs destabilize the membrane. They alter packing behavior, disrupt local protein environments, increase the likelihood of leakiness or altered receptor function, and contribute to the breakdown of the carefully organized surface conditions on which signaling depends. Signaling-wise, oxidation of PUFAs distorts the substrate pool itself. The body no longer has the same reservoir of clean, usable fatty acids available for enzymatic conversion into controlled mediator families. Instead it accumulates reactive byproducts, including aldehydes and oxidized lipid fragments, that can act as damage signals, interfere with proteins, injure nearby structures, and prolong inflammatory interpretation of the tissue. A membrane that should have been a reservoir for orderly mediator generation becomes a source of biochemical noise.

This is one reason oxidative damage to PUFAs contributes directly to failed resolution. A tissue cannot generate strong, clean pro-resolving output if its omega-3-derived substrate is being chemically degraded or if its membranes are so oxidatively unstable that they continue releasing distress chemistry faster than they can support class switching into completion. The tissue remains in a chemically ambiguous state. It carries enough PUFA content to be vulnerable, but not enough protected PUFA integrity to use that content well. Instead of moving from initiation toward resolution, the body keeps encountering oxidized lipid evidence that tells it damage is ongoing. Inflammatory signaling therefore remains justified. The site stays open, reactive, and incomplete.

Oxidative damage also makes substrate competition worse. In a tissue already dominated by omega-6-heavy initiation chemistry, damaged omega-3-derived substrate loses even more of its downstream influence. Not only is EPA and DHA underrepresented relative to arachidonic acid in many modern membrane environments, but whatever omega-3 is present may be more vulnerable to oxidative attrition if the tissue remains metabolically noisy. That means the body does not just suffer from poor omega-3 incorporation. It suffers from poor omega-3 preservation. The result is a double loss. Resolution substrate remains relatively sparse, and the portion that does arrive is less stable than it should be. Under those conditions, the balance of inflammatory chemistry tilts even more strongly toward escalation.

Seen clearly, oxidative damage to PUFAs helps explain why simply increasing intake of polyunsaturated fats, even beneficial ones, does not automatically improve tissue behavior. The question is not only whether the body contains enough EPA, DHA, or other PUFAs. The question is whether the body can protect them well enough to use them as intended. A well-supported membrane can hold polyunsaturated structure and later convert it into useful signaling. A poorly protected membrane turns that same structure into a liability. This is why membrane stability, antioxidant sufficiency, mitochondrial control, and reduction of repeated inflammatory stress are all part of the same story. The body does not resolve from fragile substrate very well. It resolves from substrate that remains intact long enough to be converted into the chemistry of completion rather than the chemistry of ongoing damage.

Loss of Resolution Capacity

Loss of resolution capacity is what happens when the body still retains the machinery to begin inflammation but no longer retains enough structural, signaling, and energetic competence to bring that inflammation to a proper end. This is one of the most important turning points in chronic disease because it marks the shift from useful inflammatory responses to repeated unfinished ones. The body can still detect disruption. It can still mobilize arachidonic acid, generate eicosanoids, recruit neutrophils, alter vascular permeability, amplify pain, and activate immune defenses. In that sense, force remains available. What is being lost is not inflammatory power. What is being lost is the ability to transition that power into cleanup, restoration, and closure. The tissue stops being good at finishing.

That loss can develop gradually. Membranes become more enriched in omega-6-dominant activation substrate and less effectively enriched in EPA and DHA. Whatever omega-3-derived substrate does enter the membrane may be more vulnerable to oxidative damage because the surrounding environment is increasingly unstable. Shared enzymatic pathways remain crowded with initiation-heavy traffic. Specialized pro-resolving mediator production becomes too weak relative to the scale of inflammatory activation. Macrophages become less effective finishers, either because their phenotype remains too inflammatory, because cleanup demand exceeds their capacity, or because the tissue environment never shifts far enough into the later phase to support efficient efferocytosis and repair. Barriers stay open. Mitochondrial output stays strained. In that setting the body does not lose resolution all at once. It loses it by attrition. Each inflammatory event becomes a little harder to close than the one before it.

The practical consequence is that tissue begins carrying forward the residue of previous inflammatory cycles. Apoptotic cells are not removed fast enough. Oxidized lipid fragments remain in place. Damaged membrane material continues signaling danger. Endothelial and epithelial surfaces fail to re-establish full control. Pain signaling remains amplified because the local environment still looks unsafe. Immune cells continue encountering evidence that the job is unfinished, so the body stays ready to re-initiate. This is what loss of resolution capacity really means. It means the site never becomes convincingly complete enough for the organism to stand down. Inflammation keeps recurring not necessarily because the original trigger is still large, but because the tissue still carries unresolved evidence of that trigger and the damage that followed it.

This is why chronic inflammatory states often feel self-sustaining. Once resolution capacity is sufficiently weakened, each new inflammatory event does more than create an immediate burden. It also worsens the tissue's future ability to resolve the next one. More oxidative damage weakens membrane integrity further. More uncleared debris increases future inflammatory signaling. More mitochondrial strain reduces energy available for later repair. More barrier dysfunction increases the probability of repeated provocation. The body becomes trapped in a compounding loop. It still knows how to start, but every cycle leaves it slightly less able to stop well. The problem is no longer only what is triggering inflammation. The problem is that the organism is losing the internal capacity required to complete inflammation as a program.

Seen clearly, loss of resolution capacity is one of the deepest ways to describe chronic illness. It explains why symptoms persist after the apparent trigger should have passed. It explains why tissues remain reactive, painful, permeable, and metabolically expensive. It explains why simply reducing inflammatory intensity often fails to restore true baseline. Most importantly, it explains why modern health problems so often involve not a failure of defense, but a failure of closure. The body is still trying to protect itself. It has simply become less able to finish that protection without remaining trapped inside it.

Chapter 12

Membrane Composition Determines Resolution Potential

Resolution potential is not created at the moment inflammation needs to end. It is built earlier, at the level of membrane composition. That is the central claim of this chapter, and it changes the way the entire inflammatory sequence has to be understood. A tissue does not wait until it is inflamed and then decide from nothing whether it will escalate cleanly and resolve well. It enters the inflammatory event carrying a preloaded structural condition. Its membranes already contain a certain balance of saturated, monounsaturated, omega-6, and omega-3 fatty acids. They already possess a certain degree of oxidative stability or oxidative fragility. They already hold a certain ratio of initiation-ready substrate to resolution-ready substrate. They already provide a certain physical environment for receptors, transporters, channels, phospholipases, cyclooxygenases, lipoxygenases, and the broader machinery of inflammatory signaling. That means a cell's capacity to resolve is partly determined before the first neutrophil arrives. The membrane is not simply where inflammatory substrate is stored. It is where inflammatory outcome is biased in advance.

This is why membrane composition has to be treated as more than a structural footnote. A membrane determines not only whether a cell can maintain gradients, host receptors, and preserve compartment boundaries. It also determines what kind of inflammatory program the cell can run under stress. A phospholipid pool enriched in arachidonic-acid-heavy omega-6-derived substrate creates one kind of future. It favors early-phase eicosanoid production, stronger recruitment logic, and greater readiness for inflammatory amplification. A membrane meaningfully enriched in EPA and DHA creates another kind of future. It still permits initiation, because the body still requires initiation, but it carries more of the precursor pool needed for mediator class switching and downstream generation of resolvins, protectins, and maresins once the tissue must stop escalating and start completing. The body therefore does not resolve from abstract nutrition. It resolves from the material built into its membranes.

The phrase resolution potential is important because it emphasizes possibility rather than guarantee. A membrane rich in omega-3-derived substrate does not automatically produce strong resolution if the tissue is severely oxidized, chronically re-triggered, energetically depleted, or trapped in a cytokine environment that never allows phase transition. But without the right membrane composition, even the possibility of strong resolution becomes weaker from the start. The tissue cannot generate what it did not store. It cannot route into later-phase lipid mediator families if the releasable pool is too skewed toward early-phase substrate. It cannot preserve signaling precision during inflammatory stress if the membrane itself is chemically fragile and structurally unstable. Resolution potential therefore depends on both what the membrane contains and how well that membrane can hold together while the inflammatory event unfolds. Composition and stability are inseparable here.

This also explains why highly unsaturated fatty acids occupy such a complex position in the story. EPA and DHA are essential to resolution potential because they provide the raw material for specialized pro-resolving mediators and alter membrane behavior in ways that can support cleaner phase transition. But they are also chemically vulnerable because their multiple double bonds make them easier targets for peroxidation. That means membrane composition determines resolution potential in two directions at once. A membrane too poor in omega-3-derived substrate is under-equipped for strong SPM generation. A membrane rich in omega-3-derived substrate but poorly protected from oxidative damage may carry theoretical resolution potential that is repeatedly degraded before it can be expressed. The body therefore needs more than omega-3 intake. It needs a membrane environment stable enough to preserve that intake as usable future biology.

The relationship with omega-6 becomes clearer inside this framework. Omega-6 is not wrong. Arachidonic acid and related substrate remain necessary because inflammation has to be able to start. But a membrane overwhelmingly dominated by omega-6-derived releasable substrate creates a biased inflammatory future. It shifts enzymatic competition, increases the relative ease of eicosanoid-heavy initiation, and makes it harder for omega-3-derived completion pathways to gain sufficient downstream influence. In that sense, membrane composition does not merely affect inflammatory intensity. It affects inflammatory direction. It determines whether the tissue is easier to push into escalation than into closure. This is why modern diet matters so much. It is not just adding inflammatory foods. It is remodeling the membranes from which future inflammatory decisions will be made.

Membrane composition also influences resolution potential through receptor behavior and signal interpretation. Inflammation is not driven only by what lipid mediators are released later. It is shaped from the beginning by how cells read the environment through membrane-bound receptors, channels, and signaling assemblies. A membrane that is too disordered, too oxidized, or too compositionally skewed can amplify danger signals more easily and normalize them more poorly. Receptors cluster differently. Microdomains behave differently. Transporters, phospholipases, and signaling proteins encounter different local conditions. The cell therefore interprets the same inflammatory cue through a different surface. This matters for resolution because a tissue that overreads danger at the receptor level will often enter more forcefully into initiation and may remain harder to shift out of it later. Membrane composition is not only setting substrate supply. It is shaping the behavior of the interpretive surface itself.

The mitochondrial dimension matters here as well. Resolution is metabolically expensive, and mitochondrial membranes are highly specialized lipid structures whose integrity determines whether repair can be paid for. A tissue with unstable or damaged mitochondrial membranes may still initiate inflammation, because initiation can be driven by acute signaling and stored substrate release, but it will struggle when the time comes to fund cleanup, efferocytosis, membrane repair, barrier restoration, and tissue rebuilding. In that sense, membrane composition determines resolution potential not only through inflammatory mediator biology, but through energy biology. A cell resolves from the membranes it stores and from the membranes it uses to generate ATP. If either level is structurally compromised, the later phase becomes harder to execute.

This chapter also helps explain why chronic illness so often looks like repeated failure rather than a single overwhelming trigger. The membrane is the place where tissue history is stored. Long-term diet, oxidative stress, inflammatory repetition, lipoprotein traffic, hormonal state, mitochondrial strain, and repair capacity all leave their mark on membrane composition over time. The body therefore accumulates a structural inflammatory memory. A tissue repeatedly remodeled under omega-6 dominance, oxidative fragility, poor omega-3 incorporation, and failed cleanup becomes a tissue with lower resolution potential before the next insult even occurs. It is easier to activate, harder to protect, and less equipped to finish. That is why inflammatory chronicity often feels disproportionate to the present moment. The tissue is not responding only from present conditions. It is responding from a membrane history that has already lowered the probability of successful closure.

Seen clearly, membrane composition determines resolution potential because the membrane decides what inflammatory future is physically possible. It stores the substrate reservoir. It shapes receptor behavior. It controls enzymatic access. It influences oxidative stability. It affects mitochondrial competence. It biases whether the tissue will be better at initiation, better at completion, or unstable in both directions. The body does not begin resolution from nowhere. It begins from the surface it already built. If that surface is rich in the right precursor material, sufficiently protected, and integrated into a broader environment capable of phase transition, then specialized pro-resolving biology can become more than theory. If it is unstable, omega-6-dominant, oxidatively damaged, and metabolically underpowered, then resolution potential remains low no matter how much the tissue might need it.

That is the deeper message of this chapter. The ability to end inflammation is not primarily a matter of willpower, not primarily a matter of one acute intervention, and not primarily a matter of suppressing the first half harder. It is a matter of what kind of membrane the body has built over time. The tissue resolves from its architecture. If the architecture has been built for escalation, then the body will escalate more easily than it finishes. If the architecture has been rebuilt to support substrate balance, structural stability, downstream conversion, and energetic sufficiency, then the body gains something much more valuable than lower inflammation. It gains the capacity to complete inflammation as a successful biological program.

EPA/DHA Incorporation into Phospholipids

EPA and DHA only become biologically decisive when they move from intake into structure. That transition happens through incorporation into phospholipids. Until then, omega-3 remains nutritionally present but physiologically shallow. Once these fatty acids are esterified into membrane phospholipids, they stop behaving like transient dietary inputs and start behaving like part of the tissue itself. They enter the bilayer, alter the physical environment surrounding receptors and enzymes, change what kinds of fatty acids can later be released during inflammatory activation, and create the precursor pool from which specialized pro-resolving mediators may eventually be derived. This is why incorporation matters more than consumption in the abstract. The body does not resolve from what was swallowed. It resolves from what was built into membranes and held there long enough to influence future signaling.

This incorporation is not uniform across all tissues, and that matters because phospholipid remodeling is one of the ways the body assigns different structural priorities to different organs. DHA becomes especially concentrated in neural and retinal membranes, where its physical properties contribute to membrane curvature behavior, excitability, vesicle dynamics, and signal fidelity. EPA tends to be discussed more heavily in relation to inflammatory signaling pools and systemic mediator balance, though it also participates structurally once incorporated. The point is that these fatty acids are not simply floating in circulation performing benefits from the bloodstream. They have to be placed into phospholipid architecture in the tissues where their later structural and signaling roles will matter. A membrane enriched with EPA and DHA is not merely chemically different. It is carrying a different future response profile.

That future profile changes because phospholipids are the storage format from which later inflammatory and pro-resolving language is generated. When phospholipase activity is triggered by tissue stress, receptor activation, microbial signals, oxidative pressure, or mechanical injury, the body releases fatty acids from the membrane positions it previously loaded. If EPA and DHA are underrepresented in those phospholipid pools, then the tissue has less omega-3-derived substrate available for downstream generation of resolvins, protectins, and maresins. If EPA and DHA are meaningfully incorporated, the tissue carries a larger reserve of completion-capable substrate. This is why incorporation into phospholipids is such a critical step. It changes not only membrane behavior in the resting state, but the biochemical options available once the membrane is mobilized during inflammation. The future mediator field is partly written into the phospholipid pool before the inflammatory event ever begins.

Incorporation also changes membrane behavior before any mediator is released. EPA and DHA alter local packing characteristics, membrane flexibility, receptor clustering behavior, and the way proteins move within the bilayer. That matters because the inflammatory response is shaped from the start by how cells interpret their environment through membrane surfaces. A phospholipid environment containing more EPA and DHA is not reading stress through the same material conditions as one dominated by omega-6-derived substrate alone. The cell is receiving the same world through a different surface. Receptor behavior, enzyme access, membrane microdomain dynamics, and downstream signaling probabilities all shift. This means omega-3 incorporation into phospholipids influences both the early interpretive phase and the later mediator phase. It affects how the tissue enters inflammation and how well it may later leave it.

This process is slow enough that it also explains why omega-3 biology is often misunderstood. People expect rapid effects from what is actually a remodeling event. Phospholipid incorporation requires digestion, absorption, transport, tissue delivery, membrane turnover, and selective replacement of existing fatty acid content. In a body long dominated by omega-6-heavy membrane composition, EPA and DHA do not immediately take command simply because intake increases. The phospholipid pool has to change over time. That means inflammatory potential is being remodeled gradually, not overridden instantly. The body is slowly replacing part of its future signaling reservoir. This is one reason the effects of omega-3 can feel delayed, partial, or dependent on broader context. The key question is not whether EPA and DHA entered the body once. The key question is whether they entered phospholipids deeply enough, broadly enough, and stably enough to alter tissue behavior in a durable way.

Oxidative stability becomes crucial at this point, because incorporation alone does not guarantee preserved function. EPA and DHA are highly unsaturated, and once placed into phospholipids they contribute both resolution potential and chemical vulnerability. If the membrane environment is heavily oxidized, metabolically unstable, or repeatedly exposed to inflammatory damage, those incorporated fatty acids may be injured before they can support strong downstream conversion into pro-resolving mediators. This creates one of the central tensions in membrane biology. The same phospholipid enrichment that increases resolution potential also requires a tissue environment capable of protecting that enrichment from peroxidative loss. The body therefore needs more than omega-3 entry into membranes. It needs membranes stable enough to preserve omega-3 as usable future substrate rather than as easily damaged material.

Seen clearly, EPA and DHA incorporation into phospholipids is the step that turns omega-3 from a dietary category into a determinant of inflammatory architecture. It places resolution substrate directly into the membrane reservoir from which future lipid mediators will be drawn. It changes receptor environment before activation and changes releasable substrate composition during activation. It is how diet becomes tissue, and how tissue becomes future inflammatory behavior. Without incorporation, omega-3 remains mostly potential outside the structure. With incorporation, the membrane itself begins carrying a different answer to the question of what kind of inflammation this tissue will be able to run and whether it will be able to finish it well.

Membrane Reservoirs for SPM Production

Specialized pro-resolving mediators are not produced out of empty chemistry. They are drawn from membrane reservoirs. This is one of the most important structural ideas in the entire resolution story, because it means the body's ability to end inflammation is partly stored in advance inside its own phospholipids. EPA and DHA do not matter only because they circulate through the blood or appear on a supplement label. They matter because, once incorporated into membranes, they become part of a tissue-level reserve that can later be mobilized when the inflammatory sequence reaches the point where completion must begin. The membrane is therefore not just the place where inflammatory signaling starts. It is also the place where the substrate for inflammatory ending is stored. A tissue can only generate meaningful SPM output if it has already built enough of the right precursor material into the right membrane pools before the need for that output becomes urgent.

This gives the membrane a dual identity. It is a structural surface in the resting state, but it is also a biochemical inventory. When phospholipase activity is triggered during inflammation, the body does not release random fatty acids. It releases what the membrane has been loaded with. If that reservoir is rich in arachidonic acid and relatively poor in EPA and DHA, then the tissue is more prepared to generate early-phase eicosanoid chemistry than later-phase pro-resolving chemistry. If EPA and DHA are more meaningfully represented, the tissue carries stronger potential for downstream production of resolvins, protectins, and maresins once inflammatory sequencing begins to shift toward closure. That is why the concept of a membrane reservoir matters so much. It moves resolution biology out of the realm of abstract nutrient theory and into the actual storage architecture of the cell.

These reservoirs are also tissue-specific. Different tissues build different phospholipid environments because they solve different structural and signaling problems. Neural membranes, retinal tissue, immune cells, endothelial surfaces, epithelial barriers, and mitochondrial membranes all handle lipids according to their own functional demands. That means the reservoir for SPM production is not identical everywhere. Some tissues may hold more DHA because of specialized membrane requirements, particularly where curvature behavior, excitability, and long-range structural stability matter. Other tissues may be more dynamically involved in inflammatory signaling and mediator generation. The body is not trying to make every membrane composition uniform. It is creating tissue-specific stored capacities for future behavior. Resolution potential therefore depends not just on total omega-3 status, but on where those fatty acids are actually being held and in what phospholipid context they are being stored.

This storage logic also explains why resolution cannot be improvised well in a body built under chronic omega-6 dominance. If the membrane reservoir has already been filled disproportionately with initiation-heavy substrate, then the tissue enters inflammatory stress carrying a stronger bias toward escalation. Even if omega-3 is later introduced, the reservoir may remain slow to change unless phospholipid remodeling becomes substantial enough to alter the releasable pool in a meaningful way. The body resolves from what it stored, not from what it wished it had stored. That is why membrane remodeling takes on such importance in chronic inflammatory states. Changing the future inflammatory outcome requires changing the reservoir from which that future outcome will be generated.

The membrane reservoir concept also makes clear why oxidative stability matters so much. A reservoir is only useful if the contents remain intact. EPA and DHA stored in phospholipids increase resolution potential, but because they are highly unsaturated, they also increase chemical vulnerability if the surrounding environment is oxidatively unstable. A tissue under chronic redox stress may technically contain omega-3-derived substrate while still failing to preserve it as clean usable precursor. Instead of serving as orderly reserve material for SPM production, those fatty acids may become damaged, fragmented, or converted into reactive byproducts that prolong inflammatory interpretation rather than support completion. The membrane reservoir must therefore be both adequately stocked and adequately protected. Resolution capacity depends on both conditions at once.

Seen clearly, membrane reservoirs for SPM production are one of the deepest reasons membrane composition determines inflammatory destiny. The body carries part of its future recovery ability inside the phospholipids from which it is built. When inflammation begins, the tissue draws from what it has already stored. When resolution should begin, the tissue again draws from what it has already stored. If the reservoir is poor, oxidatively damaged, or crowded by competing substrate, completion weakens. If the reservoir is rich in preserved EPA and DHA and the tissue environment can support downstream conversion, the body gains access to the mediator families required to stop escalating and start finishing. The membrane is therefore not only a surface under stress. It is the reserve account from which the chemistry of closure must be paid.

Structural Prerequisites for Resolution

Resolution depends on signals, but signals alone are never enough. The body can only complete inflammation if the tissue still possesses the structural conditions required to receive those signals, act on them, and survive the transition from defense into repair without collapsing back into renewed danger signaling. That is what is meant by structural prerequisites for resolution. Before specialized pro-resolving mediators can matter in a durable way, membranes have to remain intact enough to serve as stable signaling surfaces, phospholipid reservoirs have to contain usable precursor material, barriers have to retain or recover enough integrity to reduce repeated provocation, mitochondria have to maintain enough architectural coherence to fund cleanup and rebuilding, and the extracellular environment has to remain organized enough that repair is not immediately sabotaged by the residue of the inflammatory phase itself. Resolution is not just a biochemical command. It is a command that must enter a tissue still physically capable of obeying.

The membrane is the first of these prerequisites because it is both the source of substrate and the surface of interpretation. A membrane that is too oxidized, too permeable, too compositionally unstable, or too heavily dominated by initiation-heavy substrate does not simply perform worse in a generic sense. It changes the direction of inflammatory behavior. Receptors interpret danger more easily and normalize danger more poorly. Phospholipases release a substrate pool biased toward escalation. EPA and DHA, even when present, may be too sparse or too poorly protected to support strong downstream conversion into pro-resolving mediators. The tissue therefore enters the later phase already handicapped. Resolution signals may still exist, but they are being delivered into a surface environment that remains structurally committed to the front half of inflammation. The first prerequisite for resolution is therefore a membrane capable of holding both stability and usable resolution substrate at the same time.

Barrier integrity is the second major prerequisite because tissues cannot resolve while they are still being continuously re-provoked. An intestinal lining that remains too permeable keeps feeding microbial and luminal signals into immune surfaces that should be calming down. An endothelial barrier that remains too open keeps sustaining abnormal traffic, fluid shifts, and inflammatory exposure. Cellular membranes that remain damaged keep leaking distress chemistry into the surrounding environment. Resolution requires a reduction in incoming evidence that the emergency is ongoing. That reduction is not achieved through signaling alone. It requires boundaries that can close again. A tissue that cannot restore selective separation between compartments remains trapped in partial exposure, and partial exposure keeps the inflammatory program alive even when part of the later mediator environment has already begun to change.

Mitochondrial integrity is another prerequisite that is often missed because resolution is too often described as though it were mostly about the right lipids or the right cytokines. Cleanup is metabolically expensive. Efferocytosis costs ATP. Membrane repair costs ATP. Restoring gradients, rebuilding junctions, processing damaged macromolecules, and reorganizing tissue behavior all cost ATP. A cell with structurally compromised mitochondria may still initiate inflammation because initiation can run on acute signaling, stored substrate release, and emergency physiology. But it will struggle to complete the event because completion demands sustained organized energy. Mitochondrial membranes therefore matter directly to resolution potential. If oxidative phosphorylation is poorly supported because the organelle itself has lost structural coherence, the tissue may receive pro-resolving signals and still fail to execute the work those signals are directing.

There is also a mechanical prerequisite. The extracellular and local tissue environment has to remain rebuildable. Inflammatory events damage matrix structure, alter fluid dynamics, distort local signaling gradients, and generate debris that can physically interfere with restoration. If the matrix is heavily degraded, if tissue edema remains uncontrolled, if oxidized debris remains embedded in the site, or if repetitive mechanical stress keeps re-injuring the same environment before repair stabilizes, the body cannot move cleanly from inflammatory de-escalation into durable reconstruction. Resolution therefore depends not only on stopping further inflammatory recruitment, but on preserving enough structural order that restoration can take hold once recruitment slows. A tissue too thoroughly destabilized during the acute phase becomes difficult to resolve because the ground under repair keeps shifting.

Macrophage competence also belongs in this structural category, because effective cleanup is not only a signaling question. It depends on whether the cells tasked with finishing the event can physically engage, engulf, and process what has accumulated. If macrophages are metabolically strained, overwhelmed by debris burden, exposed to a persistently distorted mediator environment, or embedded in tissue whose architecture makes cleanup inefficient, then efferocytosis weakens even when some pro-resolving signals are present. The body needs more than instructions telling macrophages to finish. It needs macrophages structurally and energetically able to finish in a tissue that can actually be cleared. This is one reason chronic inflammatory states become so self-reinforcing. The site becomes progressively harder to clean, and that growing cleanup burden becomes one of the reasons the site keeps acting inflamed.

Taken together, these conditions show why resolution is never just the second half of the signaling story. It is the second half of the structural story as well. The body can only exit inflammation if the tissue has preserved enough membrane integrity, enough barrier control, enough mitochondrial function, enough matrix order, and enough cleanup capacity to convert biochemical instruction into real biological completion. Without those prerequisites, even valid pro-resolving signals remain underexpressed. The body may try to stop escalating, but the site continues behaving as though escalation is still necessary because too much structural evidence of danger remains in place. That is the deeper meaning of resolution failure. It is not simply a lack of stop signals. It is a lack of tissue conditions that allow stop signals to work.

Seen clearly, structural prerequisites for resolution explain why inflammation cannot be solved only at the level of mediator discussion. The membrane has to be built properly. The barriers have to close properly. The mitochondria have to function well enough to fund repair. The tissue has to remain cleanable and rebuildable. Only then can the chemistry of completion become the biology of completion. Resolution is therefore not just something the body wants to do. It is something the body must still be physically capable of doing.

Lipid Pools as Signal Libraries

Lipid pools function as signal libraries because the body stores future instructions inside its membranes long before those instructions are needed. This is one of the most important ways to understand inflammatory biology at a deeper level. A membrane is not only a boundary and not only a structural surface. It is also a curated archive of possible responses. The fatty acids esterified into phospholipids determine which kinds of lipid mediators can later be released, which enzymatic pathways will have meaningful substrate available, and what kinds of downstream tissue behavior will become easiest to generate once the cell is activated. In that sense, the body does not invent inflammatory language from scratch every time it encounters stress. It consults the lipid library it has already built into tissue. The quality of that library determines whether the cell is better equipped to escalate, better equipped to complete, or trapped in a chemically biased middle where escalation is always easier than resolution.

The idea of a signal library matters because it shifts the focus from momentary triggers to stored potential. Arachidonic acid-rich membrane pools represent one kind of library. They are heavily stocked with the substrate needed for eicosanoid production, vascular change, neutrophil recruitment, pain sensitization, and early inflammatory amplification. EPA- and DHA-enriched membrane pools represent another kind of library. They still permit initiation, because the body still requires initiation, but they also provide a deeper archive for resolvins, protectins, maresins, and the wider chemistry of inflammatory completion. These are not separate systems floating beside one another. They are different volumes on the same shelf. When phospholipases are activated, the body begins pulling from the collection it stored. If the library is dominated by activation-heavy substrate, then inflammatory meaning will be drawn mostly from activation-heavy pages. If the library is richer in omega-3-derived precursor pools and sufficiently protected from oxidative loss, then the body has a stronger basis for consulting the language of closure once the early phase has done enough.

This library metaphor also clarifies why membrane remodeling changes future behavior even before any obvious symptom shifts. The body is always editing its archive. Diet, oxidative stress, phospholipid turnover, lipoprotein transport, mitochondrial strain, hormonal state, and repeated inflammatory events all change what is being stocked, what is being lost, and what remains easy to retrieve later. A tissue repeatedly built from omega-6-dominant input and repeatedly exposed to inflammatory provocation will gradually accumulate a library more fluent in early-phase inflammatory grammar. A tissue that incorporates and preserves meaningful EPA and DHA in its phospholipid pools builds a broader library, one that includes more of the language needed for mediator class switching, macrophage cleanup, tissue protection, and resolution. This is why chronic inflammatory states often feel chemically repetitive. The body is drawing from the same narrow shelf over and over again because that is the shelf it has been stocked to use.

The phrase signal library also makes clear that stored lipids do not merely determine what can be released. They influence how signals are interpreted before release occurs. Membrane composition affects receptor behavior, microdomain organization, enzyme access, and the physical conditions through which extracellular information becomes intracellular action. That means the library is not only a future mediator archive. It is also a present interpretive framework. The surface of the membrane is already shaping what kinds of signals appear meaningful, how strongly they are amplified, and how easily the cell crosses the threshold into inflammatory activation. A library rich in unstable, initiation-heavy substrate does not only produce certain mediators later. It can also create a present tense bias toward overreading danger and underreading completion. The cell becomes both more fluent in escalation and less fluent in restraint.

This is why oxidative damage is so destructive to the library concept. A library only helps if its contents remain intact and legible. When PUFAs are oxidized, the stored archive begins to degrade. Clean substrate for controlled mediator generation is replaced by reactive fragments, distorted lipid signals, and membrane instability. Instead of preserving useful instructions for later resolution, the tissue begins carrying damaged text that keeps generating biochemical noise. The body can no longer consult its stored omega-3-derived potential as effectively because part of that potential has been chemically shredded. In that state, the tissue does not just lose signal options. It begins accumulating false signals as well, because oxidized lipids themselves can act as evidence of ongoing damage and help perpetuate inflammatory interpretation.

Seen clearly, lipid pools as signal libraries is one of the best ways to understand why membrane composition determines inflammatory destiny. The cell responds not only to what happens now, but to what has been stored for later use. Its membranes contain a history of previous dietary patterns, previous remodeling, previous oxidative burden, and previous inflammatory sequencing. That history becomes available the moment the tissue is activated. If the archive is rich in preserved EPA and DHA, resolution potential rises. If the archive is dominated by omega-6-heavy initiation material and damaged by oxidation, the body becomes more likely to keep repeating the first half of inflammation. The tissue does not merely react. It reads from its stored library, and what has been written into that library determines how well it can move from alarm into repair without getting trapped in alarm itself.

Chapter 13

The Threshold Problem Revisited

The threshold problem can now be seen more clearly because the earlier chapters have established what the threshold is actually sitting on. It is not just a psychological idea, not just an immune idea, and not just a signaling idea. It is a structural problem first. A threshold is the point at which a tissue decides that a given input is large enough, dangerous enough, or destabilizing enough to justify a shift from ordinary maintenance into inflammatory action. But that point is never fixed in abstraction. It is built into membranes, receptors, barriers, mitochondrial output, substrate pools, and the accumulated residue of prior inflammatory cycles. A healthy tissue has thresholds that are high enough to prevent constant false alarms and low enough to permit rapid defense when genuine disruption occurs. A chronically inflamed tissue loses that balance. It becomes easier to trigger, slower to reset, and less capable of distinguishing between ordinary biological friction and meaningful threat. The threshold drops, and once it drops, the body begins living in a world that feels more dangerous than it used to because its surfaces have become easier to disturb and harder to calm.

This is why threshold cannot be treated as a purely signaling issue. A cell does not decide to activate based only on the concentration of a cytokine, a microbial fragment, a hormone, or a mechanical input. It decides through the material state of the membrane that receives that input. If receptor clustering is altered, if microdomains are unstable, if membrane permeability is higher, if omega-6-derived activation substrate is dominant, if oxidative fragments remain embedded in the surface, or if mitochondrial stress is already generating internal danger chemistry, then the same outside event crosses threshold more easily. A food component, a stressor, a bout of exercise, a small injury, a night of poor sleep, or a transient endotoxin pulse can all produce a larger biological response than they would have in a more stable system. The event did not necessarily become more severe. The tissue became easier to push over the line that marks the transition from normal handling into defensive escalation.

The threshold problem is therefore one of the deepest ways chronic illness perpetuates itself. Every unresolved inflammatory cycle leaves behind structural evidence that lowers the threshold for the next one. Uncleared debris remains in tissue. Oxidized lipid fragments continue acting as danger-associated signals. Barriers remain slightly too open. Mitochondria remain slightly too strained. Macrophages remain slightly too incomplete in their finishing role. Membranes remain loaded with a substrate balance more prepared for initiation than completion. The next trigger then arrives in a site already leaning toward activation. That means less provocation is needed to produce more response. This is why chronic inflammatory states often feel like overreaction, but that word can be misleading. The body is not necessarily becoming irrational. It is becoming structurally preconditioned to interpret the world through lower activation thresholds.

This lowered-threshold state also explains why symptoms often seem disproportionate to the immediate trigger. A person eats a meal and flares. A small mechanical strain produces pain that lingers too long. Mild stress creates outsized fatigue, vascular reactivity, gut symptoms, or inflammatory discomfort. A poor night of sleep destabilizes the next day far more than expected. If these events are viewed in isolation, they look mysterious or psychosomatic. If they are viewed through the threshold model, they become more coherent. The tissue was already primed. The membrane was already unstable enough, the barrier already open enough, the mediator reservoir already biased enough, and the cleanup burden already high enough that a modest additional input was sufficient to reopen the inflammatory program. The trigger is real, but the scale of the response depends on the condition of the system receiving it.

This is where the relevance of specialized pro-resolving mediators becomes even sharper. SPMs are not only important because they help end ongoing inflammation. They are important because successful resolution helps restore threshold. When neutrophil infiltration stops appropriately, when macrophages clear debris efficiently, when oxidized membrane remnants are removed, when barriers regain selective control, and when tissue stops carrying so much visible evidence of unfinished danger, the threshold for reactivation rises again. The body no longer needs to defend so quickly because the tissue no longer looks so unstable. Resolution therefore does more than conclude a current event. It changes the starting conditions of the next event. It helps rebuild a body that is harder to alarm unnecessarily and easier to return to baseline after normal life stressors.

This is also why anti-inflammatory suppression so often fails to solve the deeper threshold problem. Suppression may reduce the intensity of visible inflammatory output, but if the structural residue of inflammation remains in place, the threshold often stays low. Debris remains uncleared. Barriers remain weak. Membranes remain oxidatively fragile. Mitochondria remain strained. The tissue becomes quieter for a time, but not more stable in its underlying architecture. Once suppression lifts or a new trigger appears, the low threshold reveals itself again. The person flares not because the old symptoms returned from nowhere, but because the tissue never truly regained the structural conditions that would have made it harder to trigger in the first place.

Diet becomes especially important here because threshold is partly built from long-term membrane composition. A body remodeled under omega-6 dominance, oxidative instability, poor omega-3 incorporation, glycemic volatility, and repeated inflammatory signaling will carry lower thresholds across multiple tissues. Endothelial surfaces become more reactive. Gut barriers become easier to disturb. Immune receptors become easier to activate. Nociceptive systems remain more easily sensitized. On the other side, a body with better substrate balance, better barrier integrity, preserved omega-3-derived resolution capacity, and more competent mitochondrial support can tolerate the same daily inputs without crossing into disproportionate inflammatory response. This is one reason threshold is such a useful concept. It connects the visible moment of flare to the invisible architecture built over time.

The threshold problem also clarifies why healing often feels nonlinear. A person may improve overall and still have episodes that seem out of proportion. That does not necessarily mean nothing changed. It may mean the threshold has risen, but not yet enough across all tissues, all barriers, and all membrane systems to produce stable resilience under every condition. Some reservoirs remain unresolved. Some structural prerequisites remain incomplete. Some tissues have rebuilt faster than others. Threshold is therefore not a single switch. It is a distributed property of the organism. Different tissues may have different activation points, different cleanup efficiencies, and different vulnerabilities to re-triggering. Healing means those thresholds gradually rise and synchronize into a more stable whole.

Seen clearly, revisiting the threshold problem after the full discussion of membrane composition, SPM biology, and failed resolution reveals that threshold is not just where inflammation starts. It is where structure, memory, and signal pressure meet. A body with low thresholds is not merely sensitive in a vague sense. It is a body carrying unresolved architecture. A body with restored thresholds is not simply calmer. It is a body whose membranes, barriers, substrate pools, cleanup systems, and mitochondrial support have been rebuilt enough that ordinary life no longer keeps crossing into emergency interpretation. The real solution to the threshold problem is therefore not simply fewer triggers. It is better completion, better cleanup, better membrane composition, and better structural control, so that the next input is received by a body that no longer mistakes every disturbance for a threat that cannot be finished.

Why Low Omega-3 Intake Fails to Generate SPMs

Low omega-3 intake fails to generate meaningful specialized pro-resolving mediator output for a simple reason at the most basic level: the body cannot derive a strong downstream signal from precursor material it never meaningfully stored. Resolvins, protectins, and maresins are not created from wishful physiology. They are derived from EPA and DHA that have first been absorbed, transported, incorporated into membrane phospholipids, and preserved there as part of the tissue's future signaling reserve. If intake remains low, membrane incorporation remains low. If membrane incorporation remains low, the releasable omega-3 substrate pool remains thin. And if that substrate pool remains thin, then when inflammation begins and phospholipases mobilize fatty acids from the membrane, the body has relatively little EPA and DHA available to route into pro-resolving pathways. The inflammatory sequence can still start, because omega-6-derived initiation substrate is usually plentiful. What becomes weak is the biochemical material needed to support a strong finish.

This is why low omega-3 intake is not just a dietary deficiency in the abstract. It is a structural deficiency in future inflammatory control. The membrane is the reservoir from which later lipid mediators are drawn. A tissue chronically under-supplied with omega-3 does not merely have less omega-3 in circulation. It builds a phospholipid environment that is relatively poor in the precursors required for E-series resolvins, D-series resolvins, protectins, and maresins. That means the tissue enters every inflammatory event carrying less completion-capable substrate from the beginning. It still retains access to arachidonic-acid-heavy eicosanoid initiation chemistry, so it can recruit, amplify, sensitize, and increase permeability. But it lacks comparable depth in the later-phase lipid language required to reduce continued neutrophil influx, enhance macrophage cleanup, protect tissue, and restore order. The result is not only more initiation. It is weaker closure.

Low intake also matters because short-term presence is not enough. EPA and DHA have to become part of the membrane architecture over time. A person who chronically underconsumes omega-3 is not just missing a nutrient in daily intake terms. They are failing to build and maintain the membrane reservoir from which SPM production later depends. This is one reason the effects of omega-3 status are often delayed and cumulative. The body does not generate a strong pro-resolving system from occasional exposure. It generates it from repeated incorporation and phospholipid remodeling. When intake stays low for long enough, tissues are remodeled in the opposite direction. The membrane remains more heavily defined by other fatty acid classes, especially omega-6-derived substrate, and the future mediator landscape becomes biased toward escalation rather than resolution.

There is another level to this as well, which is substrate competition. In a body with low omega-3 intake, the problem is not only that EPA and DHA are scarce. It is that the shared membrane and enzymatic spaces are filled by something else. Arachidonic-acid-related substrate continues occupying phospholipid positions and continues dominating downstream COX and LOX traffic during inflammatory activation. That means low omega-3 intake weakens SPM generation in two directions at once. It reduces the availability of the necessary precursor, and it allows competing substrate to remain relatively dominant in the same structural and enzymatic territory. The body therefore becomes increasingly practiced at generating the front half of inflammation and increasingly underbuilt in the back half.

This is especially important because SPM generation is not a luxury pathway. It is part of how the body prevents early-phase inflammatory force from becoming chronic tissue damage. Low omega-3 intake leaves the body with less material for mediator class switching, less support for downstream conversion into pro-resolving families, and less capacity to push macrophages toward efficient efferocytosis and tissue cleanup. In practical terms, the body can still call for help, but it has less biochemical authority to tell the site when enough help has arrived. It can still inflame, but it resolves with less force and less precision.

Seen clearly, low omega-3 intake fails to generate SPMs because SPM biology is built on stored precursor abundance inside membranes, not on vague nutritional virtue. If EPA and DHA are not meaningfully supplied, they are not meaningfully incorporated. If they are not meaningfully incorporated, they are not meaningfully releasable during inflammation. If they are not meaningfully releasable, downstream conversion into resolvins, protectins, and maresins remains weak. The body then enters inflammation with a full ignition system and an underbuilt braking system. That is the deeper consequence of low omega-3 intake. It does not just reduce one beneficial nutrient. It lowers the body's structural ability to complete inflammation as a successful program.

Membrane Saturation Thresholds

Membrane saturation thresholds refer to the point at which the fatty acid composition of a membrane stops being a neutral background detail and begins determining whether that membrane behaves as a stable control surface or as a structurally fragile, overly reactive, or poorly adaptable one. The term saturation here is not just about how much saturated fat is present. It is about the overall degree of fatty acid saturation versus unsaturation built into phospholipid architecture, and therefore about how tightly the membrane packs, how easily it oxidizes, how mobile its proteins remain, how permeable it becomes under stress, and how its stored lipid reservoir will behave once inflammatory activation begins. A membrane does not need to be all one thing to cross a threshold. It only needs to become compositionally weighted enough in one direction that its behavior starts changing in a decisive way.

This matters because membranes are not infinitely tolerant of compositional drift. A membrane enriched too heavily in highly unsaturated fatty acids may gain signaling flexibility and dynamic fluidity, but beyond a certain point it also becomes easier to peroxidize, easier to disturb, and easier to convert into a chemically noisy surface under oxidative or inflammatory stress. A membrane enriched too heavily in saturated structure may gain durability and resistance to oxidative injury, but beyond a certain point it may also lose some of the fluid behavior needed for receptor clustering, vesicle fusion, signal propagation, and adaptive membrane remodeling in certain tissues. The body therefore operates within functional thresholds. It is not aiming for maximal saturation or maximal unsaturation. It is aiming for enough structural firmness to preserve order and enough fluid responsiveness to preserve function. When the membrane crosses too far in either direction, tissue behavior begins to change.

The relevance to resolution biology is direct. A membrane that sits below the threshold of usable stability becomes too vulnerable to the very inflammatory sequence it is supposed to survive. Oxidative stress damages its polyunsaturated components too easily. Receptors begin reading inputs through a noisier surface. Phospholipase release draws from a reservoir that may be rich in signaling potential but chemically fragile. Under those conditions, the membrane may carry omega-3-derived substrate in theory while still failing to preserve that substrate well enough for strong downstream SPM generation in practice. Resolution potential drops because the membrane crosses a threshold where unsaturation is no longer serving mainly as strategic signaling material. It is becoming a liability under load.

At the same time, membrane saturation thresholds are tissue-specific. Neural tissue, immune cells, endothelial surfaces, epithelial barriers, and mitochondrial membranes are not solving the same structural problem. The brain and retina require membrane behavior that would not be optimal if every phospholipid surface were built for maximal rigidity. Immune cells need enough membrane adaptability to reorganize receptors, form synapses, engulf debris, and transition between activation states. Mitochondria need inner membranes capable of preserving gradients while still maintaining specialized curvature and protein organization. That means the threshold is not one global number. It is a functional boundary defined by what that tissue must do and how much chemical stress it is under while doing it.

This is why membrane saturation thresholds should be understood less as a dietary slogan and more as a systems principle. The real question is not whether a membrane is saturated or unsaturated in a simplistic sense. The real question is whether the membrane has crossed into a region where its structure now undermines its own signaling and recovery capacity. If it becomes too unsaturated relative to oxidative protection, the tissue becomes easier to inflame and harder to resolve. If it becomes too rigid relative to its signaling demands, the tissue may preserve order at the cost of responsiveness and adaptive function. Health lies in maintaining a composition that keeps the membrane below the threshold of fragility and below the threshold of maladaptive rigidity at the same time.

Seen through the lens of this book, membrane saturation thresholds help explain why lipid biology cannot be reduced to a battle between saturated fat and polyunsaturated fat. The body requires both stability and dynamic signaling substrate. It requires membranes firm enough to survive inflammatory stress and flexible enough to carry out the receptor, transport, and mediator functions that living tissues depend on. The critical issue is where the membrane sits relative to its functional threshold. When it remains inside a stable range, resolution potential is preserved because omega-3-derived substrate can be stored, protected, and later converted into meaningful pro-resolving output. When it drifts too far toward instability, that same substrate becomes too easy to damage. The body then loses not only structural coherence, but part of its ability to end inflammation from the membrane level upward.

Non-Linear Conversion to SPMs

Conversion to specialized pro-resolving mediators is non-linear because the body does not turn EPA and DHA into resolvins, protectins, and maresins in a smooth, proportional, always-on way. More precursor does not automatically produce more SPMs in a simple straight line. The pathway behaves more like a conditional system with thresholds, bottlenecks, timing gates, and phase-dependent shifts. EPA and DHA have to be present in the right membrane pools, released at the right time, routed through the right enzymes, and processed inside a tissue environment that has actually transitioned far enough beyond early inflammatory escalation to allow pro-resolving chemistry to matter. If any of those conditions are missing, more omega-3 can still increase structural potential without producing a proportionate increase in downstream SPM output. This is why people often misunderstand omega-3 biology. They assume substrate behaves like a dosage-response drug. In reality, the body treats SPM generation more like a context-sensitive phase change.

The first reason the conversion is non-linear is substrate threshold. Very low EPA and DHA incorporation produces very little meaningful SPM-generating capacity because the membrane reservoir is simply too thin. But once membrane levels rise to a more functional range, the tissue may suddenly gain much greater access to downstream mediator generation because enough precursor is now available in the releasable phospholipid pool to influence class switching and later-phase signaling. That means the early part of the curve can be flat, then a more meaningful shift appears once a certain degree of incorporation has been achieved. In other words, small increases at low tissue levels may not produce obvious resolution effects, while the same increase at a higher baseline may matter much more because the membrane has crossed from token presence into functional availability.

The second reason is enzymatic competition. EPA and DHA are not converted in isolation. They compete with omega-6-derived substrate, especially arachidonic acid, inside shared COX and LOX pathways. If a tissue remains heavily dominated by arachidonic-acid-heavy membrane composition and early-phase inflammatory signaling, then additional EPA and DHA may produce relatively modest downstream change at first because the enzymatic traffic is still crowded by initiation chemistry. Then, once membrane composition shifts enough or inflammatory tone changes enough, the same amount of added precursor may begin to exert a much larger effect because the competition landscape has changed. This is another form of non-linearity. The system can remain resistant for a while, then become more responsive once substrate balance crosses a meaningful threshold.

Timing makes the curve even less linear. SPMs are not generated as though the body were constantly trying to maximize resolution chemistry under all conditions. They belong to a later phase of the inflammatory sequence. Early in inflammation, the tissue is usually prioritizing initiation and amplification. Only later, if the event is progressing properly, does mediator class switching begin favoring pro-resolving output. That means a person can have reasonable EPA and DHA incorporation and still produce little SPM activity in a given moment if the tissue has not yet entered the phase where resolution pathways are supposed to dominate. The same substrate therefore has different consequences depending on when in the inflammatory sequence it is being mobilized. Time is built into the conversion curve.

Oxidative stability adds another layer of non-linearity. EPA and DHA are highly unsaturated and therefore vulnerable to peroxidation. In a relatively stable tissue environment, increased incorporation can raise the reservoir for SPM production. In a highly oxidized environment, however, part of that added substrate may be damaged before it can be cleanly converted into useful pro-resolving mediators. That means the relationship between stored omega-3 and actual SPM output may flatten, stall, or even become inefficient when oxidative stress is too high. The tissue may contain more precursor on paper without gaining proportionate resolution capacity in practice. The system is being pushed from one side by substrate availability and from the other by substrate fragility.

Cell type and tissue phenotype also matter. A macrophage in an effective resolving phenotype does not handle DHA and EPA the same way as a tissue still dominated by neutrophil-heavy recruitment, endothelial activation, and early cytokine escalation. The same precursor pool can therefore produce different downstream mediator behavior depending on which cells are active, what phase the tissue is in, and whether the site is organized around cleanup or continued defense. This is one reason conversion looks inconsistent from the outside. It is not inconsistent at the biological level. It is conditional. The precursor is entering different local systems with different probabilities of routing into SPM production.

This helps explain why the benefits of omega-3 often appear delayed, threshold-like, or context-dependent rather than steadily proportional. Structural incorporation may rise before mediator output changes dramatically.

Mediator output may rise before tissue-level clinical improvement becomes obvious. In another case, membrane incorporation may improve while SPM production remains weak because the person is still living inside repeated gut-triggered immune activation, oxidative overload, poor mitochondrial support, or omega-6-dominant competition. Then, once one of those constraints improves, the same precursor pool begins producing a larger biological effect. That is classic non-linear behavior. The system is not responding to one variable in isolation. It is responding to a network of gates.

Seen clearly, non-linear conversion to SPMs means the body does not resolve inflammation according to a simple input-output equation. It resolves when membrane substrate, enzymatic access, oxidative protection, inflammatory timing, immune phenotype, and tissue stability align strongly enough that EPA- and DHA-derived mediators can actually take command of the later phase. More precursor helps, but only within that larger architecture. The real lesson is that omega-3 should not be judged by a straight-line expectation. Its deepest effects emerge when enough structural and biochemical conditions are met that the system can cross from merely carrying resolution substrate to actually converting that substrate into the chemistry of completion.

The Concept of Resolution Activation

Resolution activation is the point at which the body stops treating inflammation as a problem of force generation and starts treating it as a problem of completion. That shift sounds subtle, but it marks a real biological transition. In early inflammation, the system is organized around access, recruitment, amplification, and acute defense. Blood vessels open. Neutrophils arrive. Eicosanoid cascades intensify. Pain thresholds drop. Oxidative chemistry rises. The tissue is prioritizing control of the threat. Resolution activation begins when the tissue receives and successfully acts on a different class of instruction, one that says further escalation is no longer the smartest use of energy or structure. At that point, the biology of the site changes. Recruitment begins to taper. Macrophage cleanup gains priority. Barrier restoration becomes possible. The inflammatory event stops being an expanding reaction and starts becoming a controlled dismantling of the reaction itself.

This is important because resolution is often described as though it begins automatically once the trigger fades. That is too passive. Resolution activation implies that the body must actually cross into a later phase. It has to turn on the mechanisms of closure with enough strength that they can overtake the inertia of the earlier inflammatory program. In practical terms, that means enough EPA and DHA must already be stored in membrane phospholipids, enough of that substrate must be released and converted downstream into specialized pro-resolving mediators, and the cellular environment must be ready to respond to those mediators. Neutrophil-heavy logic has to stop dominating. Macrophages must become better finishers. Endothelial and epithelial surfaces must begin closing rather than continuing to open. The tissue has to receive a credible biochemical message that the emergency phase is no longer primary. Resolution activation is that moment of phase command.

This concept helps explain why so many inflammatory conditions persist even when the body is no longer facing a major acute insult. The issue is often not that inflammation cannot decline at all. The issue is that the body never fully activates the later program strongly enough to take control. It remains in a low-grade state of initiation and amplification, repeatedly restarting the first half of inflammation because the second half never becomes dominant. Debris remains. Barriers remain weak. Oxidized membrane fragments remain visible. Pain remains justified. The tissue may show partial improvement, but it does not cross the threshold into organized closure. Resolution activation therefore means more than having some SPMs present. It means having enough pro-resolving pressure, enough structural stability, and enough metabolic support that the tissue actually switches from escalation mode into completion mode.

This also makes clear why resolution activation is a threshold phenomenon rather than a gentle linear fade. A tissue may carry some omega-3-derived substrate and still remain stuck because the inflammatory environment is too dominated by arachidonic-acid-heavy signaling, oxidative damage, enzymatic crowding, or repeated re-triggering. Then, once membrane composition improves enough, cleanup burden drops enough, barrier function improves enough, or mitochondrial support rises enough, the same tissue can begin behaving differently in a way that looks disproportionate to the size of the change. That is because the system has crossed from insufficient late-phase influence into sufficient late-phase influence. Resolution is no longer just possible in theory. It is activated in practice.

Seen clearly, the concept of resolution activation gives the back half of inflammation the same seriousness usually given to the front half. Initiation has triggers. Amplification has cascades. Resolution also has an activation point. It is not a passive settling. It is the moment when the body begins issuing a different command: stop recruiting, start clearing, stop expanding, start restoring, stop defending as though the danger is still growing, and start rebuilding as though the danger can now be finished. That is what makes resolution a real biological phase rather than just the absence of one.

PART V

EPA AND DHA THROUGH THE SPM LENS

Chapter 14

EPA-Derived Resolvins (E-Series)

EPA-derived resolvins, often grouped as the E-series, are one of the clearest examples of how omega-3 becomes biologically important only when it is understood as precursor material for phase transition rather than as a generic anti-inflammatory input. EPA by itself is not the resolution event. EPA is the stored substrate from which a family of later-phase signals can be generated once the tissue has moved far enough beyond initiation that continued escalation is no longer the correct priority. E-series resolvins matter because they help the body change the instructions governing an inflamed site. They reduce the continuation of neutrophil-heavy recruitment, alter the inflammatory environment away from repeated expansion, and support the shift toward cleanup, containment, and restored control. In that sense, EPA-derived resolvins are not merely softer inflammatory molecules. They are part of the body's machinery for deciding that enough acute force has already been used.

The distinction between EPA and the E-series it can generate is critical because it keeps the biology from collapsing into supplement language. A person can consume EPA and still fail to produce strong resolution behavior if EPA is not incorporated meaningfully into membrane phospholipids, if the releasable pool remains too small, if enzymatic competition from arachidonic-acid-heavy substrate remains too strong, or if the tissue never enters the phase in which pro-resolving mediator generation is supposed to take command. But when EPA is meaningfully incorporated and the tissue does transition, the E-series provides one of the main downstream routes by which omega-3 begins to exert true resolution influence. This is why the earlier chapters emphasized precursor logic so heavily. EPA is not the finished answer. The E-series is one of the ways the body turns EPA into an answer.

One of the most important actions of E-series resolvins is the reduction of further neutrophil recruitment. This matters because neutrophils are useful at the beginning and expensive after that. Their continued arrival brings oxidants, proteases, membrane injury, endothelial disruption, and an increased burden of apoptotic cells that must later be cleared. A tissue cannot resolve while it is still being continuously restocked with acute-phase machinery. E-series resolvins help interrupt that continuation. They reduce the conditions that keep inviting more neutrophils into a site that no longer benefits from their presence. In practice, this means the tissue begins to move away from active reinforcement and toward controlled drawdown. That is one of the most practical meanings of EPA-derived resolution. The site is no longer asking for more force. It is beginning to ask for less interference.

The E-series also helps shift macrophage behavior in the direction of cleanup rather than continued inflammatory participation. This is essential because inflammation cannot end simply by stopping new recruitment. The tissue must also remove the remains of the inflammatory event that has already occurred. Macrophages have to become better at engulfing apoptotic neutrophils and processing debris before those materials become fresh inflammatory stimulus. EPA-derived resolvins contribute to that handoff. They support the transition from an environment dominated by arrival and amplification into one dominated by clearance and closure. In this way, the E-series does not merely restrain inflammation. It helps make the site more finishable.

Another reason the E-series matters is that it changes the character of lipid mediator output without requiring the body to abandon inflammatory competence. EPA competes within the same broad biochemical landscape that otherwise heavily processes arachidonic acid, which means EPA-derived pathways can alter what kinds of signals become available when phospholipases release fatty acids from the membrane. This is important because the body does not need less signaling in the abstract. It needs different signaling once the acute phase has done enough. The E-series helps provide that difference. It does not erase the logic of host defense. It changes what the tissue is being told to do after host defense has already been launched.

This also explains why EPA-derived resolvins are especially relevant in tissues caught in chronic low-grade inflammatory repetition. Many such tissues do not lack activation signals. They are saturated with them. What they lack is enough later-phase biochemical influence to stop the repeated renewal of early-phase recruitment and vascular openness. The E-series becomes important here because it contributes to the molecular pressure required to shift the site away from perpetual reinforcement. A tissue with access to EPA-derived resolvins is better equipped to reduce further inflammatory traffic, improve cleanup efficiency, and begin reclaiming structural order after an inflammatory event. A tissue poor in that capacity may still inflame vigorously while remaining weak in the chemistry needed to stand down.

Seen clearly, Chapter 14 is not really about a niche lipid subclass. It is about one of the major ways the body turns stored EPA into the language of closure. The E-series helps stop the unnecessary continuation of inflammation without suppressing the useful fact of immune defense itself. It reduces new neutrophil entry, supports macrophage cleanup, changes the downstream mediator environment, and strengthens the shift from escalation into completion. EPA matters because it can become this. Without that downstream possibility, EPA remains just another membrane fatty acid. With it, EPA becomes part of the body's capacity to finish what inflammation began.

Eicosapentaenoic Acid Pathways

Eicosapentaenoic acid enters physiology through several linked pathways, and its importance depends on how those pathways connect structure to later signaling rather than on EPA existing as an isolated molecule in circulation. Once absorbed, transported, and incorporated into membrane phospholipids, EPA becomes part of the cell's stored lipid environment. At that stage it is already doing two things at once. It is altering membrane behavior by changing the local phospholipid composition, and it is becoming part of the releasable substrate pool that can later be mobilized during inflammatory activation. EPA therefore does not matter only because of what it can become downstream. It also matters because it changes the structural context from which downstream decisions will later be made.

The first major EPA pathway is competitive incorporation into phospholipid membranes. This matters because EPA does not enter empty tissue. It enters membranes already carrying other fatty acids, especially omega-6-derived substrate that may already dominate inflammatory potential. If EPA incorporation becomes meaningful, it changes the future composition of the releasable pool. When phospholipases are activated during tissue stress, there is now a greater chance that EPA will be among the fatty acids released from membrane phospholipids rather than the site drawing almost exclusively from arachidonic-acid-heavy stores. This is the first way EPA shifts inflammatory biology. It changes the reservoir before the event, which means it changes the probabilities during the event.

The second major pathway is EPA entry into eicosanoid-producing systems. Once liberated from membranes, EPA can compete with arachidonic acid for cyclooxygenase and lipoxygenase processing. This does not remove inflammatory signaling from the system. It changes the chemical options available within that system. The tissue can now generate EPA-derived lipid mediators rather than relying only on arachidonic-acid-derived products. That shift matters because the mediator field becomes less exclusively weighted toward the initiation-heavy language of prostaglandins, leukotrienes, thromboxanes, and related compounds produced from omega-6-dominant substrate. EPA therefore alters inflammatory output partly by changing what the enzyme systems are being asked to work on. It is not replacing signaling with silence. It is shifting signaling toward a different substrate base.

The third pathway is the generation of E-series resolvins. This is where EPA becomes especially important in the context of resolution. Once EPA has been incorporated into phospholipids, released under the right conditions, and routed through the appropriate downstream enzymatic sequences, it can be converted into E-series specialized pro-resolving mediators. These molecules are part of the later inflammatory phase. They help reduce further neutrophil recruitment, improve the shift away from repeated amplification, and support the handoff toward macrophage-led cleanup and closure. This is why EPA should not be called merely anti-inflammatory. Its deeper significance is that it feeds a pathway capable of helping inflammation finish rather than simply continue under a slightly weaker form.

EPA pathways also matter because they operate inside competition and timing, not in a vacuum. A person may increase EPA intake and still see only partial downstream effect if arachidonic-acid-heavy substrate remains dominant in membranes, if COX and LOX pathways remain crowded by early-phase inflammatory traffic, or if the tissue never truly enters the stage where mediator class switching toward resolution can take command. This makes EPA biology non-linear. Small increases in intake may produce little visible change at first. Then, once membrane incorporation rises enough or inflammatory burden shifts enough, the same EPA presence can begin exerting much stronger downstream effects because the pathway has crossed from theoretical availability into functional influence.

There is also a structural-protective dimension to EPA pathways. EPA is less unsaturated than DHA, which means it participates somewhat differently in membrane behavior and oxidative vulnerability, but it is still a highly unsaturated fatty acid and therefore still requires a tissue environment capable of preserving it. If oxidative stress remains high, if membranes are repeatedly injured, or if mitochondrial dysfunction keeps tissues chemically unstable, EPA may be present without being fully preserved as clean substrate for orderly downstream conversion. In that case the EPA pathway is not absent, but it is compromised. The tissue carries some of the precursor, yet remains too unstable to route it efficiently into strong pro-resolving output.

Seen clearly, eicosapentaenoic acid pathways begin with incorporation, continue through substrate competition, extend into altered eicosanoid production, and culminate most meaningfully in the generation of E-series resolvins. EPA changes membranes first, signaling options second, and inflammatory sequencing third. It is not a terminal molecule with one fixed function. It is part of a pathway architecture that determines whether a tissue remains fluent only in escalation or gains stronger access to the chemistry of completion.

Vascular and Immune Resolution

Vascular and immune resolution are inseparable because inflammation is never only a matter of immune cells entering tissue. It is also a matter of whether the vascular system continues behaving like an open emergency corridor or regains the selective control required for tissue to stop functioning as an inflammatory zone. Early inflammation deliberately alters blood vessels. Endothelial cells change adhesion behavior, permeability rises, local blood flow shifts, and the tissue becomes easier for neutrophils, monocytes, plasma proteins, and signaling molecules to enter. That is useful at the beginning because access is part of defense. But if vascular behavior remains locked in that state after the acute need has passed, the tissue cannot resolve. It stays too open, too exposed, too fluid-shifted, and too available for repeated immune traffic. Vascular resolution therefore means the blood-facing surfaces of the tissue stop acting as if more recruitment is still needed. They begin closing the gate without trapping unresolved debris behind it.

This matters because immune resolution cannot succeed while vascular permissiveness remains high. A tissue may begin generating some pro-resolving signals, but if endothelial surfaces still favor leukocyte adhesion and extravasation, fresh inflammatory cells keep arriving into an environment that should be transitioning into cleanup. The result is that clearance and re-entry overlap in a way that prevents completion. Specialized pro-resolving mediators help interrupt that pattern by changing both sides of the equation at once. On the immune side, they reduce continued neutrophil recruitment and improve macrophage-led cleanup. On the vascular side, they help shift the tissue away from emergency openness and toward tighter regulation of permeability, adhesion, and local inflammatory spread. This is what makes resolution a systems event rather than a single-cell event. The blood vessel has to stop supplying an acute-phase environment at the same time the immune system stops demanding one.

The vascular dimension is especially important because chronic inflammation often persists through microvascular disorder long after the original insult should have been contained. When endothelial behavior remains abnormal, tissue edema can persist, nutrient and oxygen handling become less stable, local inflammatory mediators spread more easily, and the mechanical environment of the tissue remains distorted. In that state, even good immune cleanup becomes harder because the site is still physically behaving like a place under active siege. Vascular resolution therefore is not just about less redness or less swelling. It is about restoring the physical terms under which tissue can return to orderly exchange rather than remaining a zone of exaggerated access and biochemical leakage.

Immune resolution, on the other hand, means the inflammatory cell population changes jobs. Neutrophils stop arriving in excess. Existing neutrophils proceed toward apoptosis rather than prolonged destructive persistence. Macrophages shift from amplification and inflammatory participation toward efferocytosis, debris clearance, and repair-compatible signaling. Cytokine tone changes. The tissue stops asking for reinforcement and starts processing the remains of what reinforcement already did. This is why vascular and immune resolution have to be synchronized. If the immune system shifts toward cleanup but the vessels stay open, new inflammatory cells continue entering. If the vessels begin tightening but immune cleanup remains poor, debris stays trapped and the site remains biochemically unfinished. Resolution requires that access and activity both be reprogrammed together.

This is one of the clearest places where EPA-derived and broader omega-3-derived mediator biology becomes meaningful. E-series resolvins and the wider SPM family do not merely soften inflammation in the abstract. They help change the operating logic of the vascular-immune interface. They reduce the continuation of neutrophil trafficking, support macrophage function, and help the endothelial surface stop behaving like an inflammatory invitation. That combined effect is what makes tissue more capable of leaving the front half of inflammation behind. The body is no longer just producing fewer inflammatory signals. It is reorganizing who can enter, what they do when they arrive, and when the site is allowed to stop receiving more acute-phase support.

Seen clearly, vascular and immune resolution are two sides of the same closing movement. The immune system must stop escalating and start clearing. The vasculature must stop opening and start containing. Together, they convert an inflamed tissue from a place built for emergency traffic into a place built for restoration. Without that paired transition, inflammation remains partially open even when its visible intensity drops. With it, the body gains the ability to end defense without leaving the site unfinished.

Inflammatory Tone Modulation

Inflammatory tone modulation refers to the body's ability to change the background intensity, sensitivity, and persistence of inflammatory signaling without simply switching immunity on or off. Tone is the right word because this is not about one isolated event. It is about the baseline pressure carried by the tissue before, during, and after specific triggers. A tissue with a high inflammatory tone is easier to activate, quicker to amplify, slower to calm, and more likely to interpret ordinary biological friction as meaningful threat. A tissue with a well-regulated inflammatory tone can still defend itself rapidly when needed, but it does not remain chemically tense when the threat is absent or already contained. Specialized pro-resolving mediators contribute to this modulation by changing the conditions that keep inflammatory intensity elevated beyond its useful phase. They do not abolish immune responsiveness. They lower the chronic background pressure that makes tissues feel primed for repeated escalation.

This matters because chronic illness often involves not just discrete inflammatory episodes, but a persistent elevation in inflammatory readiness. Cytokine signals remain slightly elevated, endothelial surfaces remain slightly more adhesive, nociceptive pathways remain slightly more sensitized, macrophages remain slightly more biased toward inflammatory participation, and membranes remain slightly more loaded with the evidence of unresolved danger. None of these deviations may look dramatic in isolation, but together they create a tissue climate in which the threshold for fresh inflammatory activation drops. Tone modulation is therefore one of the most important functions of the resolution phase. The body is not only trying to stop one event. It is trying to reset the background conditions that would otherwise make the next event too easy to start.

SPMs influence inflammatory tone by reducing continued neutrophil recruitment, improving macrophage cleanup, limiting collateral injury, and helping restore barrier and vascular control. Each of those actions lowers the amount of unresolved inflammatory residue a tissue carries forward. As that residue falls, the tissue stops presenting itself as chronically unfinished. Receptors encounter less damage-associated noise. Oxidized lipid fragments become less abundant. Endothelial surfaces stop behaving as though they must remain in open-access mode. Nociceptive systems lose some of the inflammatory evidence that justified sustained amplification. Tone falls not because the immune system has been weakened, but because the tissue has become less crowded with the biochemical reasons for continued alertness.

This is one reason inflammatory tone modulation is different from anti-inflammatory suppression. Suppression can reduce visible inflammatory output while leaving the tissue structurally primed for rapid reactivation. Tone modulation changes the priming itself. It raises the threshold for inappropriate activation by helping remove the conditions that keep the tissue on edge. That is why it belongs so centrally to resolution biology. The healthier body is not the body that cannot inflame. It is the body that does not remain unnecessarily inflamed between genuine needs for defense. SPMs help create that state by reducing the background pressure of unresolved inflammation and restoring a tissue environment that no longer behaves as though emergency is its default setting.

Cardiometabolic Implications

The cardiometabolic implications of failed resolution are enormous because the cardiovascular system and the metabolic system are both built on membranes, vascular surfaces, immune surveillance, and fuel-handling logic that are highly sensitive to inflammatory tone. When resolution works well, vascular tissue can mount a proportionate response to injury or stress, clear the resulting debris, restore endothelial control, and return to a lower-noise state without remaining chronically reactive. Metabolic tissues can handle substrate flux, postprandial signaling, adipose expansion, mitochondrial demand, and immune traffic without becoming locked in defensive chemistry. When resolution fails, those same tissues begin living in a state of partial alarm. Endothelial surfaces remain more adhesive and more permeable than they should be. Immune cells continue trafficking into places where cleanup never fully finished. Oxidized lipids and damaged membrane fragments remain visible. Adipose tissue continues signaling distress. The liver remains biochemically crowded. Muscle and vascular tissues become less metabolically flexible. In that environment, the body does not simply have inflammation. It develops a chronic cardiometabolic pattern built from unresolved inflammation.

The vascular side of this is especially important. Endothelium is not passive plumbing. It is a living membrane surface that constantly interprets shear stress, circulating lipids, glucose excursions, immune signals, and oxidative burden. A well-resolved vascular system maintains selective permeability, controlled leukocyte interaction, and a relatively quiet inflammatory baseline. A poorly resolved vascular system does the opposite. It remains easier for immune cells to adhere, easier for inflammatory signals to propagate, easier for oxidized lipid material to distort local behavior, and harder for the vessel wall to return to a truly resting state after repeated insults. This matters because the earliest stages of vascular dysfunction are often not dramatic obstructions but persistent low-grade endothelial irritation, altered nitric oxide handling, abnormal permeability, and repeated immune engagement with the arterial wall. Resolution biology belongs here because the vessel must be able not only to react, but to stop reacting before temporary injury becomes chronic vascular remodeling.

The metabolic side follows the same logic through different tissues. Adipose tissue is not merely a storage depot. It is an immune-active, endocrine-active tissue whose inflammatory tone shapes systemic insulin sensitivity, lipolysis, hepatic fat handling, and broader cardiometabolic stability. When adipose tissue expands under conditions of poor mitochondrial handling, oxidative stress, and repeated inflammatory signaling, it begins recruiting immune cells and generating a biochemical environment more consistent with unresolved defense than with quiet storage. The liver then receives this burden through substrate overflow, inflammatory signaling, endotoxin exposure, and altered lipoprotein traffic. Skeletal muscle receives it through impaired insulin signaling, altered substrate competition, and lower metabolic flexibility. The vascular system receives it through endothelial stress and circulating inflammatory pressure. In each case, failed resolution turns ordinary fuel management into a chronic tissue-level inflammatory problem. That is why cardiometabolic dysfunction so often presents as a cluster. The same unresolved logic is being expressed across the tissues that handle flow, storage, transport, and oxidation.

SPMs matter here because cardiometabolic disease is not only a problem of excess substrate. It is a problem of unresolved tissue response to that substrate. A body can handle large amounts of energy only if it can also maintain membrane order, preserve mitochondrial function, control inflammatory traffic, and clear the byproducts of metabolic stress before those byproducts become self-sustaining danger signals. EPA- and DHA-derived pro-resolving mediators help support that later phase. They reduce continued neutrophil recruitment, improve macrophage cleanup, limit collateral tissue injury, and help endothelial and immune behavior shift away from chronic activation.

In practical terms, this means better resolution biology may help reduce the persistence of vascular inflammation, adipose immune congestion, and liver-centered inflammatory burden that otherwise keep the entire cardiometabolic system in a half-defensive state. The issue is not that SPMs are a magic cure for metabolic disease. The issue is that without adequate resolution pressure, cardiometabolic tissues keep interpreting nutrient handling and tissue stress through the chemistry of incomplete defense.

This is also where membrane composition becomes especially relevant. Cardiometabolic disease is often discussed through glucose, insulin, triglycerides, LDL, body fat, or liver enzymes, but beneath those markers sits the question of what kind of membranes these tissues are built from and what kind of inflammatory future those membranes make possible. A vascular surface built under omega-6-dominant, oxidatively unstable conditions is easier to irritate and harder to calm. A hepatocyte membrane built under chronic inflammatory load is easier to stress and harder to restore. Adipose tissue built under poor resolution conditions becomes better at recruiting immune participation than at returning to quiet storage. Muscle tissue under chronic inflammatory tone becomes less able to transition cleanly between fuels. In all of these cases, cardiometabolic dysfunction is partly the behavior of tissues whose membrane architecture has lowered their threshold for inflammatory persistence.

Seen clearly, the cardiometabolic implications are not secondary consequences of inflammation. They are one of the main places unresolved inflammation becomes clinically visible. Endothelial dysfunction, insulin resistance, fatty liver, adipose inflammation, vascular stiffness, poor recovery from metabolic stress, abnormal postprandial responses, and chronic low-grade immune activation all make more sense when viewed as failures of closure rather than as isolated marker abnormalities. The body is still capable of responding to challenge, but it is less capable of finishing that response and returning its metabolic and vascular tissues to low-noise function. That is why resolution biology belongs at the center of cardiometabolic thinking. A system that cannot complete inflammation will eventually struggle to handle fuel, flow, and tissue maintenance without turning each of them into a chronic source of danger signaling.

Chapter 15

DHA-Derived Mediators (D-Series, Protectins, Maresins)

DHA-derived mediators represent one of the most important extensions of the resolution story because they show that omega-3 biology does not end with membrane incorporation and does not end with EPA-derived pathway effects. DHA carries its own downstream significance, and that significance is especially important in tissues where membrane architecture, excitability, longevity, and protection from collateral inflammatory injury are critical. Once DHA is incorporated into phospholipids and preserved there long enough to become part of the releasable substrate pool, it can be mobilized and converted into several families of specialized pro-resolving mediators, especially D-series resolvins, protectins, and maresins. These are not redundant copies of EPA-derived biology. They deepen the resolution phase by extending it into tissue protection, macrophage-led cleanup, and restoration-compatible signaling. If EPA helps illustrate how omega-3 can begin altering inflammatory traffic and reducing continued escalation, DHA makes even clearer how omega-3 helps defend the tissue during de-escalation and helps organize the labor of repair.

This is why DHA should never be understood only as a structural lipid for the brain or retina, though it is certainly that. DHA matters structurally because it alters membrane behavior in highly specialized tissues, but it also matters because it provides precursor material for mediator classes that become especially important once the tissue has to survive its own inflammatory response without remaining trapped in it. D-series resolvins help reduce continued inflammatory recruitment and support phase transition. Protectins help limit tissue injury and preserve function while inflammation is being wound down. Maresins help drive macrophage-led cleanup and resolution-compatible reconstruction. Taken together, these mediator families make DHA one of the body's major resources not only for signaling flexibility but for resolution intelligence. The body is not just using DHA to build sensitive membranes. It is also using DHA to create a reserve of later-phase instruction that can help those membranes survive inflammatory stress and return to order afterward.

The D-series resolvins show this clearly. Like the E-series derived from EPA, the D-series participates in reducing the continuation of acute inflammatory recruitment. But their significance often becomes especially apparent in tissues where the balance between defense and collateral injury is delicate. These mediators help the body restrain unnecessary continuation of neutrophil-heavy inflammatory activity while supporting the larger shift into cleanup and control. The point is not that D-series resolvins replace all earlier inflammatory chemistry. They help move the tissue away from the idea that more early-phase force is still the solution. This is critical because many chronic inflammatory environments remain stuck precisely because that assumption never gets overturned strongly enough. D-series resolvins provide part of the molecular logic that says the emergency has reached the stage where further escalation costs more than it protects.

Protectins add another layer by emphasizing tissue preservation. This becomes especially important in systems where inflammatory collateral damage has high long-term cost, such as the nervous system, retinal tissue, vascular interfaces, and other membranes where precise signaling and structural continuity matter. Protectins help the tissue endure inflammation without giving away more function than necessary. They reduce the chance that a useful response turns into a prolonged destructive environment. In that sense, protectins are not just anti-damage molecules. They are part of the discipline of inflammation. They help ensure that when the body defends, it does not continue sacrificing tissue integrity after the useful phase of defense has already passed. This is one reason DHA-derived pathways matter so much for chronic disease. Many chronically ill tissues are not only inflamed. They are poorly protected from the consequences of staying inflamed.

Maresins extend the story even further by linking DHA directly to macrophage-led closure. Resolution does not succeed just because recruitment slows down. It succeeds when the tissue becomes physically cleaner and more rebuildable. Maresins help support that later work by improving efferocytosis, enhancing debris clearance, and encouraging macrophages to behave as finishers rather than as lingering contributors to inflammatory continuation.

This makes maresins especially important in the transition from active defense to active repair. They do not merely help inflammation stop. They help the tissue process what inflammation left behind. In practical terms, they reduce the chance that the residue of one inflammatory event becomes the trigger for the next one. This is one of the deepest reasons DHA-derived mediator biology matters. It helps prevent inflammatory history from becoming inflammatory destiny.

These mediator families also demonstrate how much resolution depends on membrane preparedness. DHA-derived mediators cannot be generated meaningfully if DHA has not first been incorporated into phospholipids in sufficient amounts and preserved there in a usable form. That means the later protective and reparative functions of the D-series, protectins, and maresins are built upstream into tissue composition. A body low in DHA is not simply lacking a beneficial nutrient. It is building membranes with less capacity to produce some of the very signals needed to protect tissue, direct cleanup, and complete the inflammatory program later. Conversely, a body that does incorporate DHA but fails to protect it from oxidative damage, or fails to move the tissue into proper later-phase conversion, may carry theoretical resolution potential that remains underexpressed in practice. DHA-derived mediator biology therefore reinforces one of the core themes of the book: the body resolves from what it has built into itself.

This is especially important in modern chronic inflammatory environments because those environments do not merely require less initiation. They require stronger tissue-level competence in preservation and closure. A body can often still initiate inflammation powerfully. The deeper problem is that the tissue remains too vulnerable to its own defense, too poor at cleanup, too unstable at the membrane level, and too easy to re-trigger after the acute event should have passed. DHA-derived mediators address exactly those weak points. They support the protection of tissue during de-escalation, the reduction of ongoing inflammatory traffic, and the cleanup behavior needed to leave the site less chemically unfinished. That is why they matter so much in a framework built around failed resolution rather than simple inflammatory excess.

Seen clearly, DHA-derived mediators are one of the strongest arguments against reducing omega-3 biology to the phrase anti-inflammatory. D-series resolvins, protectins, and maresins are not generic dampers. They are specialized later-phase instructions for tissues that need to stop escalating, preserve function, and physically clear the remains of the inflammatory event. They explain why DHA matters not only for building specialized membranes, but for giving those membranes a better chance of surviving and recovering from inflammatory stress without being repeatedly pushed back into chronic defense. This is the deeper significance of Chapter 15. DHA is not just a structural fatty acid. It is the precursor to a family of mediators that help the body finish inflammation with more intelligence, more protection, and more effective cleanup than initiation chemistry alone could ever provide.

Neuroprotective Effects

The neuroprotective effects of DHA-derived mediators matter because nervous tissue pays a higher price for unresolved inflammation than most other tissues in the body. The brain, retina, peripheral nerves, and supporting glial environments all depend on membranes that must remain exceptionally stable while also remaining highly responsive. Neural signaling requires precise ion gradients, controlled receptor behavior, intact synaptic architecture, and membrane surfaces that can support fast electrical change without losing structural order. When inflammation enters that environment, the danger is not only the original insult. The danger is collateral damage from prolonged inflammatory chemistry, persistent oxidative stress, microglial overactivation, excitotoxic signaling, and failure to clear damaged material before it begins distorting surrounding function. Neuroprotection therefore does not mean making the nervous system inert. It means allowing defense and cleanup to occur without letting the inflammatory event degrade the very tissue that has to keep signaling accurately afterward.

This is where DHA becomes especially important. DHA is already deeply integrated into neural membranes, so its relevance begins structurally. It contributes to the physical environment of synapses, photoreceptors, and other highly specialized excitable tissues. But its deeper neuroprotective significance appears when that stored DHA becomes substrate for downstream mediator families, especially protectins and D-series resolvins. These mediators help reduce unnecessary continuation of inflammatory traffic, limit collateral injury, and support a shift away from prolonged tissue danger. In a neural context, that matters enormously because persistent inflammatory activation can destabilize membrane excitability, alter neurotransmission, impair synaptic plasticity, distort microglial behavior, and keep local signaling trapped in a defensive mode long after the initiating event should have moved into closure. DHA-derived mediators help interrupt that persistence. They do not erase neural immunity. They help stop neural defense from becoming neural damage.

The neuroprotective idea is most clear when inflammation is understood as a threat not only to neurons but to the signaling environment around them. A neuron does not function in isolation. It depends on glial regulation, vascular support, membrane integrity, mitochondrial performance, and an extracellular environment that is not chemically crowded with debris, oxidized lipids, inflammatory cytokines, or persistent danger signals. When resolution fails, that environment stays noisy. Microglia remain activated too long. Damaged membrane fragments continue signaling distress. Vascular and barrier behavior remain abnormal. Excitatory signaling can become harder to regulate. The tissue begins to lose the quiet structural conditions required for precision. Neuroprotective DHA-derived mediators matter because they help create the opposite trajectory. They support de-escalation, cleanup, and preservation of the environment in which neural signaling remains possible.

This also explains why neuroprotection is not just about reducing symptoms such as pain, fog, irritability, or hypersensitivity. Those are downstream experiences of a tissue environment that may still be carrying unresolved inflammatory evidence. A truly neuroprotective resolution response must lower the amount of ongoing structural threat to the neural membrane system itself. It must help reduce oxidative injury, improve removal of damaged cellular material, and prevent the continued recruitment or activation patterns that keep local neural tissue behaving as though the emergency is still active. Protectins are especially important here because they highlight the principle that inflammation in delicate tissues must not only be ended, but ended with minimal collateral cost. The body has to defend the nervous system while also defending it from its own defense chemistry.

Seen clearly, the neuroprotective effects of DHA-derived mediators are one of the strongest examples of why resolution is biologically more sophisticated than suppression. The nervous system does not need blunt silencing. It needs orderly exit from inflammatory stress, preservation of membrane function, and efficient cleanup of what the inflammatory event produced. DHA matters because it gives the body part of the precursor reserve required to carry out that later-phase work. In a tissue where precision is everything, the ability to resolve without shredding the signaling architecture is not a luxury. It is one of the central conditions of continued function.

Synaptic Stability and Repair

Synaptic stability and repair depend on one central fact that is too often ignored: a synapse is not just a signaling event. It is a membrane structure under repeated stress. Every round of neurotransmitter release, receptor activation, vesicle docking, membrane fusion, ion flux, and structural remodeling places demands on a highly specialized lipid environment that has to remain coherent while changing rapidly. A synapse cannot function well if its membranes are too rigid to reorganize, too unstable to preserve receptor architecture, too oxidized to maintain signaling precision, or too inflamed to return to baseline after activation. This is why synaptic biology belongs inside the larger membrane-resolution framework. The synapse does not merely transmit information. It survives transmission through structure, and when that structure is chronically exposed to unresolved inflammation, oxidative damage, and poor lipid support, signaling becomes noisier, less stable, and harder to repair once disrupted.

DHA is especially important here because synaptic membranes require a degree of dynamic flexibility and curvature control that simpler membrane models do not capture well. The presynaptic terminal has to package neurotransmitter into vesicles, traffic those vesicles, dock them, fuse them with the membrane, recover membrane material afterward, and then repeat the process continuously. The postsynaptic side has to maintain receptor organization, scaffold interactions, local membrane excitability, and the capacity to strengthen or weaken signaling over time. None of that happens in empty space. It happens in phospholipid surfaces whose composition influences receptor mobility, membrane curvature, protein conformation, and the probability that signaling complexes assemble correctly. DHA contributes to this architecture, which means it supports synaptic performance before any downstream mediator is even produced. But its importance does not stop there. Once neural tissue is stressed, DHA can also become substrate for mediator families that help reduce collateral inflammatory injury and support a tissue environment more compatible with synaptic recovery.

Repair at the synaptic level is therefore not just about replacing damaged molecules. It is about restoring signaling order after disruption. A synapse exposed to unresolved inflammatory chemistry may accumulate oxidized lipids, altered receptor trafficking, local glial overactivation, disturbed ion handling, and persistent excitatory or inhibitory imbalance. If those conditions remain in place, the synapse can stay functionally unstable even after the original insult has faded. Synaptic repair requires cleanup of inflammatory residue, stabilization of membrane structure, reduction of ongoing oxidative pressure, normalization of receptor distribution, and restoration of the energetic support needed to maintain vesicle cycling and ion gradients. This is where resolution biology becomes essential. A synapse cannot be repaired cleanly while the surrounding neural environment still behaves as though danger is actively expanding. The tissue has to stop generating the biochemical evidence of immediate threat before precise signaling can be rebuilt.

This is also why synaptic instability often shows up first as altered function rather than obvious structural damage. The person may experience brain fog, slower cognitive recovery, increased sensory sensitivity, irritability, altered mood, reduced stress tolerance, or poor sleep regulation long before any gross lesion is visible. At the synaptic level, those changes can reflect membranes that are still intact enough to signal but not intact enough to signal cleanly. Receptors may cluster less reliably. Vesicle fusion may become less efficient. Local inflammatory tone may remain too high. Microglia may stay too ready to interpret routine activity as suspicious. The system becomes noisy before it becomes broken. Synaptic repair, then, is not just about reversing severe damage. It is also about restoring enough membrane order and enough inflammatory completion that precision returns to a system that has drifted into reactivity.

Seen clearly, synaptic stability and repair depend on the same deeper logic running through the rest of the book. The nervous system does not recover from inflammatory stress by suppression alone. It recovers when membranes are protected, inflammatory debris is cleared, glial activation is brought back under control, DHA-rich structural environments are preserved well enough to support downstream neuroprotective mediator generation, and the synapse is no longer forced to operate inside a chemically unfinished tissue. A stable synapse is not just one with the right neurotransmitters. It is one built from membranes capable of surviving activity, recovering from stress, and returning to signaling order after disturbance without remaining trapped in defensive chemistry.

Tissue Regeneration Signaling

Tissue regeneration signaling begins only after the body has decided that continued escalation is no longer the main priority. That sequence matters because regeneration is not built on top of active battlefield chemistry very well. A tissue still dominated by neutrophil influx, vascular leak, oxidized lipid fragments, proteolytic activity, and unresolved debris cannot rebuild with precision because the environment is still organized around damage control rather than structure restoration. Regeneration signaling therefore belongs to the later phase of inflammation, after recruitment has begun to taper, after macrophage cleanup has become effective enough to reduce the visible residue of injury, and after specialized pro-resolving mediators have started shifting the tissue from open emergency mode into controlled reconstruction. The body does not regenerate by simply growing new material. It regenerates by changing the meaning of the injured site from one that demands defense to one that permits rebuilding.

This change in meaning is biochemical and structural at the same time. Once resolution begins to dominate, macrophages stop acting mainly as inflammatory amplifiers and become organizers of cleanup and repair-compatible signaling. That change is crucial because macrophages do more than engulf debris. They alter the local environment in ways that make neighboring cells interpret the site differently. Epithelial cells can begin restoring barrier continuity. Endothelial surfaces can begin tightening permeability and normalizing flow relationships. Fibroblasts and other local structural cells can begin rebuilding matrix architecture under conditions that are less distorted by acute inflammatory noise. Parenchymal cells in the tissue can redirect energy away from survival and alarm signaling and toward restoration of specialized function. Regeneration signaling is therefore not one molecule giving one command. It is a coordinated shift in the entire local instruction set.

DHA-derived mediator biology becomes especially important here because regeneration requires more than reduced inflammation. It requires tissue preservation during de-escalation and competent cleanup before new structure is laid down. Maresins are particularly relevant in this context because they are closely associated with macrophage-led finishing behavior and repair-compatible transitions. They help improve efferocytosis, reduce the inflammatory burden left behind by apoptotic cells and debris, and support the move from unresolved damage toward a tissue environment that can tolerate reconstruction. Protectins contribute by limiting collateral injury in sensitive tissues so the amount of structure needing replacement does not continue expanding while repair is trying to begin. D-series resolvins help reduce continued recruitment and therefore lower the amount of fresh inflammatory disruption entering the site. Together, these mediator families do not simply calm tissue. They create the signaling conditions under which regeneration becomes biologically possible.

This is one reason tissue regeneration signaling is inseparable from membrane biology. A cell can only receive repair signals through the membrane environment it has. If that membrane remains oxidized, compositionally unstable, or saturated with the biochemical evidence of continuing danger, the cell will continue reading the local environment as hostile. Under those conditions, regeneration signaling stays weak or fragmented because the tissue has not crossed the threshold into safety. But if membrane composition supports better receptor behavior, lower oxidative instability, and stronger access to omega-3-derived pro-resolving mediator production, then the same tissue can begin shifting into a different mode. The cell is no longer reading every signal through an inflammatory surface. It begins reading through a surface that can interpret closure as real. Regeneration depends on that change in interpretation as much as it depends on any individual growth-related pathway.

Energy also defines the quality of regeneration signaling. A tissue may receive signals consistent with repair, but if mitochondrial function is too compromised, those signals cannot be executed well. Regeneration is expensive. New membrane synthesis is expensive. Matrix remodeling is expensive. Re-establishing gradients, restoring specialized protein organization, rebuilding cytoskeletal integrity, and recovering tissue-level function all require ATP. This is why chronically inflamed tissue often shows poor regeneration even when some inflammatory intensity has fallen. The site may be quieter, but it is not yet energetically capable of carrying out reconstruction at the level required. Tissue regeneration signaling therefore succeeds only when cleanup, membrane stability, vascular normalization, and mitochondrial support all converge strongly enough that the repair command can be obeyed rather than merely heard.

Seen clearly, tissue regeneration signaling is the language of a site that has successfully moved beyond pure defense. It tells the tissue that recruitment can slow, debris can be removed, structure can be preserved, and rebuilding can now become the dominant task. It is not separate from resolution. It is what resolution makes possible. Without successful inflammatory completion, regeneration remains weak, distorted, or repeatedly interrupted. With it, the tissue begins to shift from surviving injury to reorganizing itself after injury, which is the real start of repair.

Nervous System Resolution

Nervous system resolution is the process by which neural tissue exits inflammatory defense without losing the signaling precision required for continued function. That distinction matters because the nervous system cannot tolerate prolonged inflammatory disorganization the way some other tissues can. A joint can swell. A muscle can stiffen. A vascular surface can remain irritated for some time. Neural tissue pays for unresolved inflammation more quickly in the currency of signal distortion. Ion gradients become less stable. Synaptic timing becomes less precise. Glial surveillance becomes more reactive. Membranes become more vulnerable to oxidative disruption. Pain pathways remain amplified. Sensory thresholds drift. Mood, cognition, sleep, attention, autonomic tone, and stress responsiveness all begin to reflect a tissue that has not truly finished its inflammatory event. Nervous system resolution therefore is not merely the reduction of inflammation in the brain or nerves.

It is the restoration of a signaling environment in which defense has ended cleanly enough that precision can return.

This is why neural inflammation has to be understood as both immune activity and membrane instability at the same time. Neurons, astrocytes, microglia, oligodendrocytes, endothelial interfaces, and extracellular signaling spaces all depend on tightly controlled lipid architecture. DHA is especially important here because neural membranes require a degree of flexibility, curvature control, receptor organization, and long-horizon structural stability that simpler tissues do not demand in the same way. But the nervous system does not only need DHA for resting structure. It also needs DHA-derived downstream mediator potential for moments when inflammatory stress threatens to push the tissue into prolonged dysfunction. Protectins and D-series resolvins become important because they help reduce unnecessary continuation of inflammatory signaling, limit collateral injury, and support the shift from neural alarm into neural recovery. Nervous system resolution depends on both the membrane and the mediator. It depends on what the tissue is built from and what that tissue can later generate under stress.

Microglia sit close to the center of this process because they are one of the main immune-surveillance populations of the nervous system, but they are not simple defenders. In a healthy context, they sample, prune, monitor, and help maintain local integrity. Under injury, infection, excitotoxic stress, vascular insult, oxidative damage, or repeated systemic inflammatory input, they can shift toward an activated state that becomes useful at first and destructive if it persists too long. Nervous system resolution requires that microglial behavior stop being organized around continued alarm and begin being organized around controlled cleanup, restraint, and restoration. If that transition fails, neural tissue stays chemically loud. Synapses are read through a threat-biased environment. Local debris and inflammatory fragments are cleared too slowly. Cytokine tone remains elevated. The result is not only ongoing inflammation. It is degraded signal quality. The nervous system begins functioning inside a field of incomplete closure.

This is one reason chronic pain, brain fog, sensory hypersensitivity, poor sleep regulation, mood instability, and autonomic dysregulation so often cluster together. These are not necessarily separate diseases in the mechanistic sense. They can be different expressions of nervous tissue that remains partially inflamed, partially sensitized, and structurally unfinished. Pain pathways stay amplified because local tissue still appears unsafe. Cognitive performance falls because synaptic environments remain noisy and less metabolically efficient. Sleep worsens because inflammatory tone alters neural timing and stress chemistry. Sensory thresholds drop because membranes and glial systems remain too ready to interpret input as threat. Nervous system resolution means reversing that background state. It means reducing the biochemical evidence that keeps neural tissue behaving defensively when the acute need for defense has already passed.

The blood-brain and blood-nerve barrier dimensions matter here as well. Neural resolution cannot proceed well if vascular interfaces remain too open, too reactive, or too exposed to repeated systemic inflammatory traffic. Endothelial stability, membrane integrity, and reduced peripheral inflammatory burden all influence whether neural tissue can quiet down after an insult. If systemic inflammation remains high, if gut-derived immune provocation remains ongoing, or if oxidative and metabolic stress continue to flood the system with danger signals, then the nervous system may remain trapped in partial activation even when no obvious local insult is expanding. This is one reason nervous system resolution cannot be isolated from whole-body resolution. The brain and nerves resolve partly from their own lipid and glial architecture, but they also resolve from the inflammatory quality of the organism surrounding them.

Seen clearly, nervous system resolution is the return of neural tissue from defended instability to signaling order. It requires reduced microglial overactivation, better cleanup of damaged material, restoration of membrane coherence, reduction of oxidative pressure, normalization of barrier behavior, and access to DHA-derived pro-resolving mediator biology strong enough to help the tissue stop protecting itself after the useful phase of protection has ended. The nervous system does not heal by being silenced. It heals when its membranes, glial systems, vascular interfaces, and synaptic environments all become stable enough that precision no longer has to compete with chronic alarm.

Chapter 16

Functional Divergence: EPA vs DHA via SPM Output

EPA and DHA are usually grouped together under the label omega-3, but that label becomes too blunt once the discussion reaches the level of specialized pro-resolving mediator output. They are related, they overlap, and they often cooperate, but they do not contribute to resolution in identical ways. The divergence begins in structure and becomes clearer in downstream signaling. EPA tends to express more of its importance through inflammatory mediator competition and through the generation of E-series resolvins, which help reduce continued recruitment and alter the direction of inflammatory traffic once the early phase has done enough. DHA carries part of that same broad resolution logic through the D-series resolvins, but it also extends much further into tissue protection and cleanup through protectins and maresins. In practical terms, EPA is often easier to understand as a modifier of inflammatory sequence, while DHA is often easier to understand as a substrate for preserving tissue and supporting the actual labor of restoration. That distinction should not be overstated into a false opposition, but it does matter. The body is not using two identical omega-3 fatty acids redundantly. It is using them to build different branches of the same later-phase intelligence.

EPA's divergence becomes visible first in the eicosanoid environment. Because EPA can compete with arachidonic acid within COX and LOX pathways, it influences the character of inflammatory mediator production closer to the point where initiation chemistry is already active. It does not remove the body's ability to inflame. It changes which inflammatory language becomes more available once membrane substrate is released. That means EPA sits closer to the interface between escalation and de-escalation. It affects how the tissue moves out of pure arachidonic-acid-dominant signaling and into a less reinforcement-heavy state. The E-series resolvins extend that effect further by helping reduce continued neutrophil recruitment and by supporting the turn away from repeated early-phase logic. EPA therefore often appears as the omega-3 fatty acid that most clearly modifies inflammatory traffic and inflammatory momentum.

DHA diverges by carrying more of the burden of tissue preservation and tissue finishing. Its role in membrane structure is already more pronounced in highly specialized tissues, especially neural and retinal tissue, where curvature, excitability, receptor behavior, and long-term signaling precision all depend on a very particular membrane environment. But the divergence becomes even more important at the SPM level. DHA does not just produce D-series resolvins. It also gives rise to protectins and maresins. Protectins emphasize tissue defense against collateral inflammatory injury, especially where preserving function during inflammation is critical. Maresins emphasize macrophage-led cleanup, efferocytosis, and repair-compatible reconstruction. This means DHA-derived output is not only about reducing further inflammatory pressure. It is also about defending delicate structures during de-escalation and making the site more physically finishable once escalation has begun to subside.

This creates a meaningful functional split. EPA-derived output is often easier to associate with reducing continued inflammatory recruitment and shifting the mediator environment away from persistent amplification. DHA-derived output is often easier to associate with preserving tissue integrity, supporting macrophage transitions, and improving the conditions required for real recovery after inflammation. EPA helps change the direction of the response. DHA helps protect the tissue and organize the cleanup through which the response can actually be completed. Again, these are differences of emphasis, not absolute separation, but they matter because they explain why the body retains both molecules and why a general statement like omega-3 reduces inflammation fails to capture the architecture of the system.

This divergence also helps explain why different tissues may appear to need different forms of omega-3 biology more strongly. Vascular and immune contexts often reveal the importance of EPA-related pathway competition and E-series output because the question there is frequently how to reduce continued inflammatory traffic and repeated reinforcement. Neural tissue, retinal tissue, and any environment where structural precision is easily lost under inflammatory stress make the importance of DHA more visible because the question is not only how to reduce continued recruitment, but how to preserve specialized membranes and support repair without sacrificing function. A macrophage-rich cleanup environment also reveals DHA's importance through maresin biology because the bottleneck there is often not only less inflammation, but more competent closure. The tissue must actually be cleared, not merely left with fewer incoming cells.

The divergence becomes even more important when resolution is viewed as a threshold problem. EPA can help push tissue away from early-phase persistence by changing substrate competition and reducing further neutrophil-heavy continuation. DHA can help push tissue across the later threshold where cleanup, preservation, and repair-compatible signaling become dominant enough to finish the event. In that sense, EPA often seems to help the body stop continuing, while DHA often seems to help the body survive and complete. Both functions are necessary. A tissue that reduces recruitment but cannot preserve structure or organize cleanup still fails. A tissue that is well-protected but remains stuck in continued inflammatory traffic also fails. Resolution requires both divergence and cooperation.

This is also why membrane composition matters so much. The body cannot express EPA and DHA divergence if neither is meaningfully incorporated into phospholipids. EPA has to be present strongly enough to affect substrate competition and support E-series generation. DHA has to be present strongly enough to support membrane behavior and provide the precursor reservoir for D-series resolvins, protectins, and maresins. A membrane poor in both remains heavily biased toward omega-6-derived initiation chemistry. A membrane richer in one but not the other may gain some part of resolution intelligence while remaining underbuilt in another part. The full architecture of completion is strongest when the membrane reservoir is broad enough to support both the traffic-modulating effects associated with EPA and the tissue-protective, cleanup-supportive effects associated with DHA.

Seen clearly, the functional divergence of EPA versus DHA through SPM output is one of the strongest arguments against treating omega-3 as one generic health signal. EPA and DHA are cooperative but not interchangeable. EPA-derived pathways are especially important in changing inflammatory momentum, competing within eicosanoid systems, and reducing continued recruitment through E-series resolvins. DHA-derived pathways are especially important in preserving tissue, supporting macrophage-led cleanup, and enabling repair-compatible resolution through D-series resolvins, protectins, and maresins. The body uses both because finishing inflammation requires more than one kind of later-phase instruction. It requires less continuation, better protection, and better cleanup all at once.

Different SPM Families, Different Outcomes

Specialized pro-resolving mediators are often grouped together as though they all perform the same general function, but that simplification hides one of the most important truths in resolution biology. They all belong to the later phase of inflammation, but they do not all solve the same problem within that phase. Different SPM families produce different outcomes because the body is not trying to do one thing when it resolves inflammation. It is trying to do several things at once. It has to stop further neutrophil recruitment, increase macrophage-driven cleanup, protect tissue from collateral injury, restore vascular and barrier control, reduce persistent pain sensitization, and create conditions compatible with repair. No single mediator family carries that whole burden equally. That is why the body derives multiple SPM classes from EPA and DHA. It is building a diversified biochemical language for completion, not repeating one molecular message in several names.

The resolvins are the clearest example of SPMs that shift inflammatory traffic and timing. Both E-series resolvins from EPA and D-series resolvins from DHA are strongly associated with reducing continued neutrophil infiltration and helping the tissue stop calling for more early-phase force once enough force has already arrived. Their outcome is directional restraint. They help the inflammatory site stop expanding. This matters because unresolved inflammation often persists through repeated reinforcement. Fresh neutrophils keep arriving, vascular openness remains too high, and the tissue stays caught in an incoming-wave logic. Resolvins change that pattern. Their main effect is not simply lowering inflammation in general, but altering the flow of the inflammatory event so that it stops behaving like something still asking for more recruitment.

Protectins produce a different outcome. Their emphasis is tissue preservation, especially in settings where collateral inflammatory damage is costly. In neural tissue, retinal tissue, and other highly specialized membrane environments, the problem is not only how to reduce continued inflammatory traffic. It is how to keep the tissue from losing too much function while inflammation is being brought under control. Protectins help limit the spread of injury within delicate structures and support a more disciplined exit from inflammatory stress. Their outcome is therefore more protective than traffic-oriented. They help the body preserve what must keep working even while cleanup and de-escalation are still underway.

Maresins generate yet another outcome, and their importance becomes especially clear once resolution is understood as physical cleanup rather than mere quieting of signals. Maresins are strongly linked to macrophage activity, especially efferocytosis, debris handling, and the tissue transition into repair-compatible organization. Their outcome is not primarily less recruitment or less inflammatory intensity, though those can be secondary effects. Their outcome is better finishing. A tissue burdened with apoptotic cells, oxidized lipid fragments, and inflammatory residue cannot truly resolve no matter how much new recruitment is reduced. Maresins matter because they improve the removal of what inflammation left behind. They make the tissue more cleanable and therefore more recoverable.

This is why different SPM families matter clinically and conceptually. A tissue can suffer from too much continued inflammatory traffic, too much collateral injury, too little cleanup, or all three at once. The body answers those problems with different later-phase mediator emphases. In one context, reducing further neutrophil entry is the urgent priority. In another, preventing damage to fragile neural membranes is the urgent priority. In another, the central bottleneck is macrophage-led clearance. Resolution is not one-dimensional, and the mediator families reflect that. Each family changes the tissue in a different way because each family is addressing a different failure point in the transition from inflammation to repair.

Seen clearly, different SPM families produce different outcomes because the body does not define healing as one act. Healing requires less incoming damage, more tissue protection, better cleanup, and a better structural foundation for repair. Resolvins, protectins, and maresins all belong to the same late-phase intelligence, but they express different parts of that intelligence. That is why omega-3-derived resolution biology is so much more sophisticated than the phrase anti-inflammatory suggests. The body is not merely turning inflammation down. It is selecting which part of unfinished inflammation must be corrected first and using different mediator families to push the tissue toward a more complete end state.

Tissue-Specific Effects

The effects of specialized pro-resolving mediators are tissue-specific because different tissues are not trying to solve the same inflammatory problem. Resolution in a blood vessel is not the same as resolution in a joint, a gut barrier, a liver lobule, a synapse, or a retinal membrane. Each tissue has different structural demands, different immune exposure, different membrane composition, different cleanup burdens, and different consequences if inflammation persists too long. The body therefore does not use SPM biology as one uniform blanket signal. It uses the same mediator families inside different local architectures, and those architectures shape what outcome matters most. In one tissue the priority is reducing continued leukocyte recruitment. In another it is protecting membrane precision. In another it is restoring barrier selectivity. In another it is improving macrophage-led debris clearance so regeneration can begin. The mediators belong to the same late-phase logic, but the tissue decides how that logic is expressed.

In vascular tissue, the dominant issue is often endothelial behavior. Early inflammation makes vessels more adhesive, more permeable, and more permissive to immune traffic. Resolution in that environment means the endothelium has to stop behaving like an emergency access point. SPM action there tends to matter through reduced leukocyte adhesion and infiltration, improved control of permeability, lower persistence of inflammatory signaling along the vessel wall, and better restoration of the surface conditions required for controlled flow and exchange. The outcome is not simply less inflammation in the blood. It is a vascular lining that becomes less reactive and less likely to keep extending the inflammatory event.

In barrier tissues such as the intestine, the skin, and other epithelial interfaces, tissue-specific effects center more heavily on selective separation. These tissues are constantly exposed to external load, microbial contact, mechanical stress, and repeated turnover. When inflammation occurs, resolution must do more than calm immune activity. It has to help the barrier close again. That means reducing continued inflammatory traffic, supporting cleanup of damaged cells, and restoring enough membrane and junctional integrity that the tissue stops leaking signals and substances that keep the immune system activated. In these tissues, SPM action becomes especially meaningful through improved barrier restoration and reduced re-triggering. The outcome is a surface that stops behaving like an open wound and starts behaving like a controlled boundary again.

In immune-rich tissues and inflamed connective environments such as joints or chronically irritated soft tissue, the tissue-specific effect is often more about managing cellular traffic and cleanup burden. These sites can accumulate apoptotic cells, oxidized membrane remnants, extracellular debris, and inflammatory byproducts that are slow to clear. There, SPM families that improve macrophage performance and efferocytosis become especially important. The outcome is not just less swelling or less pain. It is a site that becomes physically cleaner, less crowded with unresolved damage, and therefore less likely to keep re-initiating the same inflammatory sequence. Tissue-specific resolution here is heavily tied to whether the tissue can actually finish the cleanup job.

Neural tissue presents a different problem entirely because its tolerance for collateral damage is so low. In the nervous system, the issue is not only immune recruitment. It is preservation of signaling precision. Membrane instability, glial overactivation, persistent oxidative chemistry, and poor clearance of damaged material can all distort synaptic behavior, excitability, sensory thresholds, mood regulation, and cognitive performance. In that setting, DHA-derived mediators such as protectins and D-series resolvins become especially meaningful because they help reduce continued inflammatory stress while preserving function in tissue that cannot afford prolonged biochemical noise. The tissue-specific outcome is neuroprotection, lower persistence of inflammatory signaling, better cleanup, and a greater chance that the nervous system returns to signal fidelity rather than remaining trapped in defensive instability.

In the liver and broader cardiometabolic tissues, SPM effects are shaped by substrate traffic, immune pressure, and metabolic load. These tissues are constantly managing lipids, glucose, endotoxin exposure, oxidative stress, and membrane turnover. Resolution here often means improving the ability of the tissue to stop interpreting metabolic burden as ongoing injury. That includes reducing persistent inflammatory recruitment, improving cleanup of damaged cellular material, lowering the inflammatory tone of adipose and hepatic environments, and making vascular and parenchymal tissue more capable of returning to low-noise metabolic function. The tissue-specific outcome is not one dramatic repair event. It is restoration of a less inflamed operating state across fuel-handling systems.

Seen clearly, tissue-specific effects are the reason SPM biology should never be reduced to one generic statement like resolves inflammation. It does resolve inflammation, but it does so differently depending on what the tissue most needs in order to finish the event. Some tissues need less incoming traffic. Some need more preservation. Some need more cleanup. Some need better barrier restoration. Some need all of these at once. The body uses different SPM families within different membrane environments to solve those different problems. That is why the same late-phase mediator logic can produce meaningfully different outcomes across the organism. Resolution is one biological principle, but it is expressed according to the architecture of the tissue trying to recover.

Designing Intake Based on Goal

Designing intake based on goal requires abandoning the idea that omega-3 is one generic tool used the same way in every tissue, every phase, and every person. EPA and DHA do not produce identical downstream effects, and their value depends on what problem is being solved at the membrane and mediator level. If the goal is to influence inflammatory traffic more directly, reduce repeated reinforcement of early-phase signaling, and strengthen the biochemical pressure that helps stop continued neutrophil-heavy escalation, then EPA usually becomes more central because of its competition within eicosanoid pathways and its role as precursor for E-series resolvins. If the goal is to support membrane architecture in highly specialized tissues, especially the nervous system, and to increase access to mediator families more strongly associated with tissue protection, macrophage-led cleanup, and repair-compatible resolution, then DHA becomes more central because of its structural role and its downstream conversion into D-series resolvins, protectins, and maresins. This does not mean the body wants one without the other. It means intake strategy should be shaped by what kind of tissue problem is most dominant and what kind of inflammatory outcome is being sought.

When the goal is systemic inflammatory de-escalation, especially in contexts marked by repeated vascular irritation, cardiometabolic inflammation, chronic low-grade immune activation, or a tissue environment biased toward arachidonic-acid-heavy early-phase signaling, a more EPA-forward approach often makes conceptual sense. EPA sits closer to the inflammatory traffic layer. It changes substrate competition in a way that can alter downstream eicosanoid character and strengthen E-series resolvin biology once the tissue is ready to resolve. In practical terms, this makes EPA especially relevant when the body appears too fluent in escalation and too weak in the biochemical language that tells escalation to stop continuing. The intake goal there is not simply more omega-3. It is more influence over the inflammatory direction of the tissue.

When the goal is neural support, membrane precision, sensory stability, cognitive resilience, retinal support, or the preservation of tissues that cannot tolerate much collateral inflammatory damage, DHA becomes more strategically important. DHA is not only a precursor to later mediator families. It is also deeply integrated into the structure of highly specialized membranes whose function depends on very particular lipid behavior. In those settings, the question is not just how to reduce inflammatory continuation. It is how to maintain the architecture of delicate tissue while also preserving the downstream ability to generate protectins, D-series resolvins, and maresins when the tissue comes under stress. A DHA-emphasized intake strategy therefore makes the most sense when the goal is not only less inflammatory traffic, but better tissue preservation and better recovery quality in membrane-sensitive systems.

If the goal is resolution itself, rather than a narrow focus on one tissue or one symptom cluster, then intake design has to respect the fact that completion requires more than one kind of later-phase instruction. The body needs less continued recruitment, more tissue protection, and better cleanup all at once. That usually argues for a meaningful presence of both EPA and DHA rather than overcommitting to one in isolation. EPA supports the shift away from continued inflammatory reinforcement. DHA supports tissue preservation and macrophage-compatible finishing behavior. The body does not resolve well from a one-dimensional omega-3 architecture. It resolves best when the membrane reservoir is broad enough to support multiple branches of SPM output, provided the broader tissue environment is stable enough to protect and use that reservoir intelligently.

Goal-based intake design also has to account for baseline membrane conditions. A body long dominated by omega-6-heavy phospholipid composition, high oxidative stress, poor barrier control, and repeated inflammatory re-triggering may not respond to added omega-3 in a smooth or immediately proportional way. In that case, the initial goal may not be maximizing mediator output right away. The initial goal may be membrane remodeling, substrate displacement, and slow rebuilding of a more favorable phospholipid environment. That means intake strategy has to be understood over time. Early on, the objective may be changing the reservoir. Later, once the reservoir changes and the tissue becomes less chemically crowded by early-phase substrate, the objective becomes stronger downstream expression of resolvins, protectins, and maresins. Intake design should therefore match not only the tissue goal, but the phase of membrane repair the person is actually in.

Oxidative environment matters just as much as dose or ratio. A person can increase EPA and DHA intake and still fail to realize the full benefit if the membranes receiving that intake remain too chemically unstable. Highly unsaturated fatty acids are useful precisely because they enable specialized membrane and mediator behavior, but they are also vulnerable. If the goal is better resolution biology, intake design has to assume that omega-3 works best when it enters a body that is also reducing repeated oxidative damage, repeated barrier-triggered immune activation, and repeated metabolic chaos. Otherwise the intake may build potential faster than the tissue can preserve it. The design problem is therefore not only how much EPA or DHA to provide. It is what kind of membrane environment that intake is entering.

This is why designing intake based on goal should never collapse into a simplistic rule such as EPA for inflammation, DHA for brain. That shorthand points in a useful direction, but it is too flat for real physiology. The better question is what kind of resolution deficit the tissue is showing. Is the main problem excessive inflammatory traffic. Is it membrane fragility in a high-precision tissue. Is it poor macrophage cleanup. Is it broad cardiometabolic inflammatory tone. Is it a chronically low-threshold, easily reactivated organism whose membranes have lost the ability to finish what they start. Intake design becomes more intelligent when it is tied to that level of analysis, because EPA and DHA are not retail categories. They are inputs into different branches of the body's later-phase inflammatory intelligence.

Seen clearly, designing intake based on goal means designing for the kind of membrane and the kind of downstream mediator environment you are trying to build. EPA becomes more central when the priority is shifting inflammatory traffic and weakening repeated early-phase reinforcement. DHA becomes more central when the priority is preserving specialized membranes, protecting sensitive tissue, and strengthening cleanup-and-repair signaling. Both become necessary when the goal is a broader increase in resolution capacity across the organism. The deeper principle is that omega-3 should be chosen according to the phase problem being addressed. If the body is too good at continuing, EPA deserves more attention. If the body is too poor at preserving and finishing, DHA deserves more attention. If the body is broadly underbuilt in its capacity to complete inflammation, both must be treated as structural and signaling partners in the same larger project.

Strategic Application

Strategic application means using the EPA–DHA distinction on purpose rather than treating omega-3 as a single undifferentiated input. Once the structural and signaling differences are clear, the question becomes practical: what is the body failing to do, and which branch of omega-3 biology is more relevant to that failure. If the dominant problem is persistent inflammatory traffic, repeated vascular irritation, chronic low-grade immune escalation, or a body that keeps re-entering the front half of inflammation too easily, then an EPA-forward strategy makes more sense because EPA competes more directly within the inflammatory mediator landscape and feeds E-series resolvin output that helps reduce continued recruitment. If the dominant problem is neural instability, sensory overload, poor membrane resilience in high-precision tissue, slow cleanup, or poor recovery after inflammatory stress, then DHA becomes more strategically important because it supports specialized membrane architecture and feeds D-series resolvins, protectins, and maresins, which are more strongly tied to tissue preservation and macrophage-led completion.

This does not mean strategy should become reductionist. The body does not resolve through one mediator family alone, and most chronic inflammatory conditions are not pure EPA problems or pure DHA problems. They are mixed failures of traffic control, tissue protection, cleanup, barrier restoration, and membrane stability. Strategic application therefore usually means emphasis, not exclusion. In a person whose tissues are dominated by early-phase inflammatory chemistry, EPA may deserve greater emphasis at first because the immediate need is to weaken repeated reinforcement and alter the mediator direction of the site. In a person whose main burden is nervous system instability, neuroinflammatory persistence, poor recovery, and membrane fragility in sensitive tissues, DHA may deserve greater emphasis because the deeper need is preservation and higher-quality repair. In broader cardiometabolic dysfunction, systemic inflammatory tone, postprandial irritability, vascular reactivity, and adipose-immune congestion, a combined approach often makes the most sense because the body needs less continued escalation and more competent completion at the same time.

Strategic application also has to account for sequence. A tissue that is heavily omega-6 dominant, oxidatively unstable, and repeatedly re-triggered may not express the full value of either EPA or DHA immediately, no matter how intelligently the intake is designed. In that setting, the first strategic objective is often membrane remodeling and reduction of repeated provocation. The body has to become less crowded with initiation-heavy substrate, less exposed to barrier-derived immune noise, and less chemically hostile to highly unsaturated fatty acids before later-phase mediator biology can express itself strongly. This means a person may need to think in stages. First change the reservoir. Then improve the likelihood of useful downstream conversion. Then reinforce the tissue-specific branch of resolution most relevant to the dominant problem. Strategy is therefore not just choosing a fatty acid. It is choosing where in the failure sequence intervention is actually needed.

The most important principle is that omega-3 should be applied according to inflammatory architecture, not according to marketing categories. EPA is strategically useful when the body is too good at continuing. DHA is strategically useful when the body is too poor at preserving and finishing. Both are strategically useful when the organism is broadly underbuilt in resolution capacity and needs a membrane reservoir capable of supporting multiple branches of pro-resolving output. The real task is not to ask which omega-3 is better in the abstract. The real task is to identify whether the tissue most needs less continued recruitment, more tissue protection, better cleanup, or some combination of all three, and then build membrane composition in a way that makes that later biology more possible.

PART VI

DISEASE AS FAILED RESOLUTION

Chapter 17

Chronic Inflammation as Resolution Failure

Chronic inflammation is usually described as if the body were simply generating too much inflammatory force for too long. That description is not completely wrong, but it remains shallow because it places the emphasis on excess rather than on sequence. The deeper problem in many chronic conditions is not that the body can still initiate inflammation. It is that the body cannot complete inflammation well enough to restore tissue order. The machinery of initiation remains available. Membranes still release arachidonic acid. Eicosanoid cascades still form. Cytokines still rise. Neutrophils still arrive. Endothelial surfaces still open. Pain pathways still amplify. What is impaired is the later phase that should bring recruitment under control, clear apoptotic cells and oxidized debris, restore barrier function, reduce inflammatory tone, and shift tissue from emergency logic back into maintenance and repair. Chronic inflammation is therefore better understood as resolution failure than as inflammatory excess alone. The body is still entering defense. It is simply not exiting defense cleanly enough to stop defending.

That distinction matters because it changes what chronic tissue looks like mechanistically. A chronically inflamed site is not merely a place with too many inflammatory molecules floating around. It is a place where the evidence of unfinished defense remains visible. Dead cells have not been cleared efficiently enough. Oxidized membrane fragments remain in the extracellular environment. Macrophages have not completed enough efferocytosis to empty the site of inflammatory residue. Endothelial behavior has not normalized enough to stop permissive immune traffic. Epithelial barriers have not re-sealed enough to stop feeding the tissue new provocation. Mitochondria have not restored enough energetic control to fund reconstruction. In this condition, the body is not behaving irrationally when it continues inflammatory signaling. It is responding to a site that still looks unresolved. Chronic inflammation persists because the tissue remains structurally legible as unfinished danger.

This is why the concept of over-initiation remains incomplete unless it is linked to failed resolution. A body can become too easy to activate, but that ease of activation becomes especially damaging when every inflammatory event leaves behind residue that lowers the threshold for the next one. The tissue is repeatedly pushed into initiation, but each cycle also weakens its ability to complete. Neutrophil infiltration continues too long. Cleanup lags. Oxidative damage accumulates. Omega-3-derived substrate is too sparse, too weakly converted, or too poorly protected to generate enough specialized pro-resolving mediator pressure. The next trigger then lands in a tissue already carrying the debris, membrane instability, and biochemical memory of the last trigger. Chronic inflammation is not one prolonged event in the simplest sense. It is often a series of incompletely finished events layered on top of one another until the tissue never truly returns to baseline between them.

This framework also explains why so many chronic inflammatory disorders present with both activation and exhaustion at the same time. The person may have pain, swelling, fatigue, brain fog, vascular irritation, poor recovery, and exaggerated reactivity to minor inputs, yet also show signs of depleted repair capacity, metabolic fragility, and low resilience. That apparent contradiction makes sense once inflammation is seen as resolution failure. The body is still spending on defense, but it is not collecting the return that resolution would normally provide. Energy keeps being used for surveillance, recruitment, and containment, while cleanup and reconstruction remain incomplete. The tissue stays metabolically expensive because it keeps living in a state that should have been temporary. Chronic inflammation therefore is not just immune overactivity. It is chronic incomplete work.

This is where membrane composition becomes decisive. A tissue built under omega-6 dominance, poor omega-3 incorporation, oxidative instability, and repeated inflammatory stress is structurally biased toward initiation and underbuilt for completion. Its phospholipid reservoir carries more substrate for early-phase eicosanoid production and less substrate for strong downstream generation of resolvins, protectins, and maresins. Its membranes are easier to damage. Its receptors interpret danger through less stable surfaces. Its mitochondrial output becomes less reliable under load. Even before a visible flare occurs, the tissue has already lost part of its resolution potential. Chronic inflammation in that setting is not just a failure of signaling discipline. It is a failure of inflammatory architecture. The tissue does not possess enough protected later-phase capacity to finish what the earlier-phase machinery keeps starting.

This is also why chronic inflammation is so often multisystemic. Once resolution failure takes hold, the body does not merely carry local symptoms. It carries altered thresholds across multiple tissues. Gut barriers remain more permeable. Vascular surfaces remain more reactive. Adipose tissue remains more immune-active. Neural tissue remains more sensitized. Joints remain more debris-laden. Muscles recover more slowly. Sleep destabilizes more easily because nociceptive and cytokine tone remain elevated. The person experiences these as separate problems, but they are often different expressions of the same deeper pattern: inflammation entered, did not complete, and left behind a tissue environment that now behaves as though fresh escalation is still easier than closure. Chronicity spreads because unresolved tissue does not keep its costs to itself.

Seen clearly, this chapter marks a conceptual correction. Chronic inflammation should not be treated only as too much fire. It should be treated as fire that did not go out properly because the system failed to execute the phase of biology responsible for ending it. That changes what counts as progress. Lowering inflammatory markers is not enough if debris remains uncleared. Reducing pain is not enough if the tissue remains structurally unstable. Improving one symptom is not enough if the membrane reservoir still favors initiation and the barrier still leaks new triggers into the site. Real improvement means rebuilding resolution capacity. It means stronger omega-3-derived substrate pools, better downstream SPM production, better macrophage-led cleanup, better mitochondrial support, better membrane protection, and better barrier closure. Chronic inflammation is not only a problem of too much inflammatory signaling. It is a problem of too little successful completion. That is the lens through which the rest of the book must now be read.

Persistent Cytokine Signaling

Persistent cytokine signaling is one of the clearest expressions of failed resolution because cytokines are not only markers of inflammation. They are part of the reason an inflammatory site continues behaving as though the job is unfinished. In an acute, well-sequenced response, cytokines help coordinate the early and middle phases of inflammation. They amplify danger recognition, recruit immune cells, alter endothelial behavior, change tissue metabolism, and make the inflammatory event large enough to matter. That is useful at the beginning because force has to be organized quickly. But cytokines are not supposed to remain the dominant language of the tissue indefinitely. Once the useful phase has passed, their persistence means the site has not transitioned successfully into closure. The body keeps receiving biochemical messages that the emergency is still active, and tissue behavior continues to reflect those messages even when the original trigger should already be moving toward completion.

This is why persistent cytokine signaling is not best understood as a separate problem floating above the rest of the inflammatory sequence. It is tied directly to unresolved debris, unresolved membrane damage, unresolved barrier dysfunction, and unresolved immune traffic. Cytokines remain elevated because the tissue still contains the physical evidence of danger. Apoptotic cells are not cleared fast enough. Oxidized lipids remain embedded in membranes or extracellular debris. Endothelial and epithelial surfaces remain too open. Macrophages remain too incomplete in their cleanup role. Fresh immune-provoking material continues reaching the site through damaged barriers. Under those conditions, cytokines do exactly what they were designed to do. They continue coordinating an environment that still looks unfinished. The problem is not that cytokines exist. The problem is that the tissue keeps giving them reasons to remain relevant.

Persistent cytokine signaling also lowers thresholds across the system. A tissue living under ongoing cytokine pressure becomes easier to activate and harder to calm. Endothelial surfaces become more adhesive. Nociceptive pathways remain more sensitized. Hepatic metabolism remains more inflammatory in tone. Mitochondrial stress can increase because the cell is repeatedly being pushed toward defensive rather than restorative priorities. Appetite, sleep, mood, energy, vascular tone, and cognitive resilience all begin to reflect a body that is interpreting itself through chronic inflammatory messaging. This is why persistent cytokines often correlate with symptoms that seem diffuse or systemic. The person is not just dealing with one inflamed site. They are dealing with an organism whose background signaling has shifted toward unfinished defense.

This is also where specialized pro-resolving mediators become especially relevant. SPMs do not simply quiet cytokines directly as though muting a speaker. They help remove the underlying reasons cytokine signaling remains active. They reduce continued neutrophil recruitment, improve macrophage-led efferocytosis, limit collateral tissue injury, and support barrier restoration and vascular normalization. As the tissue becomes physically cleaner and less structurally dangerous, cytokine signaling loses its justification. The environment no longer needs the same level of inflammatory coordination because the evidence of unresolved threat has begun to disappear. This is why resolution biology is more powerful than blunt suppression in this context. Suppression may lower cytokine output transiently. Resolution lowers the need for that output by changing the tissue itself.

Seen clearly, persistent cytokine signaling is one of the ways chronic inflammation keeps declaring that it has not reached its end state. The tissue continues speaking the language of emergency because emergency-like conditions remain in place. Until debris is cleared, membranes stabilized, barriers repaired, and omega-3-derived resolution pathways strengthened enough to help the site complete its inflammatory sequence, cytokine signaling tends to remain part of the background. The body is not just inflamed. It is being continually instructed to stay inflamed.

Incomplete Debris Clearance

Incomplete debris clearance is one of the most important reasons inflammation becomes chronic, because tissue cannot convincingly exit defense while it is still physically carrying the remains of the event it is trying to finish. Debris is not passive residue. It includes apoptotic neutrophils that were not engulfed in time, fragments of damaged cell membranes, oxidized phospholipids, denatured proteins, extracellular matrix breakdown products, and other remnants of tissue injury and immune activity. As long as that material remains in place, the inflammatory site continues to present itself as unfinished. Receptors on macrophages, endothelial cells, epithelial cells, and other neighboring structures keep encountering evidence that something is still wrong. The body does not stand down because the tissue has not yet become quiet enough, clean enough, or structurally restored enough to justify standing down. Incomplete clearance therefore keeps the inflammatory program open from the inside.

This is why debris clearance is not a minor housekeeping detail that happens after the real immune work is done. It is part of the real immune work. Early inflammation creates disruption on purpose. Neutrophils arrive, release oxidants and enzymes, damaged host cells die, extracellular proteins are altered, lipids oxidize, and the tissue environment becomes chemically crowded. That phase can be necessary, but once the acute objective has been achieved, all of that material has to be removed if the site is going to stop behaving like a place under attack. If clearance lags, the inflammatory response becomes self-perpetuating. Yesterday's neutrophils become today's inflammatory stimulus. Yesterday's oxidized membrane fragments become today's danger signals. The body keeps reading the site through the remains of its own unfinished work.

Macrophages sit at the center of this problem because they are the main cells responsible for turning inflammatory residue into biological closure. Through efferocytosis and related cleanup functions, they remove apoptotic cells before those cells lose membrane integrity and spill their contents into the surrounding tissue. They internalize membrane remnants, oxidized lipids, and other debris that would otherwise continue stimulating inflammatory interpretation. When macrophage cleanup is efficient, the site becomes less visibly dangerous to the immune system. When macrophage cleanup is weak, overwhelmed, or mistimed, the site becomes trapped in chemical repetition. Debris remains present long enough to transform from waste into renewed provocation. This is one of the main ways resolution failure becomes chronicity.

The consequences of incomplete clearance extend beyond inflammation in the narrow sense. A debris-laden tissue remains metabolically expensive. It continues attracting immune surveillance. It keeps vascular surfaces more reactive. It prolongs nociceptive signaling because pain pathways keep receiving evidence that the area is still unsafe. It interferes with repair because new structure is being laid down into an environment still crowded with the molecular signs of old damage. A tissue cannot regenerate cleanly while it is still full of unresolved fragments from the previous phase. In that sense, incomplete debris clearance does not just delay healing. It actively contaminates the conditions required for healing.

This is also why specialized pro-resolving mediators matter so much here. Their importance is not just that they reduce future inflammatory recruitment. They improve the tissue's ability to finish the current event by enhancing macrophage cleanup, supporting efferocytosis, limiting further collateral damage, and helping the site shift away from repeated reinforcement. A body with weak SPM biology often does not simply inflame more. It clears worse. The tissue then remains full of inflammatory leftovers, which keeps cytokine signaling alive, keeps barriers unstable, and lowers the threshold for the next flare. Incomplete debris clearance is therefore one of the central physical expressions of failed resolution. The body is still inflamed because it is still surrounded by the material proof that inflammation has not actually been completed.

Tissue Damage Accumulation

Tissue damage accumulation is what happens when inflammatory events keep producing structural injury faster than the body can clear, repair, and reorganize the site back into a stable state. This is one of the main reasons chronic inflammation becomes progressive rather than merely repetitive. A single inflammatory event always carries some cost. Membranes are stressed. Proteins are oxidized or degraded. Extracellular matrix is altered. Vascular behavior shifts. Immune cells enter, act, and die. Under ideal conditions, those costs are paid back during resolution. Debris is removed, membranes are rebuilt, barriers are restored, and the tissue returns to a lower-noise state. When resolution fails, that repayment does not happen fully. The tissue carries part of the injury forward. Then the next inflammatory event begins on top of that residue. Over time, the body is no longer responding from clean baseline structure. It is responding from accumulated damage.

This accumulated damage changes the meaning of future triggers. A tissue with repeated membrane oxidation, persistent debris, altered vascular surfaces, and incomplete repair is easier to activate because it already looks partially unsafe. Receptors encounter more danger-associated material. Barriers are weaker. Macrophages are more burdened. Mitochondria are more strained. The threshold for new inflammatory activation drops because the tissue never fully stopped presenting evidence of previous injury. This is why chronic inflammatory states often intensify gradually even when no single new trigger seems dramatically worse. The body is dealing not only with the present insult, but with the layered cost of the insults that were never properly finished before it.

Tissue damage accumulation also distorts function before it produces obvious structural failure. In vascular tissue it may appear as persistent endothelial reactivity, abnormal permeability, or reduced nitric oxide handling. In joints it may appear as longer recovery, stiffness, and recurring irritation because inflammatory residue and matrix damage were not fully cleared. In the nervous system it may appear as persistent sensitization, cognitive instability, altered mood regulation, or poor stress tolerance because synaptic and glial environments remain biochemically noisy. In barrier tissues it may appear as exaggerated reactivity and repeated immune provocation because the surface never fully re-established selective control. The damage accumulates as altered behavior first. Only later does it become easier to recognize as more obvious pathology.

This is one of the deepest reasons specialized pro-resolving mediators matter. They do not just reduce the intensity of the current inflammatory response. They help prevent current inflammation from becoming future structural burden. By reducing continued neutrophil recruitment, improving macrophage cleanup, limiting collateral injury, and supporting repair-compatible tissue transitions, SPMs lower the amount of damage that gets carried into the next cycle. A body with weak resolution capacity accumulates injury because every event leaves behind more than it should. A body with stronger resolution capacity still experiences stress and still inflames when necessary, but it finishes with less residue. That difference becomes enormous over time.

Seen clearly, tissue damage accumulation is the material memory of failed resolution. It is how chronic inflammation leaves a record inside the tissue itself. The body keeps getting easier to trigger because the site keeps carrying the leftovers of previous unfinished defense. Until that accumulation is reduced through better cleanup, better membrane protection, better barrier restoration, and stronger resolution biology, each new inflammatory event starts from a worse position than the last. That is how chronic inflammation stops being just a signaling problem and becomes a structural problem.

The "Stuck Inflammation" State

The stuck inflammation state is what the body looks like when it never fully exits the inflammatory program, even if the original trigger has partially faded or changed form. It is not the same as acute inflammation, and it is not simply the presence of inflammatory markers in the blood. It is a tissue condition in which initiation remains easier than completion, cleanup remains slower than residue generation, and repair remains too weak to restore a true baseline before the next round of activation begins. The body in this state does not experience inflammation as a clean episode with a beginning, middle, and end. It experiences inflammation as a semi-permanent operating mode. The tissue is no longer fully in crisis, but it is not fully out of crisis either. It remains partially recruited, partially permeable, partially oxidized, partially sensitized, and structurally unfinished enough that normal life keeps re-triggering the same defensive logic.

What makes this state so important is that it explains why chronic illness often feels diffuse, recurring, and disproportionate. In stuck inflammation, the body still knows how to launch force. Neutrophils still arrive. Cytokines still rise. Eicosanoids still form. Pain pathways still amplify. Endothelial surfaces still open. But the back half of the sequence never takes command strongly enough. Macrophages do not clear debris efficiently enough. Specialized pro-resolving mediator output is too weak relative to the inflammatory burden. Membranes remain oxidatively unstable. Barriers remain too open. Mitochondria remain too strained to fund real completion. The result is a body that keeps defending because it never receives convincing structural evidence that the event has ended. The site still looks dangerous, so the system keeps behaving as though danger is present.

This is why the stuck inflammation state is so often mistaken for random symptom variability. A person may have days that are better and days that are worse, but the underlying tissue never becomes truly normal between them. Pain may recede but not disappear in a biologically complete way because local nociceptive amplification remains justified by unresolved debris and membrane instability. Fatigue may improve somewhat but return quickly because the body remains metabolically committed to surveillance and partial defense. Gut symptoms may quiet temporarily but flare with minor dietary stress because the barrier never fully re-stabilized. Brain fog may lighten but recur because the neural environment remains too chemically noisy to sustain precision under pressure. These fluctuations are not random. They reflect a system oscillating inside an incomplete inflammatory program rather than moving fully beyond it.

The phrase stuck is useful because it captures the fact that the body is not simply inflamed harder. It is inflamed unfinished. The machinery of escalation and the machinery of closure are no longer proportionate. Too much of the tissue's biology is still organized around the front half of the response. Omega-6-derived initiation substrate remains abundant. COX and LOX traffic remains biased toward early-phase chemistry. SPM generation remains too weak or too poorly expressed. Debris remains visible. Thresholds remain low. Each new stressor lands in a body already leaning toward activation. That is why the same tissue can feel both exhausted and overreactive at once. It is spending on defense without receiving the restoration that should follow defense.

Seen clearly, the stuck inflammation state is the lived physiology of resolution failure. It is what happens when the body loses the ability to convincingly declare an inflammatory event complete. The answer is not simply to silence symptoms harder. The deeper requirement is to rebuild the conditions that allow completion: better membrane composition, stronger omega-3-derived resolution substrate, better downstream conversion into SPMs, better macrophage cleanup, lower oxidative damage, tighter barriers, and enough mitochondrial capacity to pay for repair. Until those conditions improve, the body remains what it appears to be in this state: not fully sick in one acute moment, but not fully recovered from the last one either.

Chapter 18

Lipid Imbalance and Disease Patterns

Lipid imbalance does not produce disease in a random or isolated way. It produces recognizable patterns because lipids are not secondary inputs sprinkled onto an otherwise stable system. They are part of the physical and signaling architecture through which the system behaves in the first place. When membrane composition drifts, when omega-6-derived initiation substrate becomes overrepresented, when omega-3-derived completion substrate becomes underrepresented, when highly unsaturated lipids are exposed to chronic oxidative injury, and when structural lipids lose their ability to maintain stable boundaries under stress, the body does not simply become unhealthy in a general sense. It begins expressing a patterned physiology. Certain tissues become easier to trigger. Certain barriers become easier to breach. Certain vascular surfaces become more reactive. Certain immune responses become more prolonged. Certain neural circuits become noisier and more difficult to stabilize. The visible diseases may carry different names, but underneath them the same imbalance is often appearing through different structural contexts.

This is why disease patterns matter more than isolated biomarkers. A person may present with vascular irritation, metabolic instability, poor recovery, chronic pain, cognitive fog, gut reactivity, low stress tolerance, or skin inflammation, and each of those can be named separately. But naming is not explanation. Explanation begins lower, at the membrane and mediator level, where lipid imbalance changes what kind of body the person is carrying into daily life. A membrane enriched in unstable substrate and repeatedly exposed to inflammatory triggers does not only change one pathway. It alters threshold behavior across the system. Receptors interpret more danger. Cytokine tone remains elevated longer. Endothelial surfaces remain more permissive to inflammatory traffic. Mitochondria spend more energy on defense and less on repair. Macrophages remain more burdened by unresolved cleanup. In that setting, disease stops looking like a collection of unrelated failures and starts looking like different tissue expressions of the same unresolved structural bias.

The vascular pattern is one of the clearest examples. Lipid imbalance in vascular tissue does not begin as a catastrophic blockage. It begins as altered endothelial behavior. The vessel wall becomes easier to irritate, easier to open, easier to recruit immune traffic into, and harder to return to low-noise function after exposure to mechanical, metabolic, or inflammatory stress. Oxidized lipids and poorly resolved inflammatory residue remain in contact with surfaces that should have normalized. The result is a state of persistent vascular defensiveness. Blood vessels stop behaving like quietly regulated exchange surfaces and begin behaving more like semi-activated interfaces, prone to abnormal permeability, adhesion signaling, and inflammatory continuation. Over time that pattern can contribute to the broader cardiometabolic picture, but its roots are not only in cholesterol transport or blood pressure. Its roots are in unresolved inflammatory signaling carried through membrane imbalance.

A second pattern appears in metabolic tissues, especially liver, muscle, and adipose tissue. These tissues are constantly exposed to substrate flow, and that makes them especially vulnerable to lipid-driven mis-sequencing. Adipose tissue built under chronic caloric excess, omega-6-heavy membrane remodeling, oxidative stress, and poor resolution capacity becomes less like a passive energy reserve and more like an immune-active inflammatory organ. The liver receives this burden through altered lipoprotein traffic, endotoxin exposure, inflammatory cytokines, and excess substrate it must either oxidize, export, or store. Muscle receives it through lower metabolic flexibility and poorer recovery. What emerges is a recognizable disease pattern: insulin resistance, fatty liver, poor fuel switching, chronic fatigue after meals or stress, and a body that remains chemically defensive even when gross energy intake is abundant. This is not just too much energy. It is energy entering tissues built from poor lipid architecture and poor resolution capacity.

A third pattern appears in barrier tissues. The intestine, skin, respiratory surfaces, and epithelial interfaces more broadly depend on lipid structure for selectivity. They must remain permeable enough to exchange and absorb where appropriate, but stable enough to prevent indiscriminate passage of inflammatory triggers. Lipid imbalance disrupts that balance in both directions. Membranes become easier to irritate, easier to oxidize, and harder to restore after repeated exposure. Junctional systems lose resilience. Local immune tone remains too elevated. The tissue becomes less able to decide clearly what belongs through the barrier and what does not. Once this happens, disease patterns emerge that are often described separately: food reactivity, chronic gut irritation, exaggerated immune responses to normal exposures, repeated low-grade endotoxin burden, skin sensitivity, poor mucosal recovery. But again the pattern underneath is the same. A membrane-defined interface has lost part of its structural intelligence, and the body is now reacting through a barrier that no longer holds and filters well enough.

Neural tissue expresses lipid imbalance differently, but no less predictably. The brain, retina, and peripheral nervous system depend on membranes that are not only intact, but precise. Synaptic signaling, membrane excitability, myelin behavior, glial surveillance, and receptor organization all depend on a lipid environment that can sustain fast dynamic change without collapsing into noise. When that environment is built under chronic omega-3 insufficiency, poor DHA preservation, ongoing oxidative pressure, and unresolved inflammatory signaling, the nervous system begins expressing a recognizable pattern. The person becomes easier to overstimulate, slower to recover after stress, more vulnerable to pain amplification, more prone to cognitive drag, and less able to maintain emotional and autonomic stability under ordinary load. The nervous system is not simply malfunctioning at random. It is behaving through membranes and mediator fields that never fully leave defensive mode.

Immune tissue shows another pattern, and perhaps the most fundamental one. Lipid imbalance shifts the immune system toward initiation-heavy competence and away from cleanup-heavy competence. The body remains good at recruitment, cytokine release, eicosanoid production, and danger amplification, but becomes less effective at terminating neutrophil-heavy phases, clearing apoptotic cells, reducing collateral injury, and restoring quiet tissue conditions afterward. This creates the broad pattern of chronic inflammatory disease that underlies so many modern diagnoses. The body is not immunodeficient in the simplest sense. It is resolution-deficient. It can still react, but it reacts through a substrate environment and membrane architecture that are too heavily weighted toward beginning and too weakly built for finishing. That produces recurring disease patterns across joints, vessels, gut, liver, skin, brain, and connective tissue because every one of those tissues depends on cleanup and closure after force has been used.

This is also why lipid imbalance rarely stays local for long. A gut barrier problem changes systemic immune tone. Vascular irritation changes tissue perfusion and inflammatory trafficking elsewhere. Adipose inflammation alters liver handling, endothelial behavior, and whole-body cytokine pressure. Neural inflammatory instability changes sleep, stress signaling, appetite, and autonomic regulation. Once the body is viewed as a membrane-linked system rather than as isolated organs, disease clustering becomes easier to understand. The same lipid imbalance expresses differently according to tissue function, but the tissues are still connected. One unresolved zone raises the burden on others. One barrier failure feeds another inflammatory surface. One poorly resolved tissue shifts thresholds across the system. This is how lipid imbalance becomes a disease pattern rather than a single lesion.

The phrase disease patterns is important because it resists reductionism. It recognizes that lipid imbalance does not dictate one inevitable diagnosis. Instead, it creates a tendency, a set of structural biases, a narrowing of physiological options. It makes some responses more likely and others less available. It makes inflammation easier to start and harder to complete. It makes membranes easier to injure and harder to stabilize. It makes energy production more expensive and recovery less efficient. Which clinical label emerges first depends on tissue history, genetic context, environmental load, developmental timing, and the specific weak point in the individual system. But the pattern underneath remains recognizable: chronic activation, poor closure, low resilience, barrier weakness, oxidative fragility, and a system that keeps interpreting ordinary life through unresolved structure.

This chapter therefore marks another shift in perspective. Disease should not be viewed only as isolated pathology at the organ level. It should also be viewed as patterned expression of lipid architecture under stress. When the lipid environment is coherent, tissues maintain thresholds, resolve inflammation, preserve boundaries, and recover with less residue. When the lipid environment is incoherent, tissues begin showing the recurring signatures of failed completion. Vascular disease, metabolic disease, barrier disease, neuroinflammatory instability, chronic pain, and immune overreactivity all become easier to place inside one larger framework. The body is expressing the consequences of what it has been built from, what it has failed to clear, and what kinds of signals its membranes are now most prepared to generate. That is what lipid imbalance really is. It is not just a nutritional problem. It is a disease-pattern generator.

Cardiovascular Dysfunction

Cardiovascular dysfunction becomes much easier to understand once the vascular system is seen not as a set of passive pipes, but as a membrane-defined signaling interface that is constantly interpreting flow, substrate, immune traffic, oxidative load, and structural stress. The endothelium is the critical surface here. It lines the vascular tree, controls permeability, modulates coagulation, regulates leukocyte adhesion, shapes local inflammatory tone, and helps determine whether a vessel behaves like a quiet transport corridor or like a tissue under threat. When lipid balance is coherent and resolution capacity is strong, endothelial surfaces remain selective, relatively quiet, and capable of responding proportionately to transient insults without staying activated after the need for activation has passed. When lipid balance is distorted, especially under omega-6-dominant membrane remodeling, poor omega-3 incorporation, oxidative damage to polyunsaturated lipids, and weak specialized pro-resolving mediator output, the vascular system begins to lose that discipline. It becomes easier to irritate, easier to recruit immune traffic into, easier to permeabilize, and harder to return to baseline once inflammatory signaling has been initiated.

This is one reason cardiovascular dysfunction should not be reduced to a simple story of circulating cholesterol or mechanical obstruction. Those are downstream expressions within a much larger problem of vascular surface behavior. A dysfunctional vessel wall is often a vessel wall living in a low-grade unresolved inflammatory state. Endothelial cells remain exposed to oxidized lipids, cytokine signaling, glycemic volatility, altered shear stress interpretation, and membrane-level substrate pools that favor early-phase inflammatory mediator production more than efficient resolution. Once that condition takes hold, leukocyte adhesion becomes easier, local permeability control becomes weaker, nitric-oxide-dependent vascular regulation becomes less stable, and the vessel wall begins behaving less like a controlled interface and more like an irritated tissue boundary. The artery or microvascular bed is no longer just transporting blood. It is participating in unresolved immune-metabolic signaling.

The role of lipid imbalance becomes especially clear at the membrane level. Endothelial cells, platelets, circulating immune cells, and vascular smooth muscle all operate through phospholipid surfaces whose composition changes what kind of signals are easiest to generate under stress. A membrane reservoir heavily weighted toward arachidonic-acid-rich omega-6-derived substrate is more prepared to generate eicosanoid-heavy initiation chemistry, including signals that alter vascular tone, platelet behavior, permeability, and inflammatory recruitment. If that same environment is relatively poor in EPA and DHA, or if omega-3-derived substrate is too oxidatively fragile or too weakly converted into resolvins and related mediator families, then the vascular system becomes better at initiating inflammatory response than at completing it. In practical terms, the vessel wall develops a biochemical bias toward continued activation. That does not require dramatic acute injury. It only requires repeated low-grade insults that are never fully resolved.

This is where cardiovascular dysfunction begins to reveal itself as a resolution problem rather than just a load problem. A healthy vascular system can respond to temporary stress, immune challenge, pressure changes, or metabolic disturbance and then normalize once the event is handled. A poorly resolving vascular system cannot do that efficiently. Endothelial irritation persists. Microvascular permeability remains elevated too long. Platelet and immune interactions remain more reactive than they should be. Oxidized lipid debris remains in contact with vascular surfaces. Macrophage cleanup within the vessel wall or its surrounding microenvironment remains incomplete. The result is persistent inflammatory tone within the cardiovascular system. Over time, that pattern changes vascular behavior, tissue perfusion, nutrient exchange, clotting risk, pressure regulation, and the tendency of the vessel wall to remain chemically and immunologically unsettled.

Nitric oxide signaling belongs inside this discussion as well, because vascular dysfunction is not only about inflammation in the narrow immune sense. It is also about whether the endothelium can still function as a regulator of tone, flow, and local anti-adhesive balance. A membrane-stable, low-noise endothelial surface can respond to flow and local need with a more coherent pattern of dilation, constriction, and barrier control. A chronically inflamed, oxidatively stressed, lipid-imbalanced surface loses some of that coherence. Flow-mediated signaling becomes less reliable. Vasodilation may become less efficient. Local oxidative pressure can degrade nitric oxide availability or distort the context in which it operates. The vessel then becomes less adaptive and more brittle in its behavior. This is not only hemodynamic dysfunction. It is membrane dysfunction expressed through hemodynamics.

Platelet behavior also becomes easier to interpret through this framework. Platelets are not isolated coagulation fragments acting independently of the inflammatory environment. Their behavior is influenced by lipid mediator balance, endothelial state, membrane composition, and the broader inflammatory tone of the blood-vessel interface. In a well-regulated system, coagulation is tightly matched to actual vascular injury. In a system built under chronic inflammatory bias and weak resolution capacity, platelet reactivity may become easier to sustain in contexts that no longer justify it. The same early-phase chemistry that is useful for acute hemostatic control begins to persist in a body that is poor at shifting into closure. This contributes to a vascular environment that is not only inflamed, but more ready to combine inflammation with altered clotting behavior.

The microvascular consequences are often overlooked because they are less dramatic than large-vessel disease in the early stages, but they may be more functionally important across the whole organism. Tissues depend on small vessels and capillary interfaces for oxygen delivery, nutrient exchange, metabolite clearance, immune traffic control, and local inflammatory containment. If those surfaces remain chronically reactive, slightly permeable, slightly adhesive, and slightly oxidatively damaged, whole-body function begins to degrade even before more obvious pathology emerges. Muscles recover more slowly. Brain tissue becomes more vulnerable to inflammatory noise. Kidney filtration environments become more stressed. Peripheral tissues receive less stable flow and more inflammatory spillover. This is one reason cardiovascular dysfunction so often travels with fatigue, brain fog, poor recovery, and metabolic dysregulation. The vascular system is not simply carrying blood poorly. It is mediating unresolved inflammatory signaling poorly.

Seen clearly, cardiovascular dysfunction is one of the most important disease patterns generated by lipid imbalance because the vascular tree is one of the body's largest membrane-mediated communication systems. When membrane composition supports stability, when omega-3-derived resolution substrate is meaningfully incorporated and protected, when specialized pro-resolving mediator biology remains strong enough to help endothelial and immune behavior return to baseline, the cardiovascular system can absorb ordinary insults without becoming chronically defensive. When that architecture deteriorates, the vessel wall begins to live in a state of incomplete closure. It remains easier to activate, harder to calm, and less capable of maintaining the quiet selective control on which real vascular health depends. Cardiovascular dysfunction, in that light, is not just a circulation problem. It is the expression of a vascular membrane system that has become better at staying inflamed than at finishing inflammation well.

Metabolic Syndrome

Metabolic syndrome is often described through surface markers: abdominal fat accumulation, elevated triglycerides, low HDL, impaired glucose control, rising blood pressure, and a general picture of insulin resistance. Those markers are useful, but they do not explain why these abnormalities cluster so reliably. They cluster because metabolic syndrome is not just a calorie problem or a glucose problem. It is a tissue-organization problem built from chronic inflammatory tone, membrane imbalance, vascular reactivity, adipose immune activation, hepatic overload, and poor resolution capacity. The body in metabolic syndrome is not simply storing too much energy. It is handling energy through tissues that have become structurally and immunologically defensive. The syndrome emerges when fuel traffic, inflammatory traffic, and membrane remodeling begin reinforcing one another in a way that keeps the organism metabolically loud even at rest.

Adipose tissue is central to this pattern because once it expands under chronically poor nutritional and inflammatory conditions, it stops behaving like quiet storage and starts behaving like an active signaling organ under stress. Adipocytes enlarge, local oxygen handling worsens, immune cell infiltration rises, and macrophages accumulate around stressed or dying fat cells. The tissue begins generating a steady stream of inflammatory cues that do not remain local. Those signals influence insulin sensitivity, hepatic substrate handling, vascular tone, and systemic cytokine balance. This is one reason metabolic syndrome is so persistent. The body is not merely carrying extra stored energy. It is carrying storage tissue that has shifted from a buffering role into a chronic low-grade inflammatory role. Once that happens, the whole organism begins interpreting nutrient flow through a more defensive metabolic lens.

The liver sits directly downstream from this dysfunction and becomes one of the first major bottlenecks. It receives fatty acids from adipose tissue, dietary substrate from the gut, inflammatory signals from circulation, and endotoxin-related immune pressure when barrier function is poor. Under healthy conditions, it can oxidize, package, store, and export lipids with relative flexibility. Under metabolic syndrome conditions, that balance begins to collapse. Substrate delivery outpaces clean processing. Triglycerides accumulate. Inflammatory tone rises. Mitochondrial strain increases. Hepatocytes stop functioning as quiet coordinators of fuel traffic and begin behaving like stressed cells inside a persistently provoked environment. Fatty liver, elevated triglycerides, altered glucose output, and abnormal lipoprotein patterns make more sense from this viewpoint. The liver is not failing randomly. It is overloaded inside a body that keeps feeding it unresolved metabolic and inflammatory burden.

Insulin resistance fits naturally into this framework because insulin signaling depends on membrane function, receptor interpretation, mitochondrial competence, and low enough inflammatory tone that tissues can hear the signal without distortion. In metabolic syndrome, that entire environment is altered. Muscle tissue becomes less metabolically flexible. Adipose tissue is already sending inflammatory cues. The liver is overburdened. Endothelial surfaces are more reactive. Membranes are often remodeled under omega-6-heavy and oxidatively unstable conditions. Under those circumstances, insulin does not simply arrive at a neutral receptor waiting to respond. It arrives at tissues already preconditioned by inflammatory signaling, lipid intermediates, oxidative stress, and altered membrane behavior. The body then appears resistant to insulin, but that resistance is better understood as degraded interpretation and degraded tissue handling across multiple layers at once.

This is why metabolic syndrome is so strongly tied to failed resolution. The body is not just dealing with excess substrate. It is failing to complete the inflammatory and metabolic responses generated by that substrate. Meals create exaggerated postprandial stress. Adipose tissue remains immune-active between meals. The liver remains crowded with unresolved lipid handling burden. Vascular surfaces remain more permeable and reactive than they should be. Mitochondria remain too strained to fully restore metabolic quiet. Omega-3-derived resolution biology is often too weak relative to the scale of omega-6-heavy initiation and chronic re-triggering. The result is a body that never fully returns to low-noise fuel handling. Each new energy exposure lands in a system still carrying the residue of the last one.

The vascular component of metabolic syndrome matters just as much as the glucose component. Endothelial dysfunction is not a side effect. It is part of the syndrome itself. Blood vessels in this state are more adhesive to immune cells, less stable in nitric oxide signaling, more likely to display altered permeability, and more prone to remain chemically reactive after ordinary metabolic stress. This means nutrient delivery, tissue perfusion, inflammatory traffic, and microvascular control all begin to drift. Muscles do not receive the same quality of flow. Brain tissue can become more vulnerable to inflammatory and metabolic noise. Peripheral tissues recover more slowly. Blood pressure regulation becomes less stable. The syndrome is therefore not only about what is happening inside cells, but also about what is happening at the membrane interface between blood and tissue across the entire vascular tree.

The lipid side of metabolic syndrome is often badly oversimplified, but it is one of the deepest parts of the picture. A body remodeled under chronic omega-6-heavy intake, poor omega-3 incorporation, repeated oxidative damage to polyunsaturated lipids, and low specialized pro-resolving mediator output becomes more fluent in inflammatory escalation and less fluent in inflammatory completion. That affects adipose tissue, liver, muscle, vascular surfaces, and immune cells simultaneously. The membrane reservoir becomes more initiation-heavy. COX and LOX traffic remain biased toward early-phase chemistry. Debris clearance stays inadequate. Barriers remain weaker. Thresholds remain lower. In this setting, metabolic syndrome is not just a set of bad lab values. It is the metabolic expression of a body built from poor lipid architecture and poor resolution capacity.

Seen clearly, metabolic syndrome is what happens when the body loses the ability to manage energy through quiet tissues. Storage becomes inflammatory. Processing becomes congested. Signaling becomes distorted. Vascular control becomes unstable. Repair never fully catches up. The syndrome emerges because metabolic events keep being interpreted through unresolved inflammatory structure. That is why it clusters so predictably and why it so often travels with fatty liver, vascular dysfunction, chronic fatigue, poor exercise recovery, hunger dysregulation, and broader inflammatory symptoms. The deeper problem is not only excess calories or excess carbohydrate or excess fat. The deeper problem is that the body can no longer process abundance without turning that abundance into an ongoing unresolved defense state.

Neuroinflammation

Neuroinflammation is not just inflammation located in the nervous system. It is inflammation occurring in a tissue that has exceptionally low tolerance for structural noise, oxidative residue, and prolonged immune activation. That difference matters because the brain, spinal cord, peripheral nerves, retina, and the glial and vascular systems supporting them are built for precision. Neurons depend on membrane integrity, ion gradient stability, synaptic timing, vesicle cycling, receptor organization, and tightly controlled extracellular conditions. Glial cells depend on similarly disciplined boundaries because they regulate surveillance, cleanup, nutrient support, myelination, and signal shaping. When inflammation enters this environment, the problem is not only the inflammatory event itself. The problem is that the event unfolds in tissue where even modest failure of cleanup or phase transition can produce outsized functional consequences. Neuroinflammation therefore becomes dangerous less because it exists and more because it so easily degrades the signaling architecture on which neural function depends.

The inflammatory sequence in nervous tissue still follows the same broad logic seen elsewhere. There is detection, initiation, amplification, and, if the system is functioning well, resolution. But the actors and costs are somewhat different. Microglia serve as one of the main immune-surveillance populations, and they are constantly sampling the environment for signs of disruption, misfolded material, synaptic irregularity, vascular leak, infection, metabolic stress, and cellular injury. Astrocytes, endothelial interfaces, oligodendrocytes, and neurons themselves all participate in or respond to this inflammatory field. When the initiating event is proportionate and resolution follows cleanly, neural tissue can absorb the disturbance, clear the debris, restore membrane conditions, and return to functional order. When resolution fails, the tissue remains chemically loud. Microglia stay too activated. Cytokine signaling remains too elevated.

Oxidized lipids and damaged membrane fragments remain visible. Synaptic environments remain unstable. The result is not only an inflamed nervous system. It is a nervous system forced to signal through unresolved tissue.

This is one reason neuroinflammation often presents first as altered function rather than obvious structural catastrophe. The person may notice brain fog, sensory hypersensitivity, chronic pain, reduced stress tolerance, altered mood, poorer sleep regulation, diminished cognitive stamina, or a feeling that the nervous system no longer settles after stimulation. These are not trivial complaints layered on top of inflammation. They are the operational consequences of tissue that remains partially defensive. Synaptic membranes do not behave cleanly when they are oxidatively stressed and compositionally unstable. Microglia do not interpret ordinary neural activity calmly when the local environment still carries danger-associated residue. Nociceptive pathways remain amplified when the tissue continues to look unfinished. Autonomic tone becomes harder to regulate when neural signaling is occurring inside a field that has not successfully returned to low-noise baseline. Neuroinflammation therefore is not merely an inflammatory diagnosis applied to the brain. It is a loss of signal fidelity under conditions of incomplete inflammatory closure.

Membrane composition matters even more here than in many other tissues because nervous tissue is so lipid-dependent. DHA is deeply integrated into neural and retinal membranes, and that is important not only for baseline structure, but for future resolution potential. A nervous system poor in DHA, or rich in DHA that is insufficiently protected from oxidative damage, is carrying weaker structural and signaling capacity for later-phase inflammatory control. Protectins and D-series resolvins matter here because they help reduce continued inflammatory stress, protect delicate tissue from collateral injury, and support the shift away from persistent alarm. If those pathways are underbuilt, the nervous system becomes relatively better at mounting local inflammatory response than at restoring neural quiet afterward. That imbalance helps explain why low-grade neuroinflammation can become persistent, self-reinforcing, and difficult to reverse once membrane architecture and cleanup behavior have drifted far enough into instability.

Barrier function is also central to the neuroinflammatory picture. The blood-brain barrier and related neurovascular interfaces are not absolute walls, but they are highly selective control surfaces. When they become more reactive, more permeable, or more exposed to chronic systemic inflammatory traffic, the nervous system loses part of its immunological insulation. Peripheral inflammatory signals, endothelial dysfunction, metabolic stress, and barrier-disrupting chemistry can all increase the burden placed on neural tissue. This is one reason neuroinflammation cannot be understood in isolation from gut barrier dysfunction, adipose inflammation, cardiometabolic stress, or chronic vascular irritation. The brain may be the site of symptoms, but the body surrounding the brain is often helping create the environment in which the brain remains unable to resolve well. Neural tissue becomes stuck not only because of local events, but because the rest of the organism keeps feeding it evidence that danger remains near.

Resolution failure is therefore one of the most useful ways to understand chronic neuroinflammation. The nervous system is still capable of defense. What it loses is the ability to turn that defense off cleanly. Microglia may remain locked in a surveillance mode that is too aggressive for ordinary function. Damaged synaptic material may be cleared too slowly. Oxidized membrane fragments may remain in neural tissue long enough to perpetuate inflammatory interpretation. Pain pathways may remain sensitized after the phase of useful protection has passed. Sleep, mood, cognition, and autonomic balance become less stable because the tissue never fully stops behaving as if something still needs guarding. Neuroinflammation in that sense is not simply too much immune activity in the brain. It is a nervous system that never receives enough credible biochemical and structural evidence that the inflammatory event has ended.

Seen clearly, neuroinflammation is one of the most vivid examples of the central argument of this book. Chronic disease is not always best explained by excess initiation. It is often better explained by failed completion. In neural tissue, that failure is especially costly because function depends on signal precision, and precision is one of the first things unresolved inflammation destroys. The solution therefore cannot be framed only as suppressing inflammatory output. The deeper task is to rebuild membrane composition, strengthen DHA-derived resolution biology, reduce oxidative damage, restore barrier control, improve cleanup of neural debris, and lower the systemic inflammatory pressures that keep the nervous system trapped in low-grade defense. Until that happens, the person will continue experiencing what neuroinflammation really is at the lived level: a brain, nerve, or sensory system trying to perform through tissue that has not yet been allowed to finish healing.

Autoimmune Conditions

Autoimmune conditions are often described as problems of mistaken identity, as though the immune system simply becomes confused and attacks self-tissue for no deeper structural reason. That description captures part of the phenomenon, but it remains too shallow to explain why autoimmune activity becomes chronic, why it localizes in certain tissues more than others, why it waxes and wanes, and why barrier dysfunction, metabolic stress, membrane injury, infection history, and unresolved inflammation so often influence its course. A more useful view is that autoimmune conditions frequently involve failure of inflammatory completion in tissues that keep presenting the immune system with unresolved danger signals, altered self-material, damaged membrane fragments, oxidized lipids, persistent debris, or chronically disturbed barrier surfaces. In that environment, the distinction between ordinary self and inflamed self becomes less stable, because the immune system is not encountering tissue in its quiet resting state. It is encountering tissue that remains biochemically unfinished.

This matters because the immune system does not make decisions in an informational vacuum. It reads tissues through membrane signals, cytokine tone, damage-associated molecular patterns, altered extracellular matrix, abnormal vascular behavior, and the presence or absence of efficient cleanup. When apoptotic cells are not cleared properly, when oxidized phospholipids remain exposed, when mitochondrial stress keeps generating internal distress chemistry, and when barriers continue feeding abnormal immune stimulation into the system, the immune environment becomes much more likely to interpret self-tissue through a lens of unresolved threat. Autoimmune conditions therefore are not only problems of immune recognition. They are also problems of tissue presentation. A chronically inflamed, poorly resolved tissue looks different to the immune system than a well-resolved one. It is carrying structural evidence that something is wrong, and that evidence can keep immune engagement alive long after the original trigger should have been finished.

Barrier dysfunction is especially important here. In many autoimmune patterns, the body is not only reacting to tissue from within but also being repeatedly re-primed by abnormal exposure across gut, skin, respiratory, or vascular interfaces. Once those boundaries lose selectivity, immune cells are pushed into chronic surveillance and chronic partial activation. That ongoing stimulation lowers thresholds, broadens reactivity, and makes self-tissue living in a damaged or debris-rich environment more likely to be drawn into the same field of attack. The issue is not that barrier dysfunction alone explains autoimmunity. The issue is that an organism under constant barrier-derived immune provocation is less able to maintain the quiet discrimination that immune tolerance depends on. Tolerance requires more than the absence of pathogens. It requires tissue environments stable enough that self can remain recognizable as self.

Resolution biology fits here because autoimmune tissue is often tissue that never truly stops looking inflamed. Neutrophil-heavy or lymphocyte-heavy processes may differ by condition, but the deeper pattern is familiar: recruitment persists, cleanup lags, macrophage finishing remains incomplete, cytokine signaling stays elevated, and specialized pro-resolving mediator influence remains too weak relative to the burden of activation. The tissue is caught in repeated immune engagement because it never receives strong enough closure signals to re-establish low-noise order. In that setting, immune restraint becomes harder to sustain. The body keeps encountering its own tissues not as healed structures but as sites of repeated membrane damage, oxidative change, and inflammatory residue. Autoimmune conditions therefore are often better understood not just as attacks on self, but as self-tissue caught in a chronic state of abnormal presentation and failed completion.

This also helps explain why autoimmune conditions often involve flare patterns rather than constant uniform activity. The tissue can partially quiet, but because debris, membrane instability, barrier weakness, and unresolved inflammatory architecture remain in place, thresholds stay low. A minor infection, stressor, dietary insult, mechanical load, hormonal shift, or sleep disruption can reopen the inflammatory program because the site never fully returned to true baseline. The immune system does not have to invent a new pathology each time. It only has to re-enter a tissue already primed by unresolved structure. That is why the person experiences recurrence. The body is not simply overreacting from nowhere. It is returning to an incompletely closed site.

Seen clearly, autoimmune conditions belong inside the same larger framework as the rest of this book. They involve membranes, barriers, cleanup failure, inflammatory residue, altered thresholds, and weak completion biology. The specifics of each disease still matter, but beneath those specifics is a recurring principle: the immune system is more likely to remain engaged with tissues that have not regained structural quiet. A body that cannot clear debris well, cannot protect membranes well, cannot restore barrier control well, and cannot generate enough pro-resolving pressure to finish inflammation convincingly is a body more likely to live in chronic immune misengagement. Autoimmunity, in that sense, is not only a failure of recognition. It is often a failure of resolution severe enough that self-tissue never fully stops appearing as unfinished danger.

PART VII

OMEGA-3 AND SPM-FOCUSED INTERVENTION

Chapter 19

Why Most Omega-3 Supplementation Fails

Most omega-3 supplementation fails because people expect a signaling result from what is actually a structural and phase-dependent problem. They take fish oil as though it were a simple anti-inflammatory drug, something that should lower symptoms directly and predictably by virtue of entering the body. But omega-3 does not work that way. EPA and DHA are not finished therapeutic actions. They are precursor materials that have to be absorbed, transported, incorporated into phospholipids, preserved within membranes, released under the right conditions, and converted downstream into mediator families capable of changing the direction of inflammation. Even then, those mediators still need to enter a tissue environment that is capable of receiving late-phase signals and acting on them. If any layer in that sequence is weak, the person may still be swallowing omega-3 while failing to generate meaningful resolution biology. The supplement does not fail in a mystical sense. It fails because the body is being asked to produce completion from architecture that was never rebuilt enough to support completion.

The first reason supplementation fails is that most people are not actually dealing with an omega-3 deficiency alone. They are dealing with omega-6 dominance, oxidative membrane instability, poor barrier integrity, persistent cytokine signaling, enzymatic crowding in COX and LOX pathways, low-grade endotoxin exposure, mitochondrial strain, and chronic re-triggering of the front half of inflammation. In that environment, adding omega-3 is like adding better materials to a site that is still being actively damaged faster than it can be repaired. The body may absorb some of the EPA or DHA. Some may enter circulation. Some may even incorporate into membranes. But the tissue receiving it is still organized around escalation, not completion.

The inflammatory event keeps restarting before the later-phase mediator environment can gain control. The person then concludes that omega-3 does not work, when in reality omega-3 entered a system that was too inflamed, too unstable, or too poorly sequenced to use it well.

A second reason is poor membrane incorporation. Omega-3 only becomes biologically meaningful when it stops being a transient nutrient in circulation and becomes part of the phospholipid reservoir from which future signaling will be drawn. That takes time, turnover, and repeated remodeling. Most people evaluate omega-3 too early, or they use it in a body whose membranes remain so heavily dominated by omega-6-derived substrate that the EPA and DHA never achieve enough influence to materially change the releasable pool. In that case, the person can technically be taking omega-3 without substantially altering the architecture of future inflammatory behavior. The supplement is present, but the membrane is still mostly speaking the same old language. That is why many outcomes are weak or inconsistent. The intake occurred. The reservoir barely changed.

A third reason is that people misunderstand what kind of result omega-3 should produce. If the expectation is that symptoms will drop quickly in a smooth linear way, disappointment is almost guaranteed. Omega-3 is not a direct-volume suppressant in the way many people imagine. It changes structural conditions and future mediator potential. That means its effects are often delayed, threshold-dependent, and highly non-linear. A tissue may need to cross a certain level of EPA or DHA incorporation before SPM biology becomes meaningfully stronger. The body may need a reduction in oxidative burden or a partial repair of gut and vascular barriers before the same omega-3 intake starts producing noticeable changes. A person may feel nothing for a while and then improve once enough variables align for resolution activation to occur. Most supplementation "failure" is really a mismatch between linear consumer expectation and non-linear physiology.

The fourth reason is oxidative damage. EPA and DHA are highly unsaturated, which makes them biologically useful and chemically fragile at the same time. If the person is living in a state of repeated oxidative stress, poor antioxidant capacity, chronic glycemic volatility, inflamed adipose tissue, poor sleep, mitochondrial dysfunction, or persistent environmental inflammatory load, the omega-3 entering membranes may be damaged before it can be preserved and later converted into useful pro-resolving mediators. In that case, the person is not just low in omega-3 function. They are poor at omega-3 protection. The problem is no longer simply how much substrate is being consumed. The problem is whether the substrate can survive inside the tissue long enough to become part of a coherent resolution program.

A fifth reason is enzymatic bottleneck. EPA and DHA do not move through empty pathways. They compete with arachidonic acid inside shared COX and LOX systems, and those pathways are often already heavily occupied by initiation-heavy traffic in chronically inflamed tissues. If arachidonic-acid-derived signaling dominates the membrane reservoir and the inflammatory environment remains stuck in early-phase logic, then omega-3-derived substrate may never gain enough downstream priority to produce strong resolvin, protectin, or maresin output. The precursor is present, but the conversion is weak. This is one of the most common hidden failures in omega-3 use. People assume intake alone determines effect, when in reality the body also has to route that intake through pathways not already crowded by a more dominant inflammatory substrate culture.

The sixth reason is that many people use omega-3 while continuing to maintain the diet and tissue environment that created the problem in the first place. A body saturated with industrial omega-6 input, repeated ultra-processed food exposure, glycemic volatility, intestinal irritation, low protein sufficiency, poor micronutrient density, and constant metabolic overstimulation is continually rebuilding membranes in the wrong direction. Adding fish oil into that environment may help somewhat, but it is often being asked to swim against a much larger structural current. The membrane is still being edited daily by a system organized around instability. In that context, omega-3 supplementation becomes additive rather than transformative. It never gains enough control over the reservoir to shift the body into a truly different inflammatory future.

The seventh reason is wrong goal matching. EPA and DHA are not interchangeable, and most supplementation strategies ignore that. If the dominant problem is persistent inflammatory traffic, vascular irritation, and repeated immune escalation, then EPA-heavy strategy often makes more sense because it more directly alters inflammatory mediator competition and feeds E-series resolvin biology. If the dominant problem is neural instability, membrane fragility in high-precision tissue, poor tissue protection, and weak cleanup, then DHA becomes more important because it supports specialized membranes and generates protectins and maresins more directly. Many people take a generic omega-3 product without asking what branch of resolution biology they are actually trying to support. The result is not always no benefit, but often an underpowered or poorly targeted benefit.

The eighth reason is that the body may simply be too stuck for supplementation alone to carry the whole burden. If the person is in a true stuck-inflammation state, then omega-3 enters a system with incomplete debris clearance, persistent cytokine signaling, low thresholds, poor macrophage finishing, mitochondrial strain, and ongoing barrier-derived re-triggering. In that situation, omega-3 can still be valuable, but it is no longer the whole intervention. The body needs cleanup, not just substrate. It needs reduced provocation, not just precursor. It needs a membrane environment capable of preserving and using omega-3, not just swallowing it. Most failure in omega-3 supplementation is really failure of reductionism. The supplement was expected to solve a resolution problem that was much larger than substrate insufficiency alone.

Seen clearly, most omega-3 supplementation fails because people use it like a symptom tool when it is actually a structural input into inflammatory completion. It cannot reliably work in a body that refuses to incorporate it, cannot protect it, cannot convert it, cannot stop re-triggering the front half of inflammation, or cannot execute the metabolic labor of repair once the relevant mediators are produced. Omega-3 is real. EPA and DHA matter. SPM biology matters. But they matter inside a hierarchy. First the membrane has to change. Then the substrate pool has to change. Then the enzymatic and inflammatory environment has to allow mediator class switching. Then cleanup and repair have to become possible. If those steps never happen, the supplement appears weak. If they do happen, omega-3 stops looking like a failed supplement and starts looking like what it actually is: one of the body's major material requirements for ending inflammation intelligently.

Insufficient Substrate for SPM Production

Insufficient substrate for SPM production means the body is trying to execute the resolution phase without having stocked enough of the raw material required to do it well. This is one of the most important hidden reasons omega-3 strategies fail. Specialized pro-resolving mediators are not created from a vague anti-inflammatory tendency. They are created from actual fatty acid substrate, primarily EPA and DHA, that must first be incorporated into membrane phospholipids and preserved there as part of the tissue's future signaling reserve. If those membrane pools remain poor in EPA and DHA, then when inflammation begins and phospholipases mobilize fatty acids from the membrane, the body simply does not have enough omega-3-derived material available to generate strong downstream resolvin, protectin, and maresin output. The inflammatory program can still begin because arachidonic-acid-heavy initiation substrate is usually plentiful. What becomes weak is the chemistry of completion.

This matters because the body does not resolve from intake in the abstract. It resolves from what was actually built into tissue. A person can consume small amounts of omega-3 and still remain functionally under-supplied if those amounts never produce meaningful phospholipid remodeling. In that case the membrane reservoir remains dominated by omega-6-derived substrate, especially in tissues already shaped by long-term modern dietary patterns. The result is a body with plenty of material for eicosanoid-heavy early-phase inflammatory signaling and too little material for later-phase pro-resolving mediator generation. This is not just a nutrient shortage. It is a built asymmetry in inflammatory capability. The body is structurally prepared to start more strongly than it is prepared to finish.

Insufficient substrate also explains why low omega-3 status is more serious than a simple deficiency model suggests. If EPA and DHA are underrepresented in phospholipid pools, then not only is SPM production weakened, but membrane behavior itself is altered before any mediator is produced. Receptor environments shift, substrate competition remains tilted toward omega-6 pathways, and the tissue enters inflammatory stress already biased toward escalation. Then, when the later phase should begin, the body reaches into the membrane reservoir for completion-capable precursor and finds too little there. Resolution pressure remains weak not because the tissue does not want to resolve, but because it was underbuilt for that task from the start.

This is one reason small or inconsistent omega-3 intake so often produces disappointing results. The body usually needs more than token exposure. It needs enough repeated input to remodel membranes meaningfully, enough stability to preserve that remodeling, and enough downstream opportunity for the new substrate environment to influence inflammatory events. Until that happens, SPM production may remain functionally sparse even if some omega-3 is technically present. The tissue has not crossed the threshold from trace availability into usable reserve. From the outside, it looks like omega-3 is weak. Mechanistically, the real problem is that the substrate pool is still too thin to support a strong resolution program.

Seen clearly, insufficient substrate for SPM production means the body is trying to generate the chemistry of closure from a membrane reservoir that was never adequately stocked for closure. It still has fuel for inflammatory initiation. It lacks enough material for inflammatory completion. That is why low omega-3 status does not merely reduce one beneficial pathway. It lowers the tissue's built-in ability to produce the signals that stop continued recruitment, improve macrophage cleanup, protect structure, and bring inflammation to a real end state.

Poor Bioavailability

Poor bioavailability is one of the simplest and most overlooked reasons omega-3 supplementation fails, because the body cannot build membranes from fatty acids it never meaningfully absorbs. A capsule can be swallowed, a label can show a large milligram number, and the person can still end up with very little useful EPA or DHA reaching tissue if digestion, emulsification, absorption, transport, and incorporation all perform poorly. This matters because omega-3 does not act by symbolic intake. It acts by physical arrival. The fatty acid has to survive the digestive process, be released from its delivery form, encounter adequate bile and lipase activity, enter micelles, cross the intestinal surface, be repackaged into transport particles, and then ultimately reach the tissues where phospholipid remodeling occurs. If that sequence is weak, the person may be consuming omega-3 without actually supplying much substrate to the membrane reservoir that later supports SPM production.

The problem is especially important for people with compromised fat digestion or poor bile coordination. Omega-3 is still a lipid, and lipids require proper handling in the gut. If bile flow is weak, if pancreatic lipase function is limited, if intestinal irritation is high, if the person has gallbladder dysfunction, if digestive timing is poor, or if the supplement form is hard to liberate efficiently, then absorption may fall well below what the label implies. In that situation the body is not refusing omega-3 at the membrane level yet. It is simply not being given enough at the absorption level to matter later. Poor bioavailability therefore creates a false sense of supplementation. The person thinks they are building future resolution capacity, but the body never receives enough usable EPA and DHA to remodel tissue meaningfully.

Delivery form also matters because not all omega-3 enters digestion in the same structural state. Some forms are easier to digest, emulsify, and absorb than others. The fatty acid may be presented as triglyceride, re-esterified triglyceride, phospholipid-bound, ethyl ester, free fatty acid, or inside an emulsified system, and that influences how easily it moves through the digestive sequence. A person using a form with weaker absorption characteristics, especially in the context of already compromised fat digestion, may obtain far less tissue delivery than expected. This helps explain why some people report dramatic differences between products that seem similar on paper. The issue is not only dose. It is how much of that dose survives the route from capsule to membrane.

Poor bioavailability also interacts with timing and meal context. Fat absorption generally works better in the presence of a meal that stimulates bile flow and digestive activity than in a completely empty digestive context, especially in people whose baseline fat handling is already marginal. If the supplement is taken in a way that minimizes digestion rather than supports it, then delivered dose and absorbed dose diverge even further. Again, the relevant biology is not what was swallowed. It is what reached phospholipid architecture.

This becomes critically important in the context of SPM production because specialized pro-resolving mediators depend on actual membrane incorporation of EPA and DHA, not on nominal intake. If bioavailability is poor, then membrane remodeling remains weak, substrate competition remains tilted toward omega-6-derived pools, and the later conversion into resolvins, protectins, and maresins remains underpowered. The person may conclude that omega-3 does not help them, when the deeper problem is that the body never received enough absorbable substrate to build the reservoir from which help could later emerge.

Seen clearly, poor bioavailability means supplementation fails before membrane biology even begins. The bottleneck is upstream. The fatty acid never meaningfully enters the system, so the body cannot store it, protect it, release it, or convert it downstream into the chemistry of completion. That is why omega-3 strategy cannot be reduced to label dose alone. The real question is how much usable EPA and DHA actually makes it into tissue.

Oxidized Inputs

Oxidized inputs are one of the most damaging and least appreciated reasons omega-3 strategies fail, because the body cannot build clean resolution biology from damaged lipid material. EPA and DHA are valuable precisely because they are highly unsaturated and can serve as membrane-active structural components and later as precursor substrate for specialized pro-resolving mediators. But that same unsaturation makes them vulnerable before they ever reach tissue. If the oil itself has already undergone oxidation during processing, storage, shipping, encapsulation, light exposure, heat exposure, or time, then the person is not taking in a clean precursor pool. They are taking in a partially degraded lipid input carrying peroxides, aldehydes, and other breakdown products that no longer behave like intact membrane substrate. In that situation, the supplement is not just weaker than expected. It can become directionally wrong. Instead of supplying clean material for phospholipid remodeling and later SPM production, it adds oxidative burden to a system that already struggles to protect highly unsaturated fats.

This matters because membranes are not improved by damaged building material. The body has to absorb, transport, and handle what it is given. If the incoming omega-3 is already oxidized, then even before questions of incorporation or conversion arise, the tissue is dealing with reactive lipid fragments rather than predominantly intact fatty acid substrate. Those damaged molecules can increase oxidative stress, interfere with membrane behavior, generate additional inflammatory signaling, and burden detoxification and antioxidant systems that should have been protecting clean omega-3 after incorporation rather than cleaning up damage before incorporation. The problem is therefore not only that oxidized omega-3 fails to support resolution. It can actively worsen the background conditions that make resolution difficult in the first place.

Oxidized inputs also distort the meaning of supplementation outcomes. A person may take fish oil expecting reduced inflammatory continuation and stronger pro-resolving biology, yet experience little benefit, instability, or even worsening symptoms. In many cases, the question is asked at the wrong level. People ask whether omega-3 works, when the more relevant question is whether the omega-3 arriving at the tissue was intact enough to function as precursor substrate rather than as oxidized debris. Highly unsaturated fats entering the body in a damaged state do not simply lose potency. They alter the biochemical environment into which they are delivered. This is especially problematic in a body already living under oxidative stress, poor membrane stability, chronic inflammation, and weak antioxidant reserve. The person is then adding fragile or already-damaged lipids into a system that is already struggling to preserve clean lipid architecture.

This is one reason quality control matters so much more for omega-3 than people often realize. With a stable nutrient, some degradation may reduce effectiveness without changing the fundamental direction of the intervention. With a highly unsaturated lipid, degradation changes the substance itself. A fresh, protected EPA- or DHA-rich input gives the body a chance to absorb and incorporate intact substrate into phospholipid pools. A rancid or partially oxidized input gives the body a burden that resembles the very membrane damage and lipid peroxidation it is often already trying to resolve. The distinction is not cosmetic. It is mechanistic.

Seen clearly, oxidized inputs fail because the body does not resolve inflammation from damaged precursor. It resolves from intact precursor that can be protected, incorporated, and later converted into resolvins, protectins, and maresins. If the input is already oxidized, then the intervention is compromised before the first membrane ever gets remodeled. The body is being asked to build order from degraded material, and that usually means less structural gain, less resolution substrate, more oxidative burden, and more confusion about why omega-3 appears unreliable.

Lack of Enzymatic Conversion

Lack of enzymatic conversion is one of the central reasons omega-3 presence fails to become omega-3 function. EPA and DHA do not resolve inflammation merely by existing in circulation or even by being present in membranes. Their deeper value depends on what the body can convert them into once inflammatory sequencing reaches the point where closure should begin. That means release from phospholipids, routing through cyclooxygenase and lipoxygenase pathways in the appropriate phase, generation of E-series or D-series mediator families, and sufficient downstream influence for those mediators to actually redirect tissue behavior. If that conversion step is weak, then omega-3 remains structurally present but functionally underexpressed. The body is carrying precursor without producing enough of the later-phase chemistry that precursor is meant to support.

This problem matters because many people assume that increasing omega-3 intake automatically means increasing specialized pro-resolving mediator output. That assumption is too simple. Enzymes do not work in a vacuum, and they do not process every available fatty acid with equal timing, equal preference, or equal downstream consequence. EPA and DHA enter tissues already crowded by arachidonic-acid-rich substrate, inflammatory cytokine pressure, oxidative stress, and repeated early-phase signaling. In that environment, COX and LOX traffic may remain dominated by initiation-heavy chemistry. The tissue keeps converting what it is most prepared to convert, and that often means the front half of inflammation continues receiving biochemical priority while the back half remains comparatively weak. The result is a body with some omega-3 in storage and too little omega-3-derived resolution output in action.

Lack of enzymatic conversion can happen for several reasons at once. One is simple substrate competition. EPA and DHA may be present, but if arachidonic acid remains far more abundant in the releasable phospholipid pool, then shared enzymatic systems remain biased toward eicosanoid-heavy initiation chemistry. A second is phase failure. The body has to undergo mediator class switching for pro-resolving pathways to gain meaningful control. If the tissue never shifts convincingly out of repeated recruitment and amplification, then the enzymes continue being used as tools of escalation rather than tools of completion. A third is oxidative instability. If the membrane environment is highly oxidized, then EPA and DHA may be damaged or functionally underused before they can be cleanly routed into useful downstream mediator production. A fourth is cellular context. The same precursor pool behaves differently depending on whether macrophages are in an effective finishing phenotype, whether neutrophil-heavy logic still dominates the site, and whether the tissue environment is actually prepared to respond to pro-resolving instruction.

This is why lack of enzymatic conversion often looks like omega-3 failure from the outside. The person takes omega-3, perhaps even achieves some tissue incorporation, but little changes in a durable way because the body never translates stored substrate into strong resolvin, protectin, or maresin output. The membrane contains more potential, but the pathways needed to express that potential remain bottlenecked. The supplement appears weak, but the deeper defect is not necessarily intake. It is pathway expression. The tissue has the ingredients for completion and still behaves as though it only knows how to begin.

Seen clearly, lack of enzymatic conversion means the body is underbuilt at the precise step where structural precursor is supposed to become functional resolution. EPA and DHA matter, but they only become decisive when the body can process them into the later-phase signals that reduce continued neutrophil recruitment, improve macrophage cleanup, protect tissue, and support real closure. Without that conversion, omega-3 remains mostly stored possibility. The inflammatory program then stays biased toward initiation because the chemistry of completion never becomes strong enough to take command.

Chapter 20

Driving SPM Production Effectively

Driving specialized pro-resolving mediator production effectively does not mean forcing the body to manufacture more of one isolated molecule. It means rebuilding the conditions under which the body can actually convert inflammation into completion. That distinction matters because SPM biology sits at the end of a long chain. EPA and DHA must be absorbed, protected from oxidation, incorporated into membrane phospholipids, stored in the right tissues, released under the right conditions, routed through the right enzymatic pathways, and then received by a tissue environment capable of acting on late-phase instruction. If any part of that chain is weak, SPM production remains underpowered no matter how enthusiastically omega-3 is consumed. The real task is therefore not simply increasing intake. It is strengthening the structural, enzymatic, oxidative, and inflammatory context that allows intake to become resolution.

The first requirement is adequate precursor supply in a form the body can actually use. SPMs are derived primarily from EPA and DHA, so the membrane reservoir has to contain enough of both to make later conversion meaningful. That means the question is never just whether omega-3 is present in the diet at all. The question is whether enough intact EPA and DHA are reaching tissues to alter phospholipid composition in a durable way. Low intake fails because it never meaningfully changes the reservoir. Poor bioavailability fails because the body never receives enough usable substrate to remodel membranes. Oxidized inputs fail because damaged fats do not build clean precursor pools. Driving SPM production therefore begins with delivering intact omega-3 substrate in a way that the body can digest, absorb, transport, and preserve.

The second requirement is membrane remodeling. SPM production cannot be driven from circulation alone. The body resolves from what it has built into tissue. EPA and DHA must displace part of the existing phospholipid environment, especially in tissues that have been chronically dominated by omega-6-heavy substrate. This takes time, repeated incorporation, and enough consistency that the membrane reservoir actually changes. Until that happens, the releasable pool during inflammation remains biased toward arachidonic-acid-heavy initiation chemistry. This is why most supplementation disappoints. People try to generate a downstream resolution response from a membrane reservoir that still mostly belongs to the front half of inflammation. Effective SPM production begins when the body is no longer trying to finish inflammation with membranes still built for escalation.

The third requirement is reducing omega-6 pathway dominance. This does not mean eliminating omega-6, because the body still requires initiation chemistry. It means reducing chronic overrepresentation. If linoleic-acid-heavy intake remains excessive and membrane pools remain crowded by arachidonic-acid-rich substrate, then shared enzymatic systems remain tilted toward early-phase eicosanoid production. EPA and DHA may be present, but they will still have too little room in the membrane and too little pathway influence once phospholipases and COX/LOX activity begin. Driving SPM production effectively therefore requires not only adding precursor, but reducing the degree to which the tissue remains preloaded for early-phase inflammatory output. Otherwise the chemistry of initiation keeps drowning out the chemistry of completion.

The fourth requirement is oxidative protection. EPA and DHA are useful because they are highly unsaturated, but that same property makes them chemically fragile. A body under chronic oxidative stress will not preserve omega-3-derived precursor pools well enough to build strong SPM biology. Membranes become damaged. Peroxidation products accumulate. Reactive lipid fragments continue acting as danger signals. The tissue then loses precursor integrity before it can gain pro-resolving strength. This means that effective SPM production depends on lowering the oxidative burden surrounding highly unsaturated fatty acids. The body has to stop chewing through the very material it is trying to use for resolution. That requires a less inflammatory diet overall, better metabolic stability, better sleep, lower chronic toxic load, better barrier control, and enough antioxidant support at the tissue level that EPA and DHA remain usable instead of becoming collateral damage.

The fifth requirement is enzymatic availability and phase transition. EPA and DHA do not become resolvins, protectins, and maresins automatically. They must be routed through the appropriate enzymatic pathways at the appropriate time. That means the tissue must shift out of front-half inflammatory dominance and into mediator class switching. If neutrophil-heavy recruitment, cytokine escalation, and arachidonic-acid-driven traffic remain dominant, then COX and LOX pathways continue serving initiation logic. The person may have improved omega-3 status and still produce weak SPM output because the site never transitions into the phase where SPM generation is supposed to matter. Effective SPM production therefore depends on reducing repeated re-triggering and allowing inflammatory events to proceed far enough into closure biology that the later mediator environment can actually take command.

The sixth requirement is macrophage competence. SPMs matter because they change what macrophages do, but macrophages also matter because if they are metabolically strained, overwhelmed by debris, or trapped in mixed inflammatory phenotypes, then even good pro-resolving signaling will have weaker effects. A tissue full of uncleared apoptotic cells, oxidized lipid debris, and repeated immune residue becomes hard to finish. Driving SPM production effectively therefore also means lowering the cleanup burden enough that macrophages can succeed. Less incoming inflammatory traffic, better barrier control, lower oxidative injury, and stronger precursor supply all converge on one practical outcome: the site becomes more cleanable. That matters because SPMs are not magic molecules that erase debris. They are instructions for cells that still have to do the work.

The seventh requirement is adequate energy availability. Resolution is labor. Efferocytosis costs ATP. Membrane repair costs ATP. Restoring endothelial and epithelial control costs ATP. Mitochondrial strain is therefore one of the major hidden blocks to SPM effectiveness. A tissue can receive pro-resolving instructions and still fail to complete inflammation if it lacks the energetic organization required to carry those instructions out. This is why driving SPM production effectively is not only a lipid problem. It is also a mitochondrial problem. The body has to have enough organized energy to fund the cleanup, barrier restoration, and structural rebuilding that SPMs are trying to direct. Otherwise the chemistry of completion appears without the labor of completion following it strongly enough.

The eighth requirement is reducing chronic re-triggering. This may be the most practically important point of all. SPM biology cannot dominate in a tissue that keeps being shoved back into early-phase inflammatory logic every day. Barrier leakage, endotoxin burden, ultra-processed food exposure, mechanical overload, sleep disruption, repeated glycemic volatility, ongoing infections, poor oral health, toxic exposures, and unresolved inflammatory debris all keep the body re-entering initiation before resolution can finish. In that setting, even excellent omega-3 delivery and strong membrane remodeling may underperform. The tissue is constantly being told to start over. Driving SPM production effectively therefore means building enough physiological quiet that the body can actually stay in the later phase long enough for pro-resolving chemistry to matter.

This also means strategy should be goal-driven. If the dominant problem is persistent inflammatory traffic, vascular reactivity, or repeated cardiometabolic escalation, then EPA often deserves greater emphasis because it more directly changes substrate competition and supports E-series resolvin output. If the dominant problem is neural fragility, tissue preservation, chronic pain sensitization, poor cleanup, or membrane instability in high-precision tissue, then DHA deserves greater emphasis because it supports structural function while also feeding D-series resolvins, protectins, and maresins. If the dominant problem is broad resolution failure across multiple tissues, then both matter, because the body needs less continued recruitment, better preservation, and stronger cleanup at the same time. Effective SPM production is strongest when intake design matches the failure pattern.

Seen clearly, driving SPM production effectively is not a supplement trick. It is a reconstruction project. The body must be given enough intact EPA and DHA, enough membrane remodeling time, less omega-6 crowding, less oxidative damage, less re-triggering, better macrophage cleanup conditions, and enough mitochondrial support that late-phase mediator biology can actually be expressed. Once those conditions are in place, SPM production stops looking mysterious. The body begins doing what it was built to do all along: stop recruiting when enough recruitment has occurred, clear what inflammation produced, protect tissue during the transition, and return the site to a state that no longer behaves like unfinished danger.

Dose Thresholds for Conversion

Dose thresholds for conversion matter because omega-3 biology does not operate in a simple straight line where any increase in intake produces a proportionate increase in specialized pro-resolving mediator output. The body has to cross from symbolic exposure into functional substrate sufficiency. Below that threshold, EPA and DHA may be present in the diet or even measurable in circulation, yet still remain too weakly incorporated into phospholipid pools to materially change the releasable membrane reservoir. In that state, inflammation still draws mainly from the substrate environment it already knows, which is often dominated by omega-6-derived initiation chemistry. The person is technically taking omega-3, but the body has not yet reached the point where that intake changes the downstream probability of resolvin, protectin, or maresin production in a meaningful way. The threshold is therefore not just about amount swallowed. It is about the amount required to shift membrane composition far enough that later-phase signaling begins to notice.

This is why low or inconsistent dosing so often produces disappointment. Small amounts may be enough to create the impression of action in the bloodstream while doing very little to remodel the tissues that actually govern inflammatory behavior. Membranes turn over slowly relative to the expectations people usually bring to supplementation. If the phospholipid pool remains overwhelmingly weighted toward omega-6-derived substrate, then a low dose of EPA or DHA may never cross the level needed to alter the competitive balance of what is released during inflammatory activation. The body continues to generate the front half of inflammation from the same reservoir it had before, and the later-phase omega-3-derived pathways remain too weak to take command. What looks like omega-3 failure is often threshold failure. The intake never became large or consistent enough to change the stored material from which future inflammatory events will be built.

The threshold is also non-linear because once membrane incorporation rises past a certain point, downstream consequences can become more noticeable relatively quickly. This is one reason some people report little change for a period of time and then a more distinct shift later. The biology is not necessarily gradual in a smooth visible way. First the membrane reservoir changes quietly. Then substrate competition begins shifting. Then, when the next inflammatory event occurs, the tissue may produce a different mediator profile because enough EPA or DHA has entered the releasable pool to matter. That delayed transition is exactly what a threshold process looks like. The body does not reward every tiny increase equally. It often stays functionally similar until the structural balance changes enough to create a different inflammatory outcome.

EPA and DHA may also have different effective thresholds depending on the goal. If the objective is to alter inflammatory traffic more directly and affect eicosanoid competition, the relevant EPA threshold is the point at which EPA is incorporated strongly enough to influence the inflammatory mediator landscape rather than remaining a minor membrane presence. If the objective is neural protection, synaptic stability, or greater access to DHA-derived mediators such as protectins and maresins, then the meaningful threshold is the point at which DHA becomes sufficiently represented in specialized membrane pools to alter both structure and downstream resolution potential. These are not identical biological targets, which is why dose thresholds cannot be treated as one universal number in a mechanistic discussion. The important point is that each branch of omega-3 biology requires more than trace presence. It requires enough precursor density in tissue to build functional rather than symbolic potential.

Oxidative state, omega-6 burden, gut absorption, and inflammatory background all change where the threshold effectively sits. A person with poor bioavailability may require far more intake to achieve the same membrane remodeling another person gets with less. A person living under chronic oxidative stress may appear to reach intake targets while still failing to preserve enough clean EPA or DHA in membranes for strong downstream conversion. A person whose tissues remain heavily loaded with omega-6-derived substrate may need a larger and more consistent omega-3 input over a longer window before substrate competition begins shifting meaningfully. In that sense, the threshold is biological, not just arithmetic. It reflects what the tissue needs in order to cross from low influence to real influence inside a living inflammatory environment.

Seen clearly, dose thresholds for conversion are the point at which omega-3 stops being merely consumed and starts becoming functionally available for SPM biology. Below that threshold, the body may still be underbuilt for completion even while supplementation is technically present. Above it, the membrane reservoir begins to change enough that downstream conversion into resolvins, protectins, and maresins becomes more plausible and more influential. The central lesson is that resolution biology does not respond well to token exposure. It responds when enough intact precursor has accumulated in the right membrane pools, under conditions stable enough, to let the body finally convert stored omega-3 into the chemistry of closure.

Supporting Enzymatic Pathways

Supporting enzymatic pathways means supporting the body's ability to turn stored EPA and DHA into actual pro-resolving output rather than leaving them stranded as underused membrane substrate. This is a crucial distinction. A tissue may contain omega-3 and still fail to resolve well if the enzymes responsible for routing that omega-3 into later-phase mediator families remain crowded, mistimed, oxidatively disrupted, or functionally overshadowed by the chemistry of ongoing initiation. Cyclooxygenase and lipoxygenase pathways are not passive assembly lines waiting to do resolution work whenever substrate appears. They are dynamic systems embedded inside living inflammatory states. They respond to phase, substrate abundance, membrane composition, oxidative pressure, and the broader condition of the tissue. Supporting these pathways therefore does not mean pushing one enzyme harder in isolation. It means building the conditions under which the body can actually shift enzymatic traffic from escalation-dominant chemistry toward completion-dominant chemistry.

The first form of support is substrate clarity. Enzymes can only work with what they encounter, and if the releasable phospholipid pool remains heavily dominated by arachidonic-acid-rich substrate, then COX and LOX traffic will remain biased toward early-phase eicosanoid production. Supporting the enzymatic pathways therefore begins by changing what reaches them. EPA and DHA have to be meaningfully incorporated into phospholipids so that when phospholipases mobilize fatty acids during inflammation, the enzymes are not seeing almost exclusively omega-6-derived initiation material. This is why membrane remodeling is not separate from enzyme support. It is upstream of it. A pathway crowded with the wrong substrate cannot produce much of the right output no matter how intact the enzymes themselves may be.

The second form of support is reducing repeated inflammatory re-triggering. Enzymes remain biased toward early-phase chemistry when the tissue never exits early-phase conditions. If neutrophil-heavy recruitment, endotoxin exposure, barrier leakage, oxidative injury, and cytokine escalation keep recurring, then the body keeps using COX and LOX systems for what it believes is still urgent work: initiation, amplification, and reinforcement. In that context, omega-3-derived conversion remains weak not because the enzymes are absent, but because the tissue never reaches a convincing enough late phase for pro-resolving routing to dominate. Supporting the pathway therefore means creating enough physiological quiet that mediator class switching can actually occur. The body has to stop being forced back into the first half of inflammation every time it tries to move into the second.

The third form of support is oxidative protection. Highly unsaturated fatty acids are vulnerable, and the enzymes processing them are operating inside membranes and tissues that can become chemically disordered under high oxidative load. If EPA and DHA are being peroxidized, if membranes remain unstable, or if reactive lipid fragments keep accumulating, then the pathway loses clean substrate and clean context at the same time. Even when omega-3 is present, the conversion process becomes less efficient because the tissue is handling damaged lipids, damaged surfaces, and continued distress signaling rather than preserved resolution substrate. Supporting the enzymatic pathways therefore requires lowering the oxidative burden that would otherwise destroy precursor integrity before useful conversion can happen.

The fourth form of support is metabolic support. Resolution is not only a signaling event. It is a labor phase. Once enzymes generate late-phase mediators, cells still have to respond. Macrophages must clear debris. Endothelial surfaces must normalize. Barriers must re-close. Membranes must be rebuilt. All of that costs energy. If mitochondrial function is poor, then even successful mediator generation may produce weak biological follow-through because the tissue cannot afford the work of completion. Supporting enzymatic pathways therefore also means supporting the metabolic competence of the cells that those pathways are trying to direct. A body underpowered for repair will underexpress the value of even properly generated pro-resolving signals.

The fifth form of support is phase discipline. The body needs to maintain the distinction between initiation and resolution rather than remaining chemically smeared across both. Early inflammation requires force. Late inflammation requires closure. If that distinction is lost, the enzymatic landscape becomes confused. The tissue keeps producing some escalation signals, some attempted stop signals, and insufficient coherence in either direction. Supporting the pathways means helping the body move through the program in order. Enough initiation to contain the problem. Then enough class switching to prevent endless recruitment. Then enough cleanup and structural support to make the new mediator environment matter. Enzymes work best when the tissue's priorities are clear.

Seen clearly, supporting enzymatic pathways means supporting substrate balance, lowering omega-6 crowding, reducing re-triggering, protecting PUFAs from oxidation, maintaining mitochondrial capacity, and allowing the inflammatory sequence to move far enough into its later phase that COX and LOX systems stop being trapped in perpetual initiation logic. The deeper point is that enzymes do not fail in isolation. They fail inside tissue environments that remain too structurally biased toward escalation. Change that environment, and the same pathways become more capable of producing the chemistry of completion instead of repeating the chemistry of defense.

Reducing Omega-6 Competition

Reducing omega-6 competition is one of the most practical ways to strengthen resolution biology, because EPA and DHA do not enter an empty membrane or an empty enzyme system. They enter a body already carrying a stored phospholipid history. If that history is dominated by linoleic-acid-heavy intake and arachidonic-acid-rich downstream substrate, then the membrane reservoir, the releasable fatty acid pool, and the shared COX and LOX pathways are all biased toward the chemistry of initiation. In that setting, adding omega-3 helps, but it often helps too weakly because the body is still structurally organized around escalation. Reducing omega-6 competition means lowering the degree to which early-phase substrate controls the membrane and the downstream mediator environment. It is not about eliminating omega-6 completely. It is about reducing chronic overrepresentation so that omega-3-derived completion pathways can gain real biochemical influence.

The first place this matters is the membrane itself. Phospholipids can only hold so much fatty acid substrate. If omega-6-derived material dominates those positions, then when phospholipases are activated during inflammation, the body mainly releases substrate for arachidonic-acid-heavy eicosanoid production. Even meaningful omega-3 intake may produce only modest downstream effects if the membrane reservoir remains crowded by omega-6. Reducing omega-6 competition therefore begins with changing what is repeatedly built into tissue over time. The goal is not to abolish initiation chemistry. The goal is to stop letting initiation chemistry monopolize the reservoir from which future inflammatory behavior will be drawn.

The second place it matters is shared enzymatic traffic. EPA and DHA compete with omega-6-derived substrate for elongase, desaturase, cyclooxygenase, and lipoxygenase handling. If omega-6 remains chronically excessive, those pathways stay crowded by the work of initiation. The tissue keeps generating prostaglandin, leukotriene, thromboxane, and related early-phase outputs because that is the substrate landscape most strongly presented to the enzymes. Reducing omega-6 competition gives EPA and DHA more room to matter within the same systems. It does not create new enzymes. It changes what those enzymes are most likely to encounter and convert.

This is one reason reducing omega-6 competition often matters as much as increasing omega-3 intake. A person can add omega-3 while still maintaining a membrane environment so heavily skewed toward omega-6 that the new substrate never gains enough influence to shift inflammatory direction meaningfully. In that case, the body remains good at escalation and only slightly less poor at completion. But when omega-6 pressure falls at the same time omega-3 intake rises, the membrane can remodel more effectively, substrate competition becomes less lopsided, and the later-phase chemistry of resolvins, protectins, and maresins has a better chance of becoming biologically relevant rather than remaining theoretically possible.

Reducing competition also helps with threshold behavior. A tissue loaded with omega-6-derived inflammatory potential becomes easier to push into early-phase signaling. Less provocation is needed to release substrate, activate eicosanoid cascades, alter vascular tone, and recruit immune traffic. When omega-6 dominance is reduced, the tissue is less preloaded for automatic escalation. That does not make it defenseless. It makes it less hair-triggered. This matters because a body that starts slightly less easily is often a body that can finish more successfully, especially if omega-3-derived resolution substrate is simultaneously being rebuilt.

Seen clearly, reducing omega-6 competition is not a moral campaign against one fat family. It is a structural strategy for reopening biochemical space. It makes membrane incorporation of EPA and DHA more meaningful, makes shared enzyme pathways less crowded by initiation-heavy traffic, lowers the tissue's bias toward repeated escalation, and improves the odds that later-phase mediator biology can actually take command when inflammation should begin resolving. The body still needs omega-6. It just cannot resolve well when omega-6 dominates the entire conversation.

Time Course of SPM Upregulation

The time course of SPM upregulation is slower and more layered than most people expect because the body does not move from omega-3 intake to full resolution output in one step. Specialized pro-resolving mediators sit downstream of several structural and biochemical events that must occur in order. First EPA and DHA have to be digested, absorbed, and transported. Then they have to be incorporated into phospholipid membranes in meaningful amounts. Then those remodeled membranes have to become part of the tissue's releasable substrate pool. Then, when an inflammatory event occurs, the tissue has to reach the phase where phospholipases, COX and LOX pathways, and mediator class switching begin routing those substrates toward resolvins, protectins, and maresins rather than leaving the chemistry dominated by arachidonic-acid-heavy initiation. Only after those steps does SPM output begin to matter functionally. That means upregulation is not immediate. It unfolds across different biological clocks at once.

The first clock is absorption and circulating availability, which is relatively fast. EPA and DHA can appear in blood and transport pools within hours to days depending on dose, form, meal context, and digestive function. But this early phase is often misleading because circulation is not the same thing as resolution capacity. A person may achieve measurable exposure quickly while experiencing almost no real change in inflammatory sequencing because the membrane reservoir has not yet remodeled enough to alter what tissues will actually release and convert later. This is one reason people often overestimate short-term omega-3 effects. The body has seen the precursor, but it has not yet become built from the precursor strongly enough to behave differently under stress.

The second clock is membrane incorporation, and this is the more decisive one. Phospholipid remodeling takes longer because tissues do not replace their fatty acid composition instantly. Some tissues turn over more quickly, some more slowly, and different compartments within the same tissue remodel at different rates. Over days to weeks, and more meaningfully over weeks to months, repeated EPA and DHA input can begin shifting the phospholipid environment enough that the releasable substrate pool changes. This is the stage where future inflammatory behavior starts being rewritten in advance. The membrane is becoming less exclusively prepared for omega-6-heavy escalation and more capable of supporting omega-3-derived completion chemistry. Upregulation of SPM potential therefore begins before actual SPM production rises dramatically. The reservoir changes first.

The third clock is inflammatory phase opportunity. Even after membranes have begun to remodel, SPM biology is not constantly maximized. These mediators belong to the later phase of inflammation. That means the tissue has to actually enter an inflammatory event and also move far enough through that event that the body begins shifting from recruitment and amplification into cleanup and closure. If the tissue is constantly being re-triggered, if the site remains too dominated by early cytokine and eicosanoid logic, or if barrier dysfunction and oxidative stress keep forcing the body back into the front half of inflammation, then the full expression of SPM upregulation may lag behind membrane remodeling. The precursor is present, but the tissue has not crossed into the phase where that precursor can be converted and used strongly enough to matter. This is why people can improve their omega-3 status and still feel stuck for a time. The chemistry of completion is available in principle before it is fully expressed in practice.

The fourth clock is cleanup burden. A tissue carrying heavy inflammatory residue, uncleared apoptotic cells, oxidized lipid fragments, macrophage inefficiency, and persistent endothelial or barrier dysfunction often needs time before improved SPM biology can produce visible functional change. Even if pro-resolving mediator output begins to rise, the tissue still has to process the damage history that was already present. Resolution is labor. Less new recruitment is only one part of it. Existing debris must still be removed. Pain amplification must still be withdrawn. Membranes must still be repaired.

Barriers must still re-close. The result is that SPM upregulation may occur before symptom relief looks dramatic, because the body is first using the improved resolution environment to finish old work rather than immediately producing a clean feeling of relief.

This is why the time course is usually non-linear. Early on, there may be little noticeable change while absorption and initial membrane incorporation are occurring. Then, once membrane composition crosses a more meaningful threshold and the tissue enters conditions where mediator class switching can happen more effectively, the system may begin changing more noticeably. After that, if repeated re-triggering remains lower and cleanup burden starts falling, the body may show a broader rise in resilience rather than just a drop in one symptom. Thresholds increase. Minor triggers create less escalation. Recovery after stress improves. Pain or reactivity becomes less sticky. That later shift can seem sudden from the outside, but it is usually the visible consequence of slower invisible remodeling that happened beforehand.

The most important point is that SPM upregulation follows structural time more than supplement time. It depends on how fast tissues can remodel, how strongly omega-6 competition is reduced, how well oxidative damage is controlled, how effectively barriers are restored, and whether the body can actually enter the later phase of inflammation without being pushed back into repeated initiation. The clock therefore differs from person to person and tissue to tissue. A relatively stable body with decent digestion, lower inflammatory load, and moderate omega-6 competition may show meaningful changes earlier. A body in a true stuck-inflammation state may require much longer because the organism is not simply waiting for more precursor. It is trying to rebuild the entire context in which precursor can become resolution.

Seen clearly, the time course of SPM upregulation runs in layers: rapid exposure, slower membrane incorporation, later non-linear increases in conversion potential, and then still later improvements in cleanup, thresholds, and tissue behavior. That is why omega-3 should not be judged by whether it produces an immediate suppressive effect. Its deepest value appears when enough time has passed for the body to stop merely containing the substrate and start using it to change the inflammatory ending.

Chapter 21

Direct SPM Supplementation vs Precursor Strategy

The question of direct SPM supplementation versus precursor strategy forces a deeper clarification of what kind of biological problem is actually being addressed. If the body is struggling with inflammation because it cannot generate enough late-phase signals from its own tissue reservoirs, then the idea of providing finished or semi-finished pro-resolving mediators appears attractive. It promises to bypass slow membrane remodeling, bypass weak conversion, and deliver the stop signal more directly. But that promise has to be evaluated carefully because inflammation is not solved only by dropping a late-phase signal into the system. The body does not merely need an instruction to resolve. It needs membranes capable of storing the right substrate, tissues capable of receiving the instruction, immune cells capable of carrying out cleanup, barriers capable of re-closing, and mitochondria capable of funding repair. Direct SPM strategies and precursor strategies therefore solve different parts of the same problem. One acts closer to the downstream signal layer. The other acts at the level of structural preparation and long-horizon tissue remodeling. Neither should be confused for the whole answer.

A precursor strategy works by rebuilding the reservoir. EPA and DHA are supplied, absorbed, transported, and incorporated into phospholipid membranes, where they gradually change the structural and signaling potential of tissue. Over time this alters substrate competition, changes what phospholipases will later release during inflammatory activation, and increases the body's ability to generate resolvins, protectins, and maresins from within. The great strength of this strategy is that it respects the architecture of physiology. It does not merely add a signal. It changes the material from which future signals are built. That matters because chronic inflammatory disease is usually not only a signaling problem. It is a membrane problem, a threshold problem, a barrier problem, and a cleanup problem. Precursor strategy works more slowly, but when it works well, it changes the starting conditions of the next inflammatory event, not just the visible tone of the current one. The body becomes harder to trigger unnecessarily and better equipped to finish what it starts.

The limitation of precursor strategy is that it is indirect. EPA and DHA have to be meaningfully incorporated. They have to survive oxidative stress. They have to compete successfully with omega-6-dominant substrate pools. They have to move through COX and LOX bottlenecks. They have to be converted at the right phase. The tissue has to remain stable enough that SPM generation can actually matter once it occurs. This makes precursor strategy highly dependent on the quality of the terrain. A person can take omega-3 for a long time and still get only partial resolution benefit if membranes remain oxidatively unstable, if gut or vascular barriers keep re-triggering the inflammatory program, if the body remains too crowded by arachidonic-acid-heavy chemistry, or if macrophage cleanup and mitochondrial function remain poor. Precursor strategy is therefore powerful but conditional. It builds capacity rather than guaranteeing immediate downstream expression.

Direct SPM supplementation tries to solve the problem from the other end. Instead of waiting for tissue to absorb EPA and DHA, remodel membranes, release substrate, and convert it enzymatically, it attempts to provide later-phase mediators or mediator-like molecules more directly. The theoretical advantage is obvious. It may bypass some of the slow structural steps and some of the enzymatic bottlenecks. It may offer a way to increase pro-resolving signaling even in tissues that are poor at generating those mediators on their own. This is especially appealing in conditions marked by severe resolution failure, where the body still inflames strongly but seems chronically unable to activate the stop signal with enough force to change the direction of the event. In that context, direct SPM delivery looks like a way to inject more phase-transition pressure into a system stuck in escalation.

But the limitations are equally important. Direct SPM supplementation is downstream by design, and downstream strategies are always limited by the state of the structure receiving them. A signal can arrive in a tissue that is too oxidized, too debris-laden, too barrier-leaky, too omega-6-dominant, or too metabolically underpowered to act on that signal well. In other words, giving the body more stop signals does not necessarily rebuild the membrane reservoir, reduce omega-6 competition, correct phospholipid composition, or improve the tissue's long-term ability to generate its own resolution chemistry. It may improve later-phase instruction temporarily, but if the body remains structurally underbuilt for closure, then the intervention risks becoming dependent on repeated external supply rather than producing a durable reprogramming of tissue behavior. Direct SPMs may help tell the body what to do. They do not necessarily change what the body is made from.

This difference becomes especially important when thinking about time horizon. Precursor strategy is slower because it works through membrane remodeling and future inflammatory potential. Direct SPM strategy is conceptually faster because it works through immediate downstream signaling. That means the two approaches are not true opposites so much as they are interventions at different depths. A precursor strategy is architectural. It attempts to make the body itself more capable of generating completion signals. A direct SPM strategy is tactical. It attempts to increase completion signaling now, even if the body is not yet structurally very good at producing that signal by itself. The question is therefore not which is universally better. The question is whether the need is immediate phase correction, long-term tissue remodeling, or both.

This also reveals a hierarchy. Direct SPM supplementation may make the most sense when the body is profoundly stuck in inflammatory continuation and a stronger downstream resolution push is needed to help move the tissue out of recruitment-heavy logic. Precursor strategy may make the most sense when the core issue is poor membrane composition, long-term omega-6 dominance, weak omega-3-derived substrate pools, and chronically low resolution potential. In many real cases, the body likely needs both phases of thinking. It needs the reservoir rebuilt and the later-phase signals strengthened. But if forced to choose which strategy builds more durable physiology, precursor strategy usually has the deeper reach because it changes the substrate library from which future inflammatory events will be written. Direct SPMs may be able to shift behavior transiently. EPA and DHA incorporation can shift the architecture of the behavior itself.

Another important distinction is robustness. The body's own SPM generation occurs within tissue-specific contexts and in relationship to local phase timing. That means precursor-driven endogenous production has the advantage of being embedded in native control systems. Direct SPM supplementation, by contrast, is attempting to influence that system from the outside, which may still be useful, but it raises a different question: how well does an externally supplied pro-resolving mediator or analog match the timing, tissue localization, receptor engagement, stability, and concentration dynamics of the body's own internal mediator biology. Even if it produces benefit, it does not necessarily reproduce the full elegance of endogenous resolution signaling. The body is normally generating these mediators from local membranes in response to local events. Exogenous strategies may help, but they are not automatically identical to native physiology simply because they resemble part of its chemistry.

Seen clearly, direct SPM supplementation and precursor strategy should be understood as interventions at different levels of the inflammatory sequence. Precursor strategy rebuilds the membrane reservoir, changes substrate competition, and increases long-horizon resolution potential from within. Direct SPM strategy attempts to strengthen the downstream stop signal more immediately, especially where endogenous conversion is weak or too slow to matter in the moment. The deeper lesson is that resolution biology cannot be reduced to either one alone. If the body is underbuilt structurally, direct signals may underperform. If the body is trapped in severe chronic escalation, precursor alone may take too long or remain too weakly expressed unless the downstream phase is also supported. The best framework is therefore not binary. It is layered. Build the reservoir, reduce omega-6 crowding, protect the membrane, support conversion, reduce re-triggering, and where appropriate strengthen the later-phase instruction directly enough that the tissue can finally stop behaving as though the emergency is still open.

Exogenous SPM Products

Exogenous SPM products are products designed to supply specialized pro-resolving mediators, or closely related downstream resolution compounds, from outside the body rather than relying entirely on the body to generate them from EPA and DHA stored in membranes. In theory, they are meant to bypass one of the biggest bottlenecks in omega-3 biology, which is the long chain between precursor intake and actual later-phase mediator production. Instead of asking the body to absorb omega-3, remodel membranes, release substrate, compete through COX and LOX pathways, and then generate enough resolvins, protectins, or maresins to matter, an exogenous SPM product attempts to deliver the later-phase signal more directly. The attraction is obvious. If chronic inflammation is partly a problem of inadequate stop-signal strength, then providing the stop signal itself appears more efficient than waiting for the body to build it from precursor.

That said, these products should be understood as downstream interventions, not structural replacements for precursor strategy. They may help increase pro-resolving signaling pressure, but they do not rebuild membrane composition, do not displace omega-6-heavy phospholipid architecture, do not correct poor DHA or EPA incorporation, and do not by themselves restore the tissue reservoir from which the body is supposed to generate its own resolution chemistry over time. In other words, they can potentially influence the instruction layer without fully correcting the storage layer. That distinction matters because many chronically inflamed tissues are not suffering only from weak late-phase signaling. They are also suffering from poor membrane architecture, oxidative instability, repeated re-triggering, barrier dysfunction, and incomplete cleanup. An exogenous SPM product may help push the system toward closure, but it is still entering a tissue environment that may be structurally underprepared to obey that signal well.

This is why exogenous SPM products make the most conceptual sense in situations where the central problem is weak downstream resolution pressure relative to persistent inflammatory activation. If the body still inflames strongly but does not generate enough convincing late-phase instruction to stop continued neutrophil traffic, improve macrophage finishing, and restore tissue order, then a direct pro-resolving signal strategy is at least mechanistically coherent. But it should not be mistaken for a complete substitute for membrane remodeling. A tissue that remains loaded with omega-6-dominant substrate, chronically oxidized lipids, uncleared debris, and repeated barrier-derived immune provocation may still underperform even when given a more direct stop signal. The body can receive the instruction and still struggle to carry it out.

The deeper point is that exogenous SPM products are best understood as tactical rather than architectural. They may help change phase. They do not necessarily change the material basis from which future inflammatory phases will be built. Precursor strategy, by contrast, is slower and less direct, but it works on the reservoir itself by increasing EPA and DHA incorporation into phospholipids. So exogenous SPM products belong to the downstream end of the sequence, while omega-3 precursor strategy belongs to the upstream end. The most honest way to frame them is not as magic replacements for omega-3, but as attempts to strengthen one specific part of the resolution program, the signaling phase of closure, in bodies that may still need broader structural repair underneath.

Stability and Bioavailability Challenges

Stability and bioavailability are the two main reasons exogenous SPM products are conceptually appealing but biologically difficult. The appeal is straightforward. If chronic inflammation reflects weak resolution signaling, then supplying resolvins, protectins, maresins, or related downstream mediators directly seems like a way to bypass slow membrane remodeling and weak endogenous conversion. The difficulty is that these molecules sit at the far end of a fragile lipid pathway. They are not robust compounds in the way many ordinary nutrients are. They are highly specialized lipid mediators that must remain chemically intact, survive formulation, survive storage, survive digestion if taken orally, cross into useful biological compartments, and reach tissues in forms and concentrations that still preserve their signaling identity. That is a demanding chain, and weakness at any point can turn a theoretically elegant strategy into a practically inconsistent one.

The stability problem begins with the same feature that makes resolution biology possible in the first place. These compounds are built from highly unsaturated fatty acid precursors. That makes them chemically expressive, but it also makes them more vulnerable to degradation. Heat, light, oxygen exposure, time, manufacturing conditions, and storage conditions can all affect lipid-derived molecules long before they reach the body. With exogenous SPM-type products, that fragility matters more than it does with simple precursor oils because the goal is no longer merely to deliver fatty acids that the body can later process. The goal is to preserve a more advanced, already-structured signaling compound. If that compound degrades, the product is not simply weaker in a general sense. It may no longer be delivering the same biological instruction at all. The closer one moves to the downstream end of lipid signaling, the more demanding chemical preservation becomes.

Bioavailability is the second major problem. Even if the compound remains stable in the bottle, the body still has to receive it in a meaningful way. Oral delivery introduces immediate uncertainty. Lipid mediators must survive the digestive environment, avoid being lost to breakdown before absorption, and then enter circulation or local tissue spaces in forms that still permit useful receptor interaction. That is not trivial. A precursor strategy can tolerate some of this inefficiency because EPA and DHA are meant to be absorbed as fatty acids and then slowly incorporated into membranes over time. Exogenous SPM products are attempting something more delicate. They are trying to deliver later-phase instruction directly. If digestion, emulsification, transport, or local metabolism distort that signal too heavily, then what reaches tissue may be less than what the label implies, or less biologically coherent than what the concept promises.

Timing makes the challenge even more serious. Endogenous SPM production happens locally, in relationship to phase, in tissues that have already entered inflammatory activation and are shifting toward completion. That means natural SPM signaling is not just about the molecule itself. It is about where it appears, when it appears, and in what inflammatory context it appears. Exogenous delivery has a harder job because it must try to introduce that signal from outside the normal timing architecture. Even if some of the compound reaches circulation, it may not reproduce the same local concentration, receptor context, or phase-appropriate appearance that endogenous resolution signaling achieves. This does not mean exogenous products cannot work at all. It means they are operating at a disadvantage compared with a body generating pro-resolving mediators directly at the membrane site where inflammatory sequencing is already unfolding.

There is also a tissue-targeting problem. Different tissues express different needs, different receptor environments, and different cleanup burdens. A local inflammatory site in the gut, a vascular interface, a joint, or neural tissue does not necessarily respond identically to the same circulating pro-resolving signal. Endogenous production partly solves this by generating mediators where substrate was stored and where the event is happening. Exogenous products have to rely more heavily on systemic distribution and hope that enough intact signal reaches the right tissue at the right time. That makes consistent outcomes harder, especially in bodies carrying multiple simultaneous inflammatory burdens across several tissues.

These challenges do not make the strategy meaningless. They simply make it conditional. A well-formulated exogenous SPM product may still provide useful downstream pressure toward closure, especially in a body that is poor at generating its own pro-resolving signals. But the strategy is inherently more sensitive to chemistry, delivery form, storage conditions, digestion, timing, and tissue context than people often assume. It is also why exogenous SPM products should not be mistaken for full substitutes for precursor strategy. Precursor strategy rebuilds the membrane reservoir and changes future inflammatory potential from the structural level upward. Exogenous SPM products try to strengthen the late-phase signal more directly, but they still depend on that signal remaining stable enough to survive delivery and biologically available enough to influence tissue behavior after arrival.

Seen clearly, stability and bioavailability challenges are not side issues. They are the core practical limits of exogenous SPM strategies. The closer an intervention gets to the body's own native late-phase signaling chemistry, the more elegant it becomes in theory and the more fragile it becomes in practice. That is why direct SPM approaches may be useful as tactical tools, but why they remain difficult to rely on as complete solutions. The body does not only need the right signal. It needs that signal intact, delivered, received, and acted on inside tissue still capable of resolution.

Precursor-Based vs Direct Delivery

Precursor-based delivery and direct delivery differ at the level of where they intervene in the resolution sequence. Precursor-based delivery supplies EPA and DHA and asks the body to do the rest. Those fatty acids must be absorbed, incorporated into phospholipid membranes, preserved there as part of the tissue reservoir, released during inflammatory activation, and then converted downstream into resolvins, protectins, and maresins if the tissue reaches the later phase strongly enough to support that conversion. Direct delivery tries to skip part of that chain by supplying downstream pro-resolving molecules, or compounds positioned much closer to them, rather than relying entirely on endogenous conversion from stored membrane substrate. In simple terms, precursor strategy rebuilds the library. Direct delivery tries to supply part of the message.

The advantage of precursor-based strategy is depth. It changes the membrane itself. Over time it can alter the phospholipid reservoir, shift substrate competition away from omega-6 dominance, improve the structural environment around receptors and enzymes, and increase the body's own capacity to generate resolution signals locally when inflammation occurs. That makes it more architectural and potentially more durable. It does not merely add a later-phase instruction. It changes the tissue from which later-phase instruction will be derived in the future. The limitation is that it is slow, indirect, and highly dependent on good absorption, good membrane incorporation, low enough oxidative stress, enough enzymatic conversion, and a tissue environment that actually reaches mediator class switching rather than remaining trapped in repeated escalation.

The advantage of direct delivery is immediacy. It aims closer to the resolution signal itself, which means it may help in situations where endogenous conversion is weak, where the body is stuck in chronic inflammatory continuation, or where waiting for slow membrane remodeling is not enough by itself. Conceptually, it applies more pressure to the late phase. The limitation is that it does not rebuild the structural reservoir. It may strengthen the stop signal without correcting the membrane imbalance, omega-6 crowding, barrier instability, oxidative fragility, or mitochondrial weakness that caused poor resolution in the first place. It is also more vulnerable to formulation, stability, timing, and bioavailability problems because downstream lipid mediators are more fragile than their precursors and harder to deliver intact in a biologically meaningful way.

So the real difference is not which one is universally better. It is that precursor-based delivery works upstream and direct delivery works downstream. Precursor strategy is better at changing what kind of tissue the body is built from. Direct delivery is better at trying to change what that tissue is being told to do right now. In a body that is structurally underbuilt for resolution, precursor strategy has the deeper reach. In a body that needs stronger late-phase signaling because it is stuck in inflammatory continuation, direct delivery is more targeted in principle. The strongest framework is layered rather than binary: rebuild the membrane reservoir, reduce omega-6 competition, improve oxidative stability and barrier control, and where needed strengthen downstream resolution signaling enough that the body can finally move from escalation into completion.

Clinical Implications

The clinical implications of this entire framework are substantial because it changes what chronic inflammatory illness is understood to be. If inflammation is viewed only as excessive immune activity, then treatment naturally centers on suppression. The goal becomes reducing cytokines, reducing pain, reducing swelling, reducing visible biochemical output. Sometimes that is necessary, and sometimes it provides meaningful relief. But if chronic inflammation is more accurately understood as failed resolution, then symptom reduction alone is no longer enough to define success. A quieter tissue is not necessarily a completed tissue. The deeper clinical question becomes whether the body is actually regaining the ability to stop recruiting, clear debris, restore barriers, normalize vascular behavior, stabilize membranes, and return the site to a state that no longer keeps re-triggering inflammatory interpretation.

This changes how persistent symptoms should be read. Chronic pain, fatigue, brain fog, vascular irritability, metabolic dysfunction, autoimmune flares, gut reactivity, and poor tissue recovery stop looking like isolated clinical categories and begin looking like different expressions of unresolved inflammatory architecture. The clinician or practitioner is no longer asking only what signal is elevated. The more useful question becomes what phase is failing. Is the tissue over-initiating because thresholds are too low. Is it failing to clear debris because macrophage cleanup is inadequate. Is it remaining chemically noisy because membrane composition is poor and omega-3-derived resolution substrate is underrepresented. Is barrier dysfunction feeding fresh provocation into a site that should already be closing. Is mitochondrial strain preventing the body from paying for the labor of completion. These are clinically important distinctions because each one points to a different therapeutic leverage point.

It also changes what counts as progress. If this model is right, then true improvement is not just lower inflammatory intensity. It is stronger resolution capacity. That means fewer flares from minor triggers, faster recovery after stress, lower persistence of pain after the useful protective phase should have passed, better tolerance of ordinary foods and activities, more stable energy, and less evidence that tissues remain partially defensive between episodes. In other words, a patient is not only better when symptoms are lower in the moment. They are better when their baseline threshold has risen, their tissue quiet has improved, and their body is less likely to re-enter the same inflammatory program from small inputs. Clinically, that is a very different standard from short-term suppression.

There are also important implications for omega-3 use itself. The framework argues against treating omega-3 as a generic anti-inflammatory supplement and argues for using it as a structural and phase-specific tool. It suggests that EPA-forward strategies may be more relevant when persistent inflammatory traffic, vascular irritation, and repeated early-phase recruitment dominate, while DHA-forward strategies may be more relevant when neural instability, membrane fragility, poor tissue protection, and weak cleanup dominate. It also suggests that precursor strategy alone may be too weak in severely stuck inflammatory states unless the broader terrain is changed at the same time, especially omega-6 competition, oxidative burden, barrier leak, and mitochondrial insufficiency. Clinically, that means omega-3 should be matched to the failure pattern rather than prescribed as a one-size-fits-all nutrient.

This framework also makes clear that chronic inflammatory patients often need more than one layer of support at once. If the membrane reservoir is poor, omega-3 substrate must be rebuilt. If omega-6 dominance is high, competition must be reduced. If oxidative injury is high, membrane protection has to improve. If barriers are leaking, fresh provocation has to be lowered. If cleanup is inadequate, macrophage finishing and tissue-level resolution need support. If energy production is weak, repair capacity has to be restored or the body will continue to start reactions it cannot afford to finish. The clinical implication is that resolution failure is a systems problem. That means care has to become architecture-aware, not just marker-aware.

Perhaps the most important implication is diagnostic in spirit, even when not formalized in laboratory language. It suggests that many chronic conditions are best understood not as diseases of too much defense, but as diseases of incomplete defense. The body is still trying to protect itself. It is just doing so through tissues that have become poor at closure. That reframing matters because it changes the posture of treatment from silencing to completion, from volume control to sequence restoration, from fighting inflammation as an enemy to rebuilding the body's ability to finish inflammation as a program. Clinically, that is a more useful model because it aligns symptoms, membrane biology, lipid balance, barrier function, mitochondrial capacity, and recovery behavior into one coherent picture rather than leaving them as separate unexplained problems.

PART VIII

LIPID BALANCE AND SYSTEM RESTORATION

Chapter 22

Resolution as the Foundation of Stability

Stability in biology is often misunderstood as the absence of disturbance, as though the healthy body is simply the body that is never challenged. That is not how living systems work. A living body is always being perturbed. Nutrients enter, metabolites accumulate, microbes make contact, tissues are loaded mechanically, hormones fluctuate, temperatures shift, sleep changes, light changes, emotional stress changes, immune surveillance continues, and small injuries occur constantly. Stability is therefore not the absence of challenge. Stability is the ability to pass through challenge without remaining reorganized by it in a defensive way. That is why resolution belongs at the foundation of real physiological stability. A system is stable not because it never inflames, never activates, never adapts, or never enters emergency programs. It is stable because it can do all of those things and still return to order once the useful phase has ended. The body becomes unstable when it can still start but can no longer finish cleanly.

This point brings the entire argument of the book into focus. Membranes are not simply structural boundaries. They are the material surfaces through which the body interprets reality, stores future signaling potential, and determines whether a tissue is better equipped for escalation or better equipped for completion. Lipids are not only fuels. They are structural materials and signaling substrates that shape whether inflammatory events remain proportionate or become chronic. Omega-6 is not a villain and omega-3 is not a saint. Omega-6-heavy substrate gives the body force for initiation. Omega-3-derived substrate gives the body access to mediator families that help the body stop extending that force once it has served its purpose. Stability emerges only when these roles remain coordinated. If the body can initiate but not resolve, then every ordinary perturbation begins to leave residue. Thresholds fall. Membranes become easier to disturb. Tissues remain partially open, partially inflamed, partially unrepaired. At that point instability is no longer a matter of bad luck. It is built into the architecture.

This is why resolution has to be understood as more than the end of inflammation. It is the process by which the body preserves continuity of self across repeated disturbance. A tissue that resolves well does not merely experience less discomfort. It remains itself more effectively over time. Its membranes are not repeatedly left oxidized and structurally confused. Its macrophages do not remain burdened with old debris. Its vascular surfaces do not remain in emergency mode. Its barriers do not remain chronically permissive. Its nervous system does not remain chemically overprotective after the actual need for protection has passed. Its mitochondria do not remain trapped in the energetics of defense. Resolution is what prevents each challenge from becoming a permanent edit to the tissue's operating style. It is therefore the foundation of resilience in the deepest sense. Without it, adaptation becomes accumulation of damage. With it, adaptation becomes recovery with preserved function.

This helps explain why chronic disease so often feels like loss of stability before it looks like catastrophic failure. People usually notice this first as low-level unreliability. Recovery takes longer. Sleep becomes less restorative. Small stressors create bigger consequences. Food tolerance narrows. Exercise either feels too inflammatory or no longer produces clean adaptation. Pain lingers. Mood and cognition fluctuate more than they used to. Skin, gut, joints, blood vessels, and nerves all begin behaving as though they are easier to disturb and harder to settle. These experiences are often described separately, but they are united by one deeper fact: the body is losing the ability to resolve perturbation without carrying it forward. Stability disappears when the body no longer returns fully to baseline between events. Resolution failure is what turns life itself into cumulative inflammatory burden.

This is also why the modern environment is so effective at destabilizing physiology. The problem is not only that it creates more triggers. The deeper problem is that it creates more triggers in bodies whose membrane architecture, substrate balance, oxidative burden, barrier integrity, and metabolic reserve are already organized in a way that weakens completion. The person is repeatedly asked to absorb perturbation through tissues built for initiation-heavy response and underbuilt for return. That is the mechanism of fragility. It is not just more stress. It is more stress entering systems that cannot close loops well. Once enough loops remain open, even small events begin to feel large because the body is already carrying the unfinished remains of previous events.

The foundation of stability is therefore not stoicism, not suppression, and not mere absence of symptoms. It is the body's material ability to complete cycles. A stable vascular system can constrict, dilate, recruit, and then normalize. A stable immune system can detect, respond, clear, and then stand down. A stable nervous system can amplify protective signaling when necessary and then withdraw that amplification once the tissue is safe. A stable gut can mount defense when barrier disruption occurs and then restore selectivity without continuing to invite the immune system into the lumen-facing world. A stable metabolic system can handle fuel abundance and fuel scarcity without turning either one into chronic inflammatory signaling. Every one of those forms of stability is built on the same principle. The system must be able to end what it starts.

This is why resolution should be placed beneath the usual categories of health rather than beside them. People often think in terms of immune health, metabolic health, cardiovascular health, brain health, or gut health as though these were separate domains with separate laws. But what makes all of them possible is the same underlying capacity: the ability to pass through activation without becoming stuck in activation. Resolution is what allows the organism to remain integrated across time. It prevents the body from becoming a collage of partially defended tissues, each carrying its own unfinished emergency into the next day. Once that is understood, the hierarchy becomes clearer. Membrane composition matters because it determines what kind of inflammatory and pro-resolving language the body can speak. Omega-3 matters because it helps stock the later-phase chemistry required for completion. SPM biology matters because it turns substrate into actual instructions for closing the inflammatory loop. But stability is the deeper outcome all of this serves.

The practical meaning of this chapter is therefore not merely theoretical. If resolution is the foundation of stability, then every meaningful intervention should be judged partly by whether it improves the body's ability to complete perturbation. Does it help membranes become more coherent and less easily oxidized. Does it reduce omega-6 dominance enough for omega-3-derived completion pathways to matter. Does it improve barrier control so tissues stop being re-triggered. Does it lower the cleanup burden and strengthen macrophage finishing. Does it improve mitochondrial capacity so repair can actually be funded. Does it raise thresholds so ordinary life stops being interpreted as repeated threat. Those are stability questions, and they are all resolution questions at the same time.

Seen clearly, the body is stable not when nothing happens to it, but when what happens to it can be finished. Resolution is the reason biological experience does not have to accumulate as permanent alarm. It is the mechanism by which the body preserves order across repeated contact with a world that is never fully quiet. Without resolution, inflammation becomes identity. With resolution, inflammation remains a tool. That is why resolution is not just one phase of immunity. It is one of the deepest foundations of physiological stability itself.

Ending Inflammation Restores Order

Ending inflammation restores order because inflammation is, by design, a temporary suspension of normal tissue rules. During the early and middle phases of the response, the body deliberately relaxes boundaries, increases vascular access, amplifies immune traffic, alters local metabolism, raises pain sensitivity, and accepts a certain degree of structural disruption in order to contain threat quickly. That tradeoff is useful when the event is acute and proportionate. It becomes damaging when the body cannot reverse it. Order is what has to be rebuilt afterward. Membranes have to stop leaking distress chemistry. Neutrophils have to stop arriving. Macrophages have to clear apoptotic cells and oxidized debris. Endothelial and epithelial surfaces have to regain selectivity. Pain pathways have to stop behaving as though the site is still under active threat. Mitochondria have to shift from emergency expenditure toward repair. Until those reversals happen, the tissue is not merely less inflamed. It is still disordered.

This is why ending inflammation should never be confused with suppressing inflammatory output alone. A quieter tissue is not necessarily an ordered tissue. If the body blocks some visible inflammatory signals while leaving behind uncleared debris, unstable membranes, persistent cytokine tone, barrier leak, and low-threshold immune reactivity, then the site remains unfinished even if symptoms temporarily soften. True ending is different. It means the tissue no longer needs emergency logic to maintain control. The inflammatory state has been converted into a resolution state, and then that resolution state has done enough work to restore ordinary structure. The body stops recruiting because recruitment is no longer needed. It stops amplifying because the site no longer justifies amplification. It stops protecting in the emergency sense because the tissue has become safe enough to return to maintenance.

Order in this context is not abstract calm. It is physical coherence. Gradients are preserved again. Membrane composition becomes functionally useful instead of chemically unstable. Receptors stop reading ordinary inputs through a background of unresolved danger. Vascular surfaces return to controlled exchange rather than inflammatory openness. Barrier tissues stop letting the outside world bleed too deeply into immune space. Neural tissue stops signaling through persistent noise and regains precision. Metabolic tissues stop behaving as though every fuel exposure is a stress event. What resolution restores is not merely comfort. It restores the architecture that lets tissues behave according to their real function rather than according to temporary defensive distortion.

This is the deeper reason specialized pro-resolving mediators matter so much. They do not only turn inflammatory intensity down. They help drive the biological work through which order is rebuilt. They reduce continued neutrophil influx, strengthen macrophage cleanup, limit collateral injury, support tissue protection, and help create the conditions under which barriers can close, membranes can stabilize, and repair can proceed without being constantly interrupted by renewed alarm. In that sense, ending inflammation restores order because resolution is the process by which the body removes the physical and signaling evidence that disorder is still justified.

Seen clearly, inflammation is useful precisely because it disrupts order in a controlled way for a defined purpose. Resolution is what makes that disruption survivable. If inflammation begins and never truly ends, the body remains trapped in a half-emergency state where function is always being subordinated to defense. If inflammation ends properly, the tissue becomes itself again. That is what restored order really means. Not silence, not suppression, but the return of structure, signaling, and behavior to a state in which defense is no longer the governing principle.

Energy System Stabilization

Energy system stabilization is one of the clearest signs that resolution has succeeded, because the body cannot remain metabolically organized while it is still spending heavily on unfinished defense. Inflammation is expensive. Recruitment costs energy. Cytokine production costs energy. Oxidative bursts cost energy. Barrier leak increases metabolic inefficiency. Membrane damage has to be contained. Ion gradients become harder to maintain. Sleep quality falls, pain rises, movement changes, and mitochondrial output is redirected toward survival chemistry instead of restoration. A tissue living in persistent inflammatory activation may still produce ATP, but it does so inside an unstable priority structure. Energy is constantly being diverted into surveillance, containment, and damage management. That is why people in chronic inflammatory states so often feel both activated and exhausted at the same time. The body is not low in activity. It is metabolically trapped in expensive activity that never reaches completion.

This is where stabilization becomes more than symptom relief. A stabilized energy system is not one that simply produces more energy in the abstract. It is one that stops wasting energy on repeated incomplete inflammatory loops. Once neutrophil infiltration tapers appropriately, once macrophages begin clearing efficiently, once cytokine tone falls, once barriers stop feeding fresh provocation into tissue, and once membranes stop releasing so much distress chemistry, the body can reallocate resources. Mitochondria are no longer being asked to support a semi-permanent emergency. The tissue can begin shifting from defensive expenditure toward repair, maintenance, and normal functional output. That shift often feels like improved stamina, better recovery, more stable cognition, fewer crashes after meals or stress, and less background fatigue, but underneath those experiences is a deeper physiological change. The organism is no longer financing unresolved inflammation at the same rate.

Mitochondria sit at the center of this process because they are not only power generators. They are also participants in inflammatory biology. When tissues remain inflamed, mitochondria are exposed to altered substrate traffic, oxidative stress, cytokine pressure, calcium instability, membrane damage, and repeated demand for emergency adaptation. Under those conditions, ATP production becomes less efficient and more costly. Reactive oxygen species can rise. Fatty acid oxidation may become incomplete. Glucose handling becomes less flexible. The cell remains capable of work, but the work becomes dirtier and less stable. Resolution helps correct this not by magically upgrading mitochondria from the outside, but by reducing the inflammatory burden that keeps mitochondrial function trapped in survival mode. Energy system stabilization therefore depends on inflammatory completion because the organelle cannot return to efficient output while the tissue keeps telling it that the emergency is still active.

This also explains why metabolic flexibility improves when resolution improves. A poorly resolved tissue often becomes metabolically rigid. It overreacts to glucose, handles fatty acids poorly, accumulates intermediates, or swings between underpowered and overstimulated states because the inflammatory environment keeps distorting substrate use. A better-resolved tissue can switch fuels more cleanly because the signaling environment is quieter, membrane transport and receptor behavior are more coherent, and mitochondrial membranes are operating under less oxidative and cytokine-driven interference. Stability at the energy level therefore is not only a matter of having enough calories or enough fuel substrate. It is a matter of whether the tissue has stopped behaving as though every substrate exposure is part of an unresolved threat state.

Seen clearly, energy system stabilization is one of the practical outcomes of successful resolution. The body stops burning resources to hold open a process that should have ended. Mitochondria become less burdened by defense chemistry and more available for repair and ordinary function. Tissues regain the ability to produce energy without coupling that production so tightly to inflammatory distress. That is why restored energy is not a superficial benefit of resolution biology. It is one of its deepest consequences. A body that can finish inflammation well is a body that can finally afford to use its energy for living instead of for remaining half-defended.

Nervous System Calm

Nervous system calm is not the absence of stimulation. It is the return of the nervous system to a state in which stimulation no longer has to be interpreted through unresolved threat. That distinction matters because a calm nervous system is often described in emotional or psychological language, when in reality it is also a membrane, immune, and energy problem. Neurons, glial cells, vascular interfaces, and synaptic membranes all have to stop behaving as though danger is still present. Pain pathways have to stop amplifying. Microglia have to stop maintaining a surveillance posture that is too aggressive for ordinary life. Synaptic environments have to become less chemically noisy. Membrane excitability has to stabilize. Sleep and autonomic tone have to stop being dragged around by unresolved inflammatory signaling. Calm, in this deeper sense, is not a mood. It is the restoration of signaling order.

This is why nervous system calm depends so heavily on successful resolution. A nervous system still carrying oxidized lipid fragments, persistent cytokine pressure, low-threshold nociceptive signaling, glial overactivation, and unstable DHA-dependent membrane structure cannot truly settle, even if the person tries to rest. The tissue is still broadcasting unfinished danger. The brain and peripheral nerves continue reading ordinary inputs through a background of defensive chemistry. Small stressors feel bigger. Sensory input becomes harder to filter. Sleep becomes lighter or less restorative. Mood becomes more fragile. Attention becomes less stable. The person experiences this as anxiety, tension, overstimulation, or poor recovery from stress, but underneath those experiences the biology is often the same. The nervous system has not finished its inflammatory event well enough to trust the environment again.

DHA-derived mediator biology matters here because calm in the nervous system requires more than less inflammation. It requires protection of the signaling surfaces themselves. Protectins, D-series resolvins, and related later-phase signals help reduce continued inflammatory pressure, support cleanup, and preserve delicate tissue from collateral injury during de-escalation. That is essential in neural tissue because precision is the function. A nervous system becomes calm not when it is suppressed into silence, but when its membranes, synapses, glial cells, and vascular interfaces no longer have to keep operating inside a field of unresolved danger. Once that happens, sensory thresholds normalize, pain amplification can withdraw, autonomic tone becomes less defensive, and the person experiences what calm actually is at the physiological level: a nervous system that no longer needs to stay half-guarded between ordinary events.

Seen clearly, nervous system calm is one of the lived outcomes of restored resolution capacity. It appears when the body can stop protecting after the useful phase of protection has passed. That means fewer lingering inflammatory signals, better cleanup of neural debris, stronger membrane stability, lower oxidative noise, and less repeated re-triggering from the rest of the organism. Calm is not passivity. It is the return of the nervous system to a state where precision no longer has to compete with chronic alarm.

Hormonal Normalization

Hormonal normalization is one of the clearest downstream consequences of successful resolution because hormones do not operate in isolation from membrane structure, inflammatory tone, vascular control, and mitochondrial status. A hormone can be present in circulation and still be poorly interpreted if the membrane receiving it is unstable, the receptor environment is distorted, cytokine signaling is chronically elevated, or the tissue remains metabolically trapped in defense. This is why chronic inflammatory states so often look hormonal from the outside. Cortisol rhythms become less stable. Insulin signaling becomes less reliable. Thyroid signaling becomes less effectively expressed at the tissue level. Reproductive hormones may be present yet poorly translated into stable function. Appetite hormones become noisier. Sleep and circadian signals lose precision. The body begins to look hormonally dysregulated, but in many cases the deeper problem is that endocrine signaling is being forced through tissues that have not completed inflammation well enough to return to low-noise interpretation.

The membrane matters here because receptors for insulin, thyroid hormone-related downstream effects, steroid signals, leptin, and many other endocrine inputs operate through surfaces whose composition determines clustering, mobility, signal propagation, and downstream coupling. A chronically inflamed membrane does not read hormonal information cleanly. If omega-6-derived initiation substrate dominates, if oxidative damage has altered phospholipid behavior, if cytokine tone remains high, or if mitochondrial strain keeps the tissue locked in emergency priorities, the same hormone can produce weaker, less stable, or more distorted downstream effects. The body then compensates with more signal, different timing, or altered set points, and what emerges clinically is called dysregulation. But the hormone is often not the only thing that has changed. The interpretive surface has changed.

Inflammatory persistence also directly reshapes endocrine priorities. In a body trapped in partial defense, cortisol and other stress-related systems remain more engaged because tissue still appears unresolved. Insulin handling becomes less stable because metabolic tissues remain inflamed, adipose signaling remains abnormal, and mitochondrial throughput remains inefficient. Reproductive signaling often degrades because the body does not invest in long-horizon anabolic and reproductive stability while local tissues still behave as though repair and defense are unfinished. Thyroid output or tissue responsiveness may look inconsistent because the system is continuously reallocating toward survival chemistry rather than confident baseline function. Hormonal normalization therefore is not just a matter of producing the right hormones. It is a matter of restoring a body state in which hormones can resume governing ordinary physiology instead of constantly negotiating with unresolved inflammation.

This is why resolution is so central. Once neutrophil-heavy continuation falls, once macrophage cleanup improves, once barriers stop feeding fresh provocation into tissue, once vascular surfaces calm, and once membranes become more coherent and less oxidatively noisy, endocrine signaling has a different landscape to work through. Receptors become easier to interpret cleanly. Energy availability improves because less ATP is being wasted on chronic incomplete defense. Sleep often improves because cytokine and nociceptive tone fall. Appetite and satiety signals become less distorted by inflammatory traffic. Stress hormones no longer have to cover for constant unresolved tissue burden. In that sense, hormonal normalization is not separate from resolution biology. It is one of the organism-level signs that resolution has become strong enough to restore ordinary command hierarchy.

Seen clearly, hormones normalize when the body no longer has to keep translating every endocrine signal through an inflammatory emergency filter. The endocrine system does not become healthier by hormone concentration alone. It becomes healthier when tissues regain the structural quiet, membrane stability, and lower inflammatory tone required to hear hormones accurately again. That is why chronic inflammatory illness so often looks endocrine, and why real endocrine recovery so often depends on far more than adding or suppressing one signal. The body has to become less defended before it can become more hormonally coherent.

Chapter 23

Why Omega-3 Alone Is Not Enough

Omega-3 matters profoundly, but it does not operate in isolation from the architecture into which it is introduced. This has to be said plainly because much of the modern conversation has turned omega-3 into a symbolic nutrient, a kind of biochemical hero expected to correct inflammatory instability by its mere presence. That expectation is too small for the problem and too large for the molecule. EPA and DHA can alter membrane composition, improve substrate availability for specialized pro-resolving mediators, support tissue protection, and help shift inflammatory sequencing toward completion. All of that is real. But none of it means omega-3 can override a body that remains structurally organized around repeated initiation, oxidative damage, barrier failure, mitochondrial strain, poor cleanup, and chronic re-triggering. The body does not resolve from one input alone. It resolves from a coordinated environment in which membranes, enzymes, immune cells, barriers, and energy systems can all participate in closure at the same time. If those surrounding conditions remain broken, omega-3 becomes an underexpressed good rather than a decisive correction.

This is the core reason omega-3 supplementation disappoints so many people. They are often trying to solve a phase problem with a single substrate. The tissue still carries omega-6-dominant phospholipid pools, still releases arachidonic-acid-heavy substrate easily, still sits in an oxidative environment that damages highly unsaturated fats, still receives continual immune provocation across the gut or other barriers, and still lacks the energetic reserve required to fund cleanup and repair. In that setting, omega-3 enters a system that may absorb it imperfectly, incorporate it weakly, oxidize part of it prematurely, convert too little of it into resolvins, protectins, and maresins, and then ask too much of the small downstream signal that remains. The supplement appears weak, but the real weakness is the architecture surrounding it. The body is not merely deficient in omega-3. It is resolution-deficient in a much broader sense.

Barrier integrity is one of the clearest examples of why omega-3 alone cannot carry the whole burden. A tissue cannot resolve while fresh provocation keeps arriving faster than old provocation is being cleared. If the intestinal lining remains too permeable, microbial products and luminal irritants continue entering immune space and sustaining cytokine tone. If endothelial barriers remain too reactive, inflammatory traffic and plasma-derived stress signals keep reaching tissues that should already be closing down. If cellular membranes remain damaged, danger-associated chemistry keeps leaking into the surrounding environment. Omega-3 can improve resolution potential, but it cannot make resolution dominant while the tissue still receives continuous evidence that danger is ongoing. The body has to reduce incoming trigger load as well as improve later-phase signaling. Otherwise the stop signal is constantly being drowned out by fresh reasons to keep going.

Oxidative state creates the same limitation from another angle. EPA and DHA are valuable because their multiple double bonds allow specialized membrane behavior and downstream pro-resolving chemistry, but those same double bonds also make them more chemically vulnerable. If the tissue remains under high oxidative stress, if mitochondria are leaking excess reactive species, if glucose handling is volatile, if inflammatory burden is constant, or if antioxidant and repair systems remain insufficient, then omega-3 may be damaged before it can be used properly. In that case, the person is not merely lacking more omega-3. They are lacking a membrane environment capable of protecting omega-3 once it arrives. This is one reason the body needs more than precursor supply. It needs lower oxidative chaos so that highly unsaturated substrate can remain intact long enough to become useful structure and useful later-phase mediator biology rather than simply additional lipid debris.

Mitochondrial function is another major reason omega-3 alone is not enough. Resolution is labor. Macrophages have to engulf apoptotic cells. Membranes have to be rebuilt. Junctions have to be restored. Ion gradients have to be re-established. Oxidized material has to be processed and removed. A tissue under mitochondrial strain can still initiate inflammation because initiation runs on stored substrate release, stress signals, and emergency immune logic. But that same tissue may fail to complete the event because it cannot fund the work required for closure. Omega-3 can improve membrane conditions and later-phase signaling potential, but it cannot fully substitute for the ATP needed to execute repair. A body can have a better stop signal and still remain stuck if it lacks the metabolic competence to obey that signal. Completion requires fuel availability, mitochondrial integrity, and enough energy margin that the tissue can afford to do something more than defend.

Macrophage competence presents the same principle at the cellular level. Specialized pro-resolving mediators matter partly because they improve efferocytosis and cleanup, but if macrophages are overwhelmed, metabolically dysfunctional, persistently driven into mixed inflammatory states, or buried in an environment full of oxidized debris and repeated incoming provocation, then even good SPM signaling may not produce sufficient closure. The body needs omega-3-derived substrate to build the language of completion, but it also needs cells capable of speaking that language into real tissue-level action. If the cleanup burden is too high, if the debris field is too persistent, or if repeated neutrophil-heavy escalation continues faster than macrophages can clear what is left behind, then omega-3 remains one contributor inside a system still structurally tilted toward unfinished work.

This also explains why reducing omega-6 dominance matters alongside increasing omega-3. The body does not process these substrates independently. They compete for phospholipid space, for release during inflammation, and for shared enzymatic pathways downstream. A person can add omega-3 while continuing to rebuild membranes from an overwhelmingly omega-6-heavy food environment, and in that case the new precursor may never gain enough structural or enzymatic influence to change inflammatory direction meaningfully. Omega-3 alone is then forced to work inside a reservoir still mostly defined by escalation substrate. The body remains fluent in the front half of inflammation and only weakly improved in the back half. Real change usually requires both sides of the equation: more completion-capable substrate and less chronic overrepresentation of initiation-heavy substrate.

There is also a behavioral and temporal dimension to this problem. A body repeatedly exposed to ultra-processed food, irregular sleep, chronic stress, sedentary recovery, repeated endotoxin burden, and constant metabolic noise is never being given enough uninterrupted physiological quiet to let late-phase biology dominate. Resolution takes time. It requires the inflammatory event to reach a point where recruitment can fall, cleanup can rise, and the site can stop being chemically re-opened every few hours by new disruption. Omega-3 alone cannot create that temporal window if the rest of life keeps hammering the system back into early-phase signaling. This is one reason some people take large amounts of omega-3 and still feel stuck. The substrate is present, but the body never stays in the right phase long enough to use it fully.

The deeper truth is that omega-3 should be understood as necessary but not sovereign. It is one of the major structural and signaling requirements for successful resolution, but it is not the whole architecture of resolution. The body also requires adequate barrier control, lower oxidative burden, sufficient mitochondrial output, effective macrophage cleanup, lower omega-6 crowding, less repeated re-triggering, and membranes stable enough to preserve highly unsaturated precursor without turning it into collateral damage. When those conditions are absent, omega-3 tends to behave like a partially expressed possibility. When those conditions improve, the same omega-3 can suddenly appear much more powerful because it is no longer being asked to solve problems that belong to the rest of the system.

This chapter therefore exists to protect the argument of the book from reductionism. Omega-3 matters enormously, but the point is not to replace one simplistic villain story with one simplistic hero story. The point is to understand that resolution is a coordinated achievement. EPA and DHA help build the later-phase chemistry through which the body can stop extending inflammation unnecessarily, protect tissue during de-escalation, and improve cleanup and restoration. But if the body remains structurally chaotic, metabolically strained, oxidatively unstable, and continuously re-provoked, then omega-3 will remain real but insufficient. It can contribute to the answer without becoming the whole answer. That is not a weakness of omega-3. It is a recognition of how complex the body's return to order actually is.

Seen clearly, omega-3 alone is not enough because inflammation is not sustained by one missing ingredient. It is sustained by a whole terrain that has become easier to activate and harder to complete. Omega-3 helps rebuild one of the most important parts of that terrain, the substrate basis of closure. But completion also requires membranes that can hold, barriers that can seal, mitochondria that can fund, macrophages that can finish, and tissues that can stop being reintroduced to threat before they have processed the last one. The body needs omega-3, but it also needs the rest of the conditions that allow omega-3 to become more than a supplement and finally become part of a successful biological ending.

Structural Lipid Requirements

Omega-3 alone is not enough because the body does not resolve inflammation from omega-3 alone. It resolves from membranes built with enough overall structural competence to remain stable under stress while still supporting the signaling transitions required for completion. That means the question is not only whether EPA and DHA are present. The question is whether the membrane as a whole has been built from the right classes of lipids in the right proportions for the tissue involved. A membrane needs phospholipids to form the basic bilayer architecture, cholesterol to stabilize and organize that architecture, sphingolipids to help create ordered domains and maintain signal sorting, saturated and monounsaturated fatty acids to provide structural resilience, and omega-3-derived polyunsaturated fatty acids to expand later-phase signaling options and support specialized tissue behavior. Resolution depends on this broader lipid architecture because the body cannot generate clean completion signals from membranes that are too fragile, too disordered, too permeable, or too structurally incoherent to survive the inflammatory event in the first place.

This is one of the most important corrections to simplistic omega-3 thinking. A membrane built with inadequate structural support may still contain some EPA and DHA, but if the surrounding lipid environment is poorly organized, then those omega-3 molecules are being asked to function inside a surface that is already unstable. Cholesterol distribution may be poor. Sphingolipid-supported domains may be weak. Saturated and monounsaturated components may be insufficient to provide adequate packing stability. The result is a membrane that becomes easier to oxidize, easier to distort under inflammatory stress, and less able to preserve the receptor behavior, transport control, and phospholipid integrity required for strong resolution signaling later. In that setting, the problem is not simply lack of omega-3. The problem is lack of structural lipid sufficiency at the membrane level. The body needs completion substrate, but it also needs a membrane stable enough to store that substrate and use it without falling apart.

Phospholipid head groups matter here as well, because structural lipid requirements are not only about fatty acid tails. Phosphatidylcholine, phosphatidylethanolamine, phosphatidylserine, phosphatidylinositol, cardiolipin, and related phospholipids create different local membrane properties and different functional environments in different tissues and organelles. Mitochondria require their own structural lipid organization. Neural membranes require theirs. Barrier tissues require theirs. If these structural foundations are weak, then later-phase inflammatory biology becomes weak with them because the body is trying to execute cleanup, signaling restraint, and tissue reconstruction through poorly built surfaces. Resolution is not just a matter of generating resolvins, protectins, and maresins. It is also a matter of whether those mediators are acting on cells whose membranes still possess the architecture needed to respond coherently.

This is why monounsaturated and more saturated structural inputs retain importance even in a book centered on omega-3 and resolution. A membrane cannot be composed entirely around signaling flexibility without paying a price in fragility. Polyunsaturated fatty acids expand signaling potential, but they also increase oxidative vulnerability. More saturated and monounsaturated fatty acids help provide the firmness and resilience that keep the membrane from becoming too chemically unstable under load. The body therefore does not need maximum unsaturation. It needs a composition that allows EPA and DHA to perform their role inside a structure capable of holding them safely. Structural lipid requirements are the requirements of balance. The membrane must be fluid enough to signal and stable enough to survive.

This is especially important in tissues exposed to repeated stress. Endothelial cells experience continuous shear and inflammatory contact. Gut epithelial cells experience repeated chemical, microbial, and mechanical challenge. Immune cells must constantly reorganize membranes during activation and cleanup. Neurons must preserve signaling precision over enormous time scales. In each case, the membrane must do more than merely exist. It must remain functionally composed under pressure. If the broader structural lipid environment is weak, then any attempt to strengthen resolution through omega-3 alone becomes limited because the body is still asking a fragile surface to carry the work of closure. Structural lipid sufficiency therefore is not a secondary nutritional refinement. It is one of the preconditions for omega-3-derived biology to become fully effective.

Seen clearly, structural lipid requirements explain why successful resolution depends on membrane quality as a whole rather than on one favored fatty acid class in isolation. EPA and DHA are indispensable because they supply part of the chemistry of completion, but completion also requires membranes built from enough phospholipid architecture, enough ordered-domain support, enough cholesterol-mediated organization, and enough structural resilience that the tissue can stay coherent while inflammatory force is being wound down. Without that broader lipid sufficiency, omega-3 remains an important input working inside an underbuilt system. With it, the membrane becomes not only a place where inflammation starts, but a place capable of carrying inflammation all the way through to a clean end.

Saturated Fat and Membrane Integrity

Saturated fat matters to membrane integrity because membranes do not only need flexibility. They also need structural firmness. A phospholipid bilayer built entirely around maximum fluidity would not become more intelligent. It would become less controlled. Membranes must hold gradients, preserve receptor organization, regulate permeability, resist mechanical disruption, and survive oxidative stress long enough for signaling to remain precise. Saturated fatty acids contribute to that stability by packing more tightly than polyunsaturated fatty acids and by providing surfaces that are less chemically vulnerable to peroxidation. This does not make saturated fat the whole answer, but it does make it an essential part of the structural problem. A membrane that contains no meaningful stable lipid architecture is easier to damage, easier to leak, and easier to push into signaling noise.

This becomes especially important in the context of inflammation and resolution. Polyunsaturated fats such as EPA and DHA are valuable because they expand signaling possibilities and provide substrate for specialized pro-resolving mediators, but their multiple double bonds also make them chemically fragile. If a membrane is built too heavily around highly unsaturated structure without enough stabilizing architecture around it, then the same membrane that is theoretically rich in resolution potential may become too easy to oxidize under stress. Saturated fatty acids help counter that vulnerability by contributing durability. They reduce the degree to which the membrane behaves like a chemically unstable field waiting to fragment under inflammatory pressure. In that sense, saturated fat does not oppose resolution. It helps create the stable background in which resolution-capable lipids can actually be preserved and used.

The key point, however, is that membrane integrity is not produced by saturated fat alone. Too much rigidity in the wrong tissue can impair receptor movement, vesicle fusion, membrane curvature dynamics, and adaptive signaling behavior. The body is not trying to make every membrane hard. It is trying to make every membrane usable. Some tissues, especially neural tissue, retinal tissue, and highly dynamic immune membranes, require more fluid and specialized phospholipid environments than others. What saturated fat contributes is not universal superiority, but structural restraint. It helps prevent the membrane from becoming too disordered, too oxidizable, or too permeable. That restraint matters more when the surrounding tissue is under chronic inflammatory or oxidative stress, because under those conditions a structurally weak membrane degrades quickly.

This is why saturated fat should be understood in architectural rather than ideological terms. It is not simply fuel and it is not simply a cardiovascular villain or hero. It is part of the material logic by which the body keeps membranes coherent. In combination with monounsaturated fats, cholesterol, phospholipid head-group organization, sphingolipid domains, and controlled inclusion of polyunsaturated fats, saturated fatty acids help create a membrane that can both function and endure. A body built only for signaling flexibility becomes fragile. A body built only for rigidity becomes inflexible. Membrane integrity emerges when saturated fat contributes enough firmness that the membrane can survive stress without losing the dynamic properties required for life.

Energy Availability and Safety Signaling

Energy availability and safety signaling are tightly linked because the body does not interpret energy as a neutral quantity. It interprets energy through context. A tissue with abundant fuel but poor mitochondrial function, chronic cytokine pressure, unresolved debris, barrier leak, and membrane instability does not experience that abundance as safety. It experiences it as burden. By contrast, a tissue with adequate fuel, coherent hormonal signaling, low inflammatory noise, stable membranes, and functioning mitochondria can interpret the same basic energetic input as permission to repair, restore, and maintain. This is one of the most important reasons chronic inflammation so often coexists with fatigue, poor recovery, and stress sensitivity. The body is not only asking whether energy is present. It is asking whether the environment is safe enough to invest that energy in rebuilding rather than reserving it for defense.

Safety signaling in physiology is therefore not psychological metaphor. It is a material state. It emerges when membranes are stable enough to interpret signals accurately, when cytokine tone is low enough that tissues are not being told danger is still active, when barriers are closed enough that fresh provocation is not constantly entering immune space, and when mitochondria can produce ATP without doing so inside a chronically stressed redox environment. Under those conditions, the organism begins reallocating resources. Repair becomes more possible. Digestion becomes more coordinated. Sleep becomes more restorative. Hormonal signaling becomes more coherent. Immune surveillance can remain competent without staying amplified. The body begins acting like a system that expects continuity rather than interruption. That is what safety signaling really is. It is the biochemical permission structure for ordinary function.

This is why energy availability alone is never enough. A person may eat adequately and still remain trapped in a low-energy state if too much of that energy is being consumed by incomplete inflammatory loops. Recruitment, cytokine production, oxidative stress management, membrane repair, pain amplification, autonomic overactivation, and barrier defense all drain ATP and distort fuel handling. The body then appears underpowered not because fuel is absent, but because the energy economy is dominated by unresolved costs. Until inflammation is completed well enough for those costs to fall, additional intake often produces less benefit than expected. The energy enters a system that still behaves as though it is under threat, so the organism keeps channeling resources toward protection rather than toward restoration.

This is also where resolution biology becomes central. Successful resolution improves safety signaling by removing the evidence that keeps tissues in defensive interpretation. Neutrophil-heavy continuation falls. Macrophages clear apoptotic cells and oxidized debris. Barrier integrity improves. Vascular surfaces become less reactive. Membranes stop leaking so much distress chemistry. As that happens, the body no longer has to hold the same level of metabolic reserve against ongoing danger. Energy becomes more usable because the tissue environment becomes more trustworthy. The organism begins shifting from survival prioritization into maintenance, repair, and adaptation. In practical terms, that often feels like better resilience, more stable energy, less post-stress collapse, improved warmth, steadier appetite regulation, and less exaggerated reaction to minor demands. But underneath those experiences is a deeper transition. The body is beginning to believe, biochemically, that it is safe enough to spend on life instead of constantly hedging against unfinished threat.

Seen clearly, energy availability and safety signaling are two sides of the same physiological reality. The body needs enough energy to resolve inflammation, but it also needs enough resolution to experience energy as usable safety rather than as fuel trapped inside a defensive system. When the membrane environment is coherent, when omega-3-derived completion pathways are stronger, when barriers are tighter, and when inflammatory residue is lower, energy stops being consumed mainly by emergency maintenance and starts becoming available for real recovery. That is one of the deepest meanings of healing. The body no longer just has energy. It trusts itself enough to use it.

Full-System Lipid Design

Full-system lipid design means thinking about fats the way the body actually uses them: not as isolated nutrients, not as moral categories, and not as single-target interventions, but as a distributed structural language that shapes every major layer of physiology at once. Membranes, mitochondria, barriers, vascular surfaces, immune cells, endocrine signaling interfaces, synapses, and storage tissues are all built from lipids, and each of those tissues solves a different problem with the lipid environment it is given. This means the body cannot be stabilized by focusing only on one fatty acid in isolation. A coherent system requires structural lipids that create durable membranes, signaling lipids that allow phase-appropriate inflammatory communication, energetic lipids that can be mobilized without overwhelming oxidation and immune tone, and enough omega-3-derived substrate to support actual completion once inflammatory activation has served its purpose. Full-system lipid design is therefore the idea that health depends on building the whole organism from a lipid architecture that can initiate, adapt, and resolve without falling into chronic distortion.

At the membrane level, this means every tissue needs the right combination of firmness, fluidity, and signaling reserve for its specific function. Endothelial surfaces need to remain selectively permeable rather than chronically reactive. Gut and epithelial barriers need membranes capable of resisting irritation while still supporting controlled exchange. Immune cells need enough dynamic membrane behavior to detect, cluster, engulf, and transition between activation states without remaining trapped in escalation. Neural tissue needs highly specialized phospholipid environments that can sustain excitability and synaptic precision without becoming chemically unstable under stress. Mitochondria need membranes that can hold gradients, organize respiratory complexes, and survive repeated metabolic demand. Full-system lipid design therefore is not about maximizing one property. It is about building each tissue with the kind of lipid environment that lets it remain itself during stress instead of becoming easier to trigger and harder to restore.

This also means correcting one of the central mistakes of modern nutrition, which is the idea that a body can be built successfully from chronic omega-6 excess, unstable polyunsaturated overload, poor omega-3 incorporation, low structural resilience, and then later be fixed by adding a single corrective supplement. That is not design. That is patching. Full-system lipid design begins earlier. It asks what kinds of phospholipid pools are being built into tissues over time, what kinds of fatty acids dominate releasable membrane substrate, what kinds of mediator families those tissues will be most prepared to generate during stress, and whether those tissues are being built with enough structural support that highly unsaturated fats can remain useful rather than becoming liabilities. In practical terms, it means reducing chronic omega-6 dominance, improving EPA and DHA incorporation, preserving cholesterol and sphingolipid-supported membrane order, and ensuring enough structural resilience that membranes can hold the chemistry of completion without collapsing into oxidation.

The energy system has to be included in this design or the whole strategy remains incomplete. Lipids do not only shape signaling surfaces. They shape the organelles that determine whether repair can be funded. A body can carry omega-3-derived substrate for resolution and still fail if mitochondrial membranes are disorganized, if redox burden remains too high, or if fuel handling remains so unstable that ATP is continually diverted into emergency maintenance. Full-system lipid design therefore means designing not only for inflammation control, but for energy coherence. The membranes that store signal substrate and the membranes that generate ATP have to be aligned. Otherwise the body receives late-phase instructions without having the energetic capacity to execute them. The result is always the same: good theory, poor closure.

This is why full-system lipid design ultimately becomes a stability strategy, not a supplement strategy. The question is no longer whether omega-3 is good, whether saturated fat is bad, or whether one oil should replace another in a vacuum. The better question is whether the organism is being built from lipids that support durable thresholds, competent initiation, low-noise signaling, barrier integrity, mitochondrial output, macrophage cleanup, and strong resolution potential across the whole body at once. If the answer is no, then disease patterns emerge because each tissue begins expressing the same architectural weakness according to its own function. If the answer is yes, then the body becomes harder to destabilize because its membranes, mediator reserves, and energy systems are no longer working against one another. Full-system lipid design, then, is the recognition that inflammation, recovery, resilience, metabolism, cognition, vascular function, and hormonal coherence all sit downstream of what kind of lipid-built body exists in the first place.

Chapter 24

Restoring the Lipid-Controlled Body

Restoring the lipid-controlled body means restoring a body whose behavior is once again governed by stable membrane architecture rather than by chronic biochemical improvisation. That distinction matters because the body is never truly controlled by isolated molecules moving through empty space. It is controlled through surfaces. Receptors read through membranes. Mitochondria produce energy through membranes. Barriers maintain separation through membranes. Immune cells decide whether to recruit or clear through membranes. The nervous system preserves precision through membranes. When those surfaces are compositionally coherent, the body behaves as though it has command over its own thresholds, its own inflammatory timing, and its own transitions between stress and repair. When those surfaces are structurally degraded, oxidatively unstable, overloaded with initiation-heavy substrate, and poor in the later-phase chemistry of completion, the body begins acting less like an organized system and more like a collection of tissues reacting to one another's unfinished emergencies. Restoring the lipid-controlled body is therefore not about adding one "good fat" to an otherwise unchanged physiology. It is about rebuilding the material architecture through which the body regains control over itself.

The first principle of restoration is that the body must stop being built from chronic contradiction. It cannot remain overloaded with omega-6-dominant initiation substrate, repeatedly exposed to oxidized lipid damage, continually re-triggered through barrier leak and metabolic volatility, and then be expected to resolve cleanly simply because some omega-3 has been introduced. That is not restoration. That is biochemical conflict. The lipid-controlled body emerges when the membrane reservoir is no longer dominated by escalation chemistry, when EPA and DHA are meaningfully incorporated into phospholipids, when cholesterol and sphingolipid-supported order are preserved rather than pathologized in abstraction, when saturated and monounsaturated fats provide enough structural resilience that highly unsaturated lipids can be held and used without turning the membrane into a chemically fragile field, and when the system as a whole is no longer being asked to operate under continuous oxidative and inflammatory assault. Restoration begins when lipids stop fighting one another inside the same tissue and begin serving their proper roles in hierarchy.

This means the project is architectural before it is symptomatic. The body must first regain stable membranes, because stable membranes are what allow receptors to interpret accurately, what allow gradients to hold, what allow inflammatory activation to remain proportionate, and what allow later-phase resolution substrate to exist as something more than theoretical chemistry. Once those membranes are rebuilt, the body gains a different future. Phospholipases no longer release only the language of escalation. COX and LOX pathways are no longer crowded only by initiation-heavy traffic. The nervous system is no longer trying to signal through chronically oxidized surfaces. Endothelial and epithelial barriers are no longer as easy to destabilize. Mitochondrial membranes are more capable of preserving the structural conditions for ATP generation. This is the real meaning of lipid control. The body is no longer improvising from damaged materials. It is acting from designed materials.

The second principle of restoration is that inflammatory completion must be rebuilt as a normal expectation of physiology rather than as an exceptional event. In the unresolved body, inflammation becomes sticky. It starts quickly, lingers unnecessarily, leaves residue, lowers thresholds, and turns ordinary life into repeated partial emergencies. In the lipid-controlled body, inflammation regains sequence. It initiates when needed, amplifies when necessary, and then resolves because the body once again carries the substrate, the membrane environment, the enzymatic flexibility, the barrier integrity, the macrophage competence, and the mitochondrial reserve required to finish what it starts. This is one of the deepest signs of restoration. The person stops feeling hijacked by every perturbation. Stress still happens, but it does not become as adhesive. Recovery becomes more believable. Small triggers stop producing outsized aftermath. Pain becomes less sticky. Sleep becomes more restorative. Food becomes less inflammatory by consequence, not only by rule. Stability begins returning not because life became easier, but because the body became better at closing loops.

The third principle is that the lipid-controlled body cannot be rebuilt through suppression alone. Suppression can reduce visible inflammatory output, but it does not automatically restore order. Order is restored when inflammatory debris is cleared, when oxidized membrane fragments stop accumulating, when apoptotic cells are removed before they become fresh inflammatory fuel, when barriers close, when vascular surfaces stop behaving as emergency corridors, and when neural tissue stops interpreting ordinary inputs through the chemistry of unresolved danger. That means restoration requires active resolution. EPA and DHA must not only enter membranes. They must become part of a tissue environment capable of generating E-series resolvins, D-series resolvins, protectins, and maresins strongly enough that the later phase becomes more than a weak afterthought. The body must once again believe, in biochemical terms, that events can end. Without that conviction built into its membranes and mediator systems, it will continue acting as though defense is the only trustworthy mode.

The fourth principle is that restoration must include energy. A body cannot become lipid-controlled if it remains ATP-poor at the level that matters. Mitochondria must be able to fund cleanup, membrane repair, barrier reconstruction, and ordinary function without remaining trapped in emergency expenditure. This is why repair often fails in chronically inflamed people even when they begin supplying better lipids. The new material arrives, but the system still lacks the energetic coherence to use it fully. Restoring the lipid-controlled body therefore means restoring both the substrate architecture of resolution and the energy architecture of resolution. The membranes storing the language of completion and the organelles funding the labor of completion must both be repaired. Otherwise the body receives better instructions but remains too exhausted to obey them. Real control emerges when signal and fuel stop working against each other.

The fifth principle is that restoration is tissue-wide, not local. The gut must stop feeding fresh provocation into circulation. The vascular system must stop carrying chronic inflammatory tone from barrier to barrier. Adipose tissue must stop behaving like unresolved immune burden. The liver must stop handling every nutrient load through inflammatory congestion. The nervous system must stop interpreting ordinary life as continued injury. These are not separate projects. They are all expressions of the same larger repair: rebuilding a body whose tissues once again trust their own boundaries, their own membranes, and their own ability to return to baseline after disturbance. The lipid-controlled body is therefore not simply a body with better blood omega-3 levels. It is a body whose tissues have regained enough structural coherence that they no longer spread unfinished danger signals to one another so easily.

This chapter must also end where the whole book has been moving from the beginning: toward the idea that control in physiology is not primarily top-down. It is not imposed by will, nor by one hormone, nor by one nutrient, nor by one signaling pathway. Control is distributed through material structure. The body becomes governable again when the membranes governing sensation, immunity, energy, permeability, vascular behavior, and repair are rebuilt into forms that can support proper timing. That is why lipids have occupied the center of this entire book. The body is built from them, reads through them, stores inflammatory futures inside them, and resolves through them. When they are arranged well, the organism becomes calmer, stronger, harder to trigger unnecessarily, and more capable of repairing without residue. When they are arranged badly, every system becomes noisier, more defensive, and less able to finish what it begins.

Restoring the lipid-controlled body, then, is not a narrow nutritional intervention. It is the reconstruction of the body as a system that once again behaves according to designed sequence rather than accumulated damage. It is the return of the membrane as a trustworthy surface. It is the return of omega-3 as real resolution substrate rather than decorative supplementation. It is the return of macrophages as competent finishers, of mitochondria as dependable funders of repair, of barriers as meaningful separators, of vascular tissue as quiet control surface, of the nervous system as a signaling environment no longer trapped in chronic alarm. Above all, it is the return of the body's ability to end things properly. That is what control really means. Not the prevention of all disturbance, but the restoration of a biological architecture in which disturbance no longer has to become identity.

Rebuilding Membrane Composition

Rebuilding membrane composition means rebuilding the physical surface from which the body interprets, reacts, protects, and recovers. That has to be stated with full weight because membrane change is not a cosmetic nutritional adjustment. It is a change in the material basis of physiology. A membrane is where receptors sit, where gradients are held, where phospholipases later pull inflammatory substrate, where mitochondria organize energy production, where barriers decide what stays in and what stays out, and where the body stores part of its future signaling language. If that surface has been built for years under omega-6 dominance, oxidative instability, poor omega-3 incorporation, repeated inflammatory remodeling, and weak structural lipid support, then the body does not just become deficient in one nutrient. It becomes physically biased toward lower thresholds, stronger initiation, and weaker completion. Rebuilding membrane composition therefore is the process of changing what kinds of futures the tissue is structurally prepared to generate.

The first part of that rebuilding is displacement. EPA and DHA do not float above membranes as abstract benefits. They have to replace part of what is already there. If phospholipid pools are crowded by omega-6-derived substrate, especially in tissues repeatedly shaped by modern processed fat exposure, then the body is storing too much of the chemistry of initiation and too little of the chemistry of completion. Rebuilding means changing the stored reservoir.

That requires repeated delivery of intact omega-3 in amounts sufficient to matter, enough time for phospholipid turnover, and enough reduction in competing omega-6 pressure that the new fatty acids can gain real structural ground rather than remaining token additions inside the same old architecture. The membrane has to begin carrying different material before it can produce different behavior.

But rebuilding is not simply about increasing unsaturation. A membrane rebuilt intelligently is not one flooded with highly fragile polyunsaturated structure in a chemically hostile environment. It is one rebuilt into balanced competence. EPA and DHA have to be there because they provide substrate for resolvins, protectins, and maresins and change membrane signaling properties in ways that matter deeply for resolution. But they need to be held inside a broader architecture that includes enough saturated and monounsaturated structural support, enough cholesterol-mediated organization, and enough sphingolipid order that the membrane can remain coherent under stress instead of turning into a peroxidation-prone surface that carries good intentions and poor durability. Rebuilding membrane composition therefore means building a membrane that can both signal and survive.

The oxidative environment determines whether this rebuilding holds. A person can increase omega-3 intake and still fail to rebuild useful membranes if the body remains under high oxidative stress, poor sleep, repeated glycemic volatility, ongoing endotoxin exposure, barrier leak, and chronic inflammatory burden. In that case, the new membrane material is being laid into a hostile construction zone. Highly unsaturated fatty acids may be damaged before they can become durable structural reserve. The tissue then appears resistant to change, but the deeper truth is that the new composition is not being preserved. Real rebuilding requires enough reduction in oxidative burden that the membrane can keep what it is gaining. Otherwise the body keeps trying to construct better surfaces while tearing them down at the same time.

Rebuilding membrane composition also changes thresholds. This is one of the most important outcomes. A membrane enriched in more stable and more resolution-capable substrate begins reading the environment differently. Receptors sit in a different physical field. Microdomains behave differently. Ion channels and transporters operate through a less noisy surface. Phospholipases release a different substrate balance when activation occurs. That means the body begins reacting differently not because a command was imposed from above, but because the surface through which it makes decisions has changed. Ordinary inputs stop crossing threshold so easily. Minor inflammatory triggers stop producing so much aftermath. Recovery after strain becomes less chemically expensive. The body becomes harder to push into escalation and better equipped to finish escalation when it does occur. That is what membrane rebuilding looks like when it becomes physiology instead of theory.

The tissue-specific nature of this rebuilding matters as well. Neural tissue, vascular tissue, barrier tissue, immune cells, and mitochondria are not all remodeling for the same reason. In the nervous system, rebuilding membrane composition means preserving DHA-rich structural precision and future neuroprotective mediator capacity. In the vasculature, it means reducing endothelial reactivity and restoring selective control over traffic and permeability. In barrier tissues, it means strengthening membranes and junctional behavior so outside signals stop crossing inward so easily. In immune cells, it means reducing initiation-heavy substrate dominance and increasing the capacity to transition into cleanup and closure. In mitochondria, it means restoring membranes capable of holding gradients and funding repair without so much oxidative spillover. The body is not rebuilding one membrane. It is rebuilding an entire membrane-defined civilization.

Seen clearly, rebuilding membrane composition is one of the deepest acts of restoration in the whole system. It changes what the body is made from, what it can store, what it can release, how it interprets signals, how it funds recovery, and whether inflammation is more likely to become a successful sequence or a chronic identity. This is why omega-3 matters, why omega-6 competition matters, why oxidative protection matters, and why structural lipid support matters. The body does not heal only by reducing what hurts it. It heals by rebuilding the surfaces through which it becomes itself again.

Re-establishing Resolution Capacity

Re-establishing resolution capacity means restoring the body's ability to finish inflammation as a normal part of physiology rather than leaving every inflammatory event half-complete. That is the real goal. The body does not become healthy by never activating. It becomes healthy by activating proportionately, clearing efficiently, and returning to order without carrying forward a residue of danger that lowers thresholds for the next event. When resolution capacity is weak, the body can still inflame, sometimes very well, but it cannot stop inflaming convincingly. Debris remains. Membranes remain unstable. Barriers remain too open. Cytokine tone remains too high. Macrophages remain too burdened or too poorly directed. Mitochondria remain too strained to pay for repair. Re-establishing resolution capacity therefore is not one intervention. It is the rebuilding of the entire chain that turns force into closure.

The first requirement is rebuilding the membrane reservoir. The body cannot produce strong late-phase mediator biology from membranes that remain poor in EPA and DHA and overloaded with omega-6-dominant initiation substrate. Resolution begins with what the tissue is made from. That means enough intact omega-3 has to be absorbed, incorporated into phospholipids, protected from oxidation, and retained long enough to become part of the releasable pool from which resolvins, protectins, and maresins can later be generated. But rebuilding the reservoir alone is not enough. The body must also reduce chronic omega-6 competition so that when phospholipases mobilize substrate during inflammatory activation, the tissue is no longer drawing almost entirely from escalation-heavy stores. Re-establishing resolution capacity therefore begins by changing what kind of inflammatory future the membrane is prepared to produce.

The second requirement is reducing repeated re-triggering. A body cannot regain resolution while it is being pushed back into initiation every day. Gut barrier leak, endotoxin exposure, ultra-processed food intake, glycemic volatility, poor sleep, chronic stress, toxic load, mechanical overuse, and unresolved inflammatory debris all keep the system from staying in the later phase long enough to complete it. This is one reason so many people appear resistant to otherwise rational interventions. The body is not failing to respond in the abstract. It is being interrupted before closure can take hold. Re-establishing resolution capacity means lowering the number of signals telling the tissue that emergency is still active, so that the stop signal has room to become more than a whisper.

The third requirement is restoring macrophage finishing. The body does not resolve just because recruitment falls. It resolves because cleanup succeeds. Macrophages must be able to engulf apoptotic cells, clear oxidized membrane fragments, process tissue debris, and help shift the site from inflammatory activity into reconstruction. If that cleanup phase remains weak, then every inflammatory event leaves behind a residue that justifies the next one. Re-establishing resolution capacity therefore means making the tissue more cleanable. That includes lowering incoming inflammatory traffic, improving membrane stability so less damage accumulates, and improving the conditions in which macrophages can work, energetically, structurally, and immunologically.

The fourth requirement is energy availability. Resolution is labor. Efferocytosis costs ATP. Membrane repair costs ATP. Rebuilding barriers costs ATP. Returning mitochondria, endothelium, epithelium, and neural tissue to ordinary function costs ATP. If mitochondrial function remains poor, the body may continue starting inflammatory events it cannot afford to finish. That is one of the defining asymmetries of chronic disease. There is enough energy for defense and not enough organized energy for closure. Re-establishing resolution capacity therefore requires more than better lipids. It requires a body that can use energy for completion rather than spending nearly all of it on partial defense.

The fifth requirement is lowering oxidative instability. EPA and DHA are essential to resolution, but they are also vulnerable. A body that remains highly oxidized will keep degrading the very substrate it needs for later-phase mediator production. Membranes rich in highly unsaturated fats only improve physiology when those fats are protected well enough to remain intact and function as stored precursor rather than as fresh oxidative debris. Re-establishing resolution capacity therefore requires a less hostile chemical environment, one in which omega-3 can be preserved, not merely ingested.

Seen clearly, re-establishing resolution capacity is the return of biological trust. The body stops assuming every perturbation will become permanent damage. It stops holding tissues in chronic partial defense. It stops treating ordinary life as a string of unfinished emergencies. Membranes become better reservoirs for closure. Macrophages become better finishers. Barriers become better separators. Mitochondria become better funders of repair. Thresholds rise. Recovery shortens. Inflammatory events stop leaving so much residue behind. That is what restored resolution capacity really is. It is the body regaining the ability to end what it starts and return to itself without carrying every disturbance forward as identity.

Predictable Signaling

Predictable signaling is what the body regains when membrane composition, inflammatory timing, and resolution capacity are restored strongly enough that tissues stop interpreting the same input in wildly unstable ways. A healthy system is not one that never changes. It is one that changes proportionately. The same meal, the same mechanical load, the same immune exposure, the same stressor, or the same night of sleep loss should not produce radically different physiological outcomes from one day to the next unless the underlying context has truly changed. When signaling becomes unpredictable, it usually means the body is no longer operating from stable architecture. Membranes have become too reactive, cytokine tone remains too elevated, barriers remain too open, substrate pools remain too biased toward initiation, and the nervous, vascular, immune, and metabolic systems are all reading the world through partially unresolved tissue. The result is not just inflammation. It is variability. The organism becomes harder to anticipate because it is no longer signaling from order.

This is one of the deepest consequences of failed resolution. A tissue that never fully clears debris, never fully restores membrane integrity, and never fully exits emergency mode does not merely stay somewhat inflamed. It becomes inconsistent. Receptors behave in a noisier environment. Vascular surfaces become more conditionally reactive. Pain pathways amplify on some days far more than others. Appetite and satiety signals become less trustworthy. Stress responses become exaggerated or blunted in ways that no longer feel proportional to the trigger. The body stops producing clean outputs from ordinary inputs because too much inflammatory residue remains between the input and the response. Predictable signaling, then, is not just convenience. It is one of the clearest signs that the organism is once again being governed by coherent structure rather than by unfinished defense.

Resolution restores predictability because it removes the biochemical and structural noise that distorts interpretation. When neutrophil-heavy recruitment actually ends, when macrophages clear efficiently, when membranes stop leaking distress chemistry, when omega-3-derived later-phase signaling becomes strong enough to matter, and when barriers regain selective control, the same inputs stop producing so much random aftermath. The body becomes easier to read because it has become easier for itself to read. Signals begin traveling through cleaner surfaces, cleaner mediator environments, and cleaner thresholds. That is what predictable signaling really means. Not rigidity, but reliability. The system can still adapt, but its adaptations once again follow understandable rules instead of reflecting whatever unfinished inflammation happened to be carried forward from the last unresolved event.

Long-Term Biological Stability

Long-term biological stability is what emerges when the body no longer has to spend so much of its future defending against the unfinished remains of its past. That is the deepest pattern running underneath everything in this book. Stability is not produced by holding the body in a fixed state, and it is not produced by eliminating every stressor. It is produced by the ability to pass through stress, activation, injury, immune challenge, and metabolic fluctuation without allowing those events to permanently lower thresholds, distort membranes, destabilize barriers, overload cleanup systems, and bias the tissue toward repeated re-initiation. A stable organism is not one that never changes. It is one that returns. It returns from perturbation, from inflammatory activation, from oxidative challenge, from immune stress, from nutrient excess, from nutrient scarcity, from neural strain. It does not have to remain in the chemistry of the event after the useful phase of the event has ended.

This is why long-term stability is impossible without resolution. A body that still knows how to initiate but has lost the ability to complete will gradually become less stable no matter how normal it may appear in snapshots. Membranes accumulate damage. Oxidized fragments remain visible. Macrophages remain burdened. Vascular surfaces remain reactive. Barriers remain easier to breach. Mitochondria keep spending on defense. The nervous system keeps interpreting ordinary life through chronic partial alarm. Hormonal signals become harder to translate cleanly. The person may still function, but function begins requiring more compensation and less true resilience. Over time, that compensation is what people often mistake for aging, fragility, poor stress tolerance, or inexplicable chronic symptoms. In reality, much of it reflects the accumulation of incompletely finished biology. Long-term stability fails when too many loops stay open.

A stable body therefore has to be built from membranes that can preserve order under load, from lipid pools that do not force every inflammatory event toward escalation, from omega-3-derived substrate sufficient to support later-phase completion, from barriers that can re-close after they open, and from mitochondria capable of funding recovery once defense has done enough. This is not a narrow nutritional statement. It is a systems statement. The body remains stable across years when its tissues do not keep carrying forward the residue of prior activation as if that residue were a permanent feature of life. That means fewer low-threshold flares, less sticky pain, fewer exaggerated responses to ordinary inputs, better metabolic flexibility, more reliable vascular control, more coherent endocrine signaling, and a nervous system that does not stay overprotective after the need for protection has passed. These are not separate wins. They are what stability looks like when it becomes embodied.

Long-term biological stability is therefore the cumulative outcome of successful completion. Every time the body finishes well, it protects the future from the present. Every time it fails to finish, it drags the present forward into the future as structural burden. That is why resolution belongs at the center of health rather than at the edge of inflammation. It is the mechanism by which the organism prevents normal life from becoming chronic damage. A body that resolves well does not merely feel better now. It stays more itself over time.

Made in the USA
Monee, IL
05 November 2026

67914361R00190